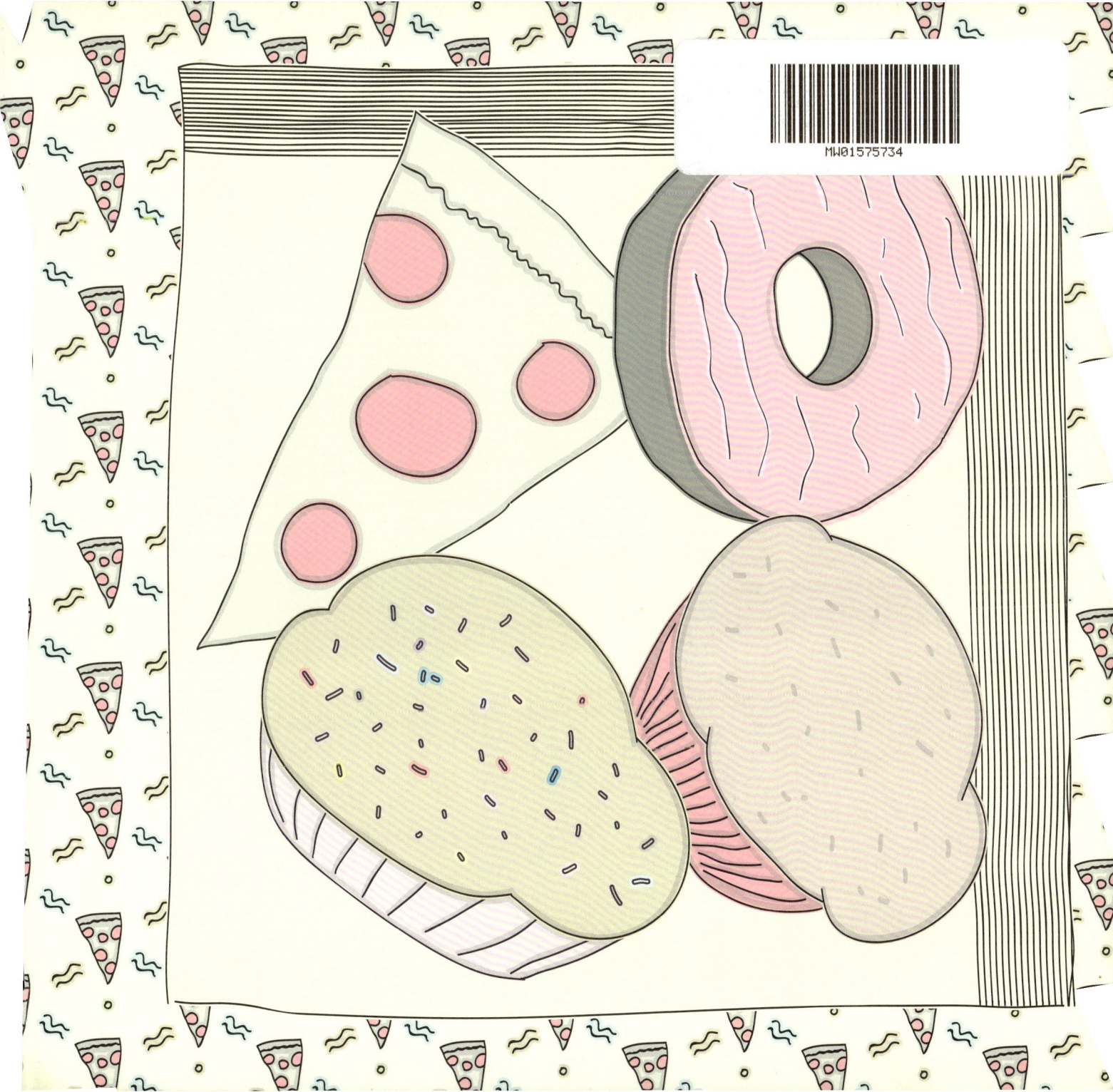

LEGAL STUFF, SMALL PRINT, AND COPYRIGHT

This is a cookbook. I make no health claims or medical claims, at all... ever. Even if I do happen to make something that *looks* like a claim of some kind, I didn't. It was an accident. I *do* claim, however, that the recipes are both lovely *and* delicious. While the whole book is mired in a specific philosophy I've picked up and massaged over the years, I only claim that they've benefitted me. Because this is a litigious world, I cannot claim these recipes will benefit you in any way, short of bringing a satisfying smile to your face 'cause they're just so karfalootin' yummy!

Point being: I'm not a doctor, nutritionist, naturopath, or any kind of chemist or biological specialist. My degree is from the Culinary Institute of America. It essentially qualifies me to peel carrots, very quickly (and I *am* quite fast!).

Listen to your doctors!

Copyright © 2017 by Kenneth Eric Williams

All rights reserved. This book or any portion thereof may not be reproduced or used in any manner whatsoever without the express written permission of the publisher except for the use of brief quotations in a book review.

~ ElDuderino@djfoodie.com

Assembled in the United States of America and Mexico

First Printing, 2017

ISBN – 978-0-9863444-1-1

www.djfoodie.com

ABOUT THE NUTRITION

I take great pride in offering the most thorough nutritional analyses I've ever seen... anywhere. I do my best to give accurate nutritional information for each ingredient. In addition to adding the values and offering a total, a total per serving is also included. I want people to feel that they can tweak the recipes and know how the removal or adjustment of a single ingredient will impact the overall nutritional value. I also feel it encourages the understanding of individual ingredients and where the macronutrients are coming from.

This is a good-faith promise that the information is as accurate as I know how to make it. The majority of the information comes from the United States Department of Agriculture's Nutrient Database for Standard Reference, Release 21 (also known as USDA SR-21). When the information is unavailable from the USDA, I do my best to find current information. However, I make no promises of the accuracy of the information, just that it's as good as I'm able to make it and that it's very honorably presented.

TABLE OF CONTENTS

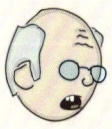

Legal Stuff, Small Print, and Copyright	2
About the Nutrition	3
Framing "The Fakery"	6
Introduction	12
Ok, So Why "The Fakery"?	16
What Is a "Quick" Bread, Anyway?	17
Ratios	19
Sweet Quick-Bread Ratio	23
Savory Quick-Bread Ratio	23
Stuff You'll Need	27
Flours	31
Almond and Other Nut Flours	31
Coconut Flour – Less is More	33
Chia Seed Flour	36
Orange-Blueberry Chia Pudding	38
Flaxseed Meal	41
Protein Powder	42
Gluten Replacers	44
Xanthan Gum	45
Guar Gum	49
Gelatin	49
Glucomannan	50
Agar-Agar	51
Psyllium Seed Husk Fiber	51
Starch	53
Tapioca Starch/Flour	53
Arrowroot Starch/Flour	55
Leavening Agents	57
Air	57
Water	57
Baking Soda	58
Baking Powder	59
Baker's Yeast	60
Brief Mention of Sweeteners	62
Tasty vs. Goodness	63
Basic Tasty Smappy	64
Basic Smappy Goodness	64
Tasty Smappy: Baking Blend	64
Smappy Goodness: Baking Blend	65
Light Brown Smappy: Baking Blend	65
Dark Brown Smappy: Baking Blend	65
Visualize	66
Substitutions	80
Grind Your Own	82
Further Tips	88

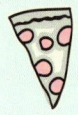

Savory — 91
Deep-Dish Pizza — 92
Cheesy Bacon-Chive Muffins — 96
Chorizo, Cilantro and Cotija Muffins — 98
Muffin aux Fines Herbes — 100
Pesto, Sausage and Parmesan Muffins — 102
Jalapeño Cheddar Muffins — 104
Grain-Free, Nut-Free Fauxcaccia — 106

Sweet — 109
Cream Cheese-Filled Spiced Apple Muffins — 110
Blueberry, Lemon and Poppy Seed Muffins — 114
Mini Carrot Cakes with Cream Cheese Frosting — 116
Brown Butter Ginger-Spice "Riddles & Games" — 118
Carrot, Coconut and Macadamia Mega-Muffin — 122
Chocolate-Banana Muffcakes — 124
Chocolate-Chocolate Chunk with Ganache — 126
Crunchy Mocha-Zucchini Muffins — 128
Mini Coconut Muffaroons — 130
Sour Cream Coffee Cake with Hazelnut Streusel — 132
Eggnog Chantilly — 134
Mini Gingerbread Loaves — 138
Fried Blob — 140
Mexican Chocolate Muffins — 142
Mocha Mint Muffins — 144
Mini Notella Muffnuts — 146
Bacon and Orange Muffins with Pecan Streusel — 148
Orange-Cranberry Muffins — 152
Pear, Walnut and Blue Cheese Tart Fauxtan — 154
Pumpkin Cheesecake Swirl — 156
Spiced Pumpkin-Sour Cream Muffin Pies — 158
Strawberry Yogurt Muffins — 160
Vanilla Bean Muffcakes — 162

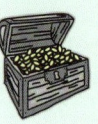

Bonus Recipes — 165
Chocolate OMM — 166
Cinnamon Roll OMM — 168
OMM French Toast — 170
One-Minute Cheddar Bread and Buns — 172
Bacon-Cheddar BBQ Pork Sliders — 174
Sweet 'n' Creamy Coleslaw — 176
Blue Cheese Lamburger with Poppy Seed OMM — 178
Greasy Fried Pork Sandwich — 180
Frosted Carrot Cake OMM with Pecans — 182
Pumpkin-Spice OMM with Maple Butter — 184
Savory Zucchini, Bacon and Herb OMM — 186
Spiced Zucchini Bread OMM — 188
Herby Sandwich Bread (Focaccia) — 190
Italian Turkey Club Sandwich — 192
Pesto alla Genovese — 194
Cream Cheese Frosting — 196
Notella — 198
Chocolate Ganache — 200
Luxurious Eggnog — 202

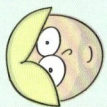
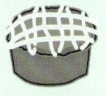

The Back of the Book — 204
Deeper Nutritional Grids — 205
Index — 230
Shameless Plug — 238

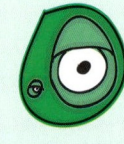

FRAMING "THE FAKERY"

I met a lovely young woman named Karina Arana about 2 years ago. She's the eldest sister of my good friend Melina. Melina was my workout buddy at the time. Karina moved to town right as her sister was traveling for work, standing me up and leaving me all alone and witnessless at the gym. Karina stepped right in (or should I say, "step up... step down... step up... step down") to take her sister's place. We became fast friends!

Being that I live, eat, and breathe this low-primal thing, it's common for me to blather on about it. Apparently, I splattered some on Karina. Since she's adopted this way of eating, she's dropped nearly half her weight; she's an absolute shadow of the Karina I met just a short while ago.

Karina moved to Mexico to become the next JK Rowling. She's a delicious writer, focusing on young adults and the wellbeing of the planet. She's highly educated, an educator, an educator's educator and an expert on language. As I was writing this book, I was watching her shrink, just as I noticed an increased bounce in her step.

My own story is plastered all over my blog, as well as my first book. I hate to be repetitive if I don't have to be. However, I *also* felt the book needed to be kicked off with *some* kind of story, as well. Something that suggests this *does* work and that I wasn't an anomaly with my 150 pound weight loss. Inspiration is a great way to start a book! Karina's a good friend. She has watched me do a thousand sit ups and listened to even more complaints about lunges. She's also my editor. Like me, she's got skin in the game. It seemed only fitting to have her share her story!

I asked her to dredge it all up, *including* all the painful stuff, often best left swept under the carpet. Then, I requested she help frame my new book through her eyes. Y'all will get *plenty* of me!

Let's hear from Karina!

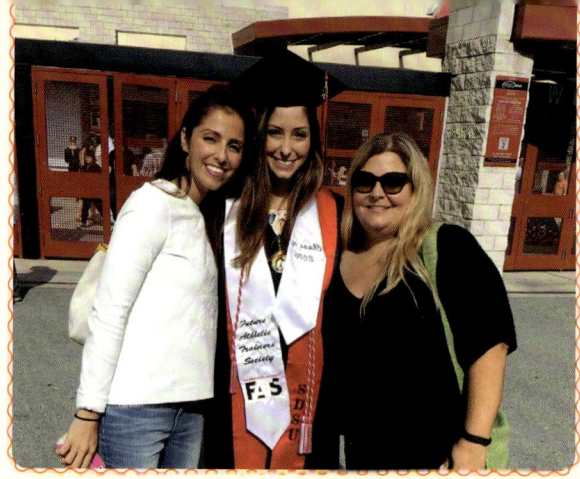

Being overweight, significantly overweight, can be devastating to the ego, emotional well-being, and of course one's physical health. Most people who are lucky enough not to have struggled with such a curse don't think about the emotional toll this can take on a person. It seems they only see the physical, and believe they have all the answers, because they are thin and you aren't.

Why tell my story? To be honest, this is probably the most painful thing I've ever written about, but if it helps even one person, then it was worth the torture.

You see, to put this out there, I have to "come out" as a formerly fat person. While this sounds ridiculous, because everyone could obviously *see* I was fat, it represents something else to me. For so long being fat equaled failure. Failure to maintain self-control, failure to eat correctly, failure to exercise enough, failure to be as good as the rest of my family, failure, failure, failure. Coming out feels like admitting failure, even though I know it's not true.

I come from a ridiculously beautiful family. I am the eldest of seven children. So, not only do I get to do everything first (e.g., turn 40, wrinkle, dye my grays, etc.), but I'm also constantly compared to my younger, beautiful, *skinny* siblings (who I love with all my heart). People either compared me, said things like "she'd be so pretty *if* she lost weight," ignored me completely, or they forgot they'd met me multiple times (a super pet peeve to this day).

I tried hiding. I tried hiding behind people in every photo. I tried hiding in my house, especially when visiting my hometown where people knew me when I was thin. I tried living in a city where I was anonymous. I tried pretending that if I just loved myself as I was, then others would too. I hid from mirrors, I hid in giant, loose-fitting clothes, I hid behind pillows, I hid under long, long hair. Sometimes I even hid within myself, in total denial.

With all this inner turmoil, I still tried to live a full life. I lost weight on many occasions with crazy diets. Sometimes I was successful, but then something horrible would happen in my life and I would just

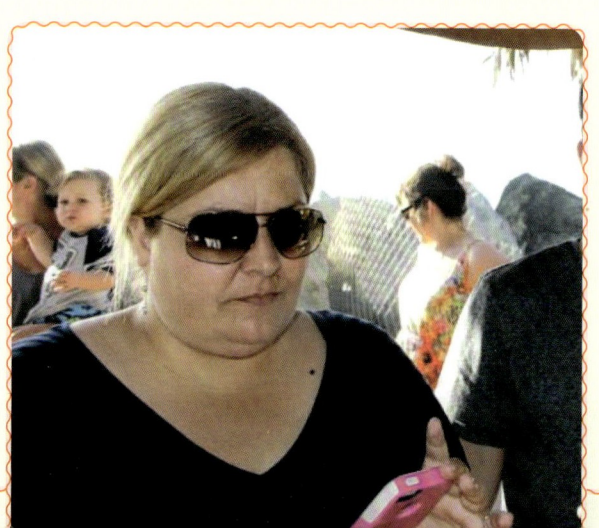

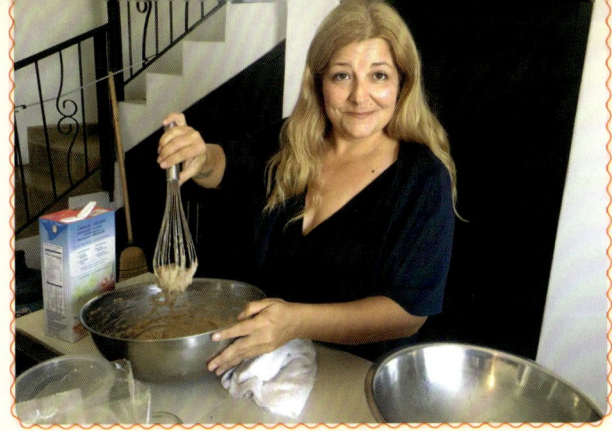

revert back to old habits, often gaining even *more* weight, hiding myself away again.

My guru of sorts, DJ, asked me if anyone ever gave me diet books as "gifts." That didn't happen exactly, but I understood what he meant. I have a fit, energetic, and iron-willed mother. I also have a gorgeous fitness instructor sister-in-law, both of whom have tried to help in their own ways. My mother once went as far as buying me a weight-loss program (without my consent), one of those mammoth programs where they send a giant box containing months' worth of prepackaged food. It was horrible, *terrible*, and TORTUROUS. She had spent so much money on it that I felt guilty, almost *forced* to do it.

I did it.

The food tasted like crap, ranging from cardboard to dog food. It was also miniscule amounts. I was hungry and grumpy all the time. Total misery. I lost weight and she was happy and then, of course, I gained it all back, plus some extra. I failed again. Once again, I was a disappointment.

My sister-in-law trained me for free. I went to her classes and she pushed me and encouraged me, but she told me (and I knew) that if I didn't change how I ate, I wouldn't really lose weight. Sometimes I was an exercise *fiend*, but still fat. I have had so many failures, it would be redundant to tell about them all. You get the gist.

In all this fatness, I was quite successful at my job. As successful as I was, the job was killing me. It

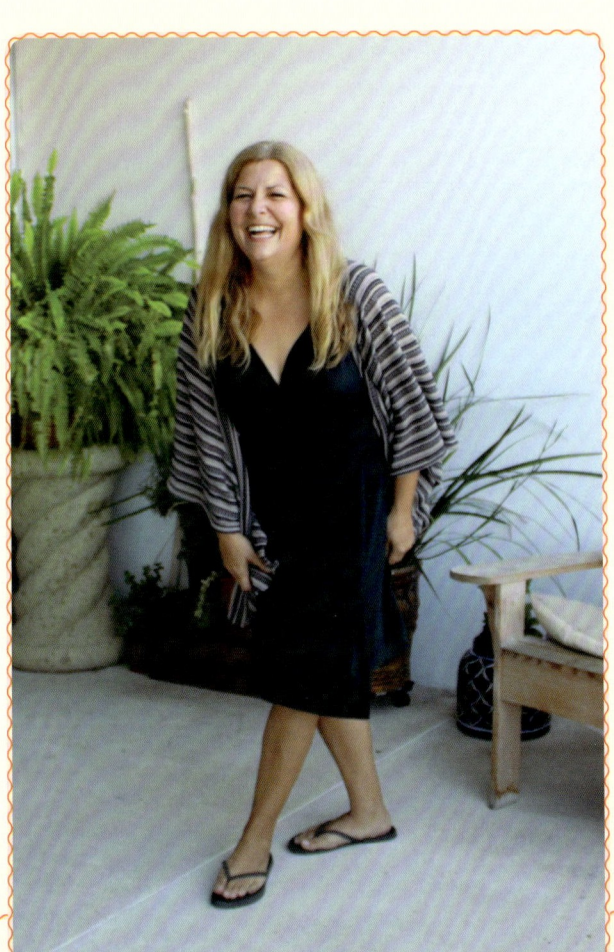

was a *major* contributor to my weight. I see that now. Inside, I was as big of a mess as outside and I hid that too. Weight gain, for me, was an effect, not a cause. I had an important position, with the most horrific boss on the planet (in my opinion). The job itself was incredibly stressful. I was constantly shielding the people that I worked with from the boss. The stress was killing me. I kept gaining weight. It took about 12 years to get to my heaviest point. I ate *tons* of fast food, processed food, sugary things, you name it. Sometimes I would be at a family gathering, eating my mom's delicious dinner. While eating, I'd be thinking about what I was going to eat when I got home, or what I'd grab at Jack in the Box for my "real" dinner. If it was bad for me, I probably ate it, *in abundance*. It was my only comfort, or so I thought.

It all came to a head when two days after a glowing employee review with my boss, I was demoted. It came out of nowhere. It was humiliating. The worst part was that I had to finish out my contract. So, I put a smile on my face every day, pretended I wasn't completely humiliated and embarrassed and forced to lie and act as though it was my choice. I just tried to focus on something else and survive until I didn't have to anymore. I was dying, inside and out. I knew that a 20-year career was over and I wouldn't be able to continue in the field anymore. I was burnt out and devastated.

So, there I was, super fat, still single, 40ish, and faced with an uncertain future.

What was one to do?

Well, I chose an unconventional route for sure. I quit everything. I left my beloved city, I moved to a different country and started a new life with basically nothing. Once semi-settled in, I found myself a gym buddy, my sister's friend (and now mine), the one and only DJ FOODIE.

During our daily gym routine, DJ started to talk to me about the way he eats and what low-primal is all about. He did it in a way that wasn't intrusive or overstepping and he never told me to do it. I'm not sure if he knew that I HATE being told what to do or that I wasn't quite ready, but he didn't ever *push* anything on me, except maybe holding a plank, doing sets of burpees, or going on a hike. Then one day, he just stated that if I ever wanted to try it out, he would help.

One day I was ready! I had sort of figured out my emotional issues, "shed some emotional weight" if you will, and I was ready to take on the *physical* weight. Here is why I was successful:

- I determined when I was ready and willing.
- I'd eliminated major stressors in my life and I'd worked on my emotional well-being.

- I prepared. I cooked, with help (did I mention I'm not much of a cook?), for two days using recipes from DJ's first book. I set myself up for a month's worth of meals: breakfast, lunch, dinner, snacks, and homemade, sugar-free ice cream. My freezer was *bloated*. I wouldn't have to even think, I'd just reheat or toss together a salad.

- The food was so good.

- I was never hungry. That first month I ate whenever I wanted (still do, I'm just not as hungry), whenever I craved, whenever I felt like I couldn't do it (which really didn't happen). I allowed myself to eat, eat, eat, but just the low-primal stuff.

- I chose to start during a month I knew I would be home more, I had less going on, and I could really dedicate myself to this. It would never have worked for me if I started in December.

- I had a guide, a friend, someone who really understood: DJ.

I've lost 70 pounds in about 7 months. I don't focus on the numbers and I don't check often, but my clothes don't fit and I feel GREAT. The best I've felt in 20 years! I'd like to lose another 30, and it will happen, because I will eat this way for life. I'm not going back. I'll remember the pain of it all and know that a sweet potato fry is better than a regular one. I know that sugar and wheat are triggers and I need to be conscious of that when I have my once a month pizza-night treat.

Once I kicked the physical addiction to sugar (and maybe wheat too?), I didn't crave all the crap anymore. I still don't. I don't miss anything I used to eat. Either there is a version of it I eat now or I just don't care. I'm not only lighter on the outside, I'm lighter on the inside. I still have my issues, but the "big fat failure" issue is gone. I can go out to eat and always find something to eat. I can do little, tiny "cheats" like a cold beer on a hot day or regular ketchup in a restaurant and still maintain. I can physically keep up with "normal" people. I can shop at a normal store. I can borrow clothes from people. In fact, that's how I feel, like a *normal* person, not a fat one, not a skinny one, not a formerly skinny, formerly fat and now-within-the-normal-weight-range person, just a person as important or unimportant as everyone else. **No more hiding.** I *don't* thank my evil ex-boss for anything. She would be the type to think she "did me a favor," but she didn't. I did it. I did it all myself. I couldn't have done it without DJ, but I definitely owe myself all the credit, because in the end **I DID IT.**

I'm super excited about this book. It adds to my repertoire. It enhances what I already find an appealing way to eat. It adds a little something-something...

As part of the editing process, I agreed to help DJ by trying out one of the recipes in this book. I've referred to my limited/lacking cooking skills, but really, it's even worse than I've implied, though I'm doing a lot better and gaining confidence. I decided to try out the mini carrot cakes. The 20-minute prep time turned into like three hours!!! When I was grinding the walnuts, they started to turn to nut butter; I'd pulsed one too many times. When the walnuts weren't working the way DJ described, I tasted them. They were old and rancid! So, I had to start over again with pecans. *That* did the trick. It WAS easy!

When I was mixing the blob together, I could already tell it was really thick, so I added some almond milk, just a little, and that worked well. I had started to scoop my blob into the little mini cake molds randomly and thought, "Duh, I should use an ice cream scooper to make them all the same." So the first couple were a slightly different size. But the *biggest* mistake I made was only making a half-recipe batch, because they were soooooooooo goooooooood!!!!!! Delightfully delectable, enjoyable, yummy!!!

I can't believe I made carrot cake AND frosting and it was DELICIOUS. I'm confident I can make all of the recipes in this book and even make up my own using

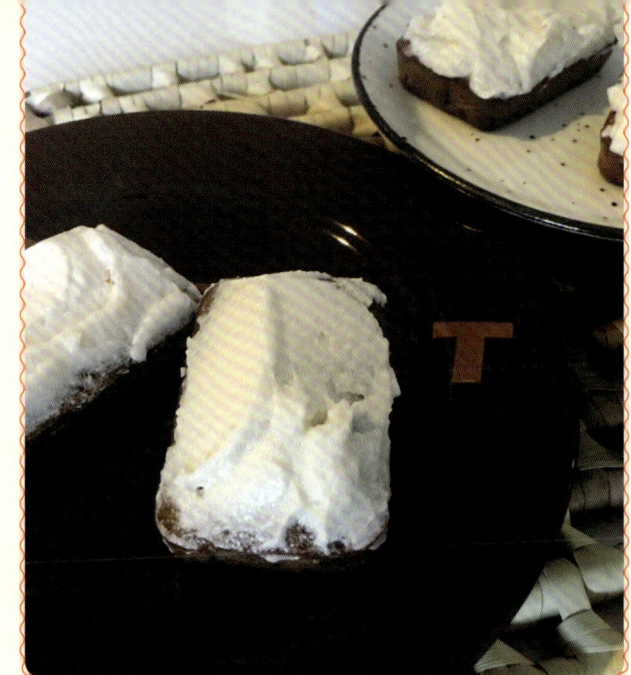

the ratios/formulas. I *also* know I can probably do it in the time suggested, especially as I gain confidence through practice.

I'm excited to be a FAKER!!!

INTRODUCTION

It's funny that I sit here writing a book and primer on grain-free, sugar-free quick breads. Or, maybe it's ironic? It's not something I ever sought to do. Twists and turns in life's experience have brought me to a house on the coast of La Paz, Mexico... to weave the following collection of recipes together and to package them with thoughts, lessons, stories, techniques, a skosh of philosophy, and loads of information.

Why is it funny or ironic? I'm glad you asked!

Two reasons...

One: I was a baker in a former life. Twenty-five years ago, it was my job to arrive at the bakery *hours* before sunrise, to roll sheets of booked dough for fresh, piping-hot, flaky, golden, buttery croissants, spiced-apple pinwheels, and filbert-stuffed bear claws. I would churn out massive Texas-sized muffins with a variety of toppings, including the kind of streusel that must have inspired the term "nooks and crannies." I made mint-infused dinner rolls, sesame steam buns, and all manner of bread loaves made from buckets of natural San Francisco yeast, known as Starters.

Yes, my friends, I was once the problem. I was once a pusher. I was once both a manufacturer and proud promoter of all things sweet, starchy, and gluteny.

Don't tell anyone. Shhhh...

People *can* change!

Two: The inception of this book comes in the form of a "One-Minute Muffin," also often known as a "Muffin in a Minute," or a "Mug Cake." I typically refer to them as OMMs, but they're all more or less the same kind of animal. They are all a quick-bread batter, loaded into a microwave-safe container (typically a coffee mug), then "nuked" for 60 to 90 seconds, resulting in a fresh, hot, and super quick little goodie to be devoured with glee!

One-Minute Muffins have been around for a very long time. I was aware of them within minutes of reading about low-carb diets and philosophies. They're *that* prominent in this culture. The two are inextricably intertwined.

When I first discovered low-carb, I didn't own a microwave.

Well... that's not *entirely* true. I lived in a rented beachfront condo in Los Cabos, Mexico. It had one of those permanent microwaves designed and built snugly into the cabinetry. It looked like it had been a very nice microwave, but by the time I got to it, it had been reduced to telling time and taking up space. It was little more than a nonfunctional prop, occasionally tricking friends into warming nothing with it, in increments of 1 and 2 minutes. It didn't perform; it simply lived in the cabinet, taunting me, leaving me to read about One-Minute Muffins, but rendering me unable to nuke one up and sample it.

I lost almost 150 pounds within that first year. Sadly, I never *once* enjoyed the famous OMM during this time.

About a year later, I moved to a modern building in Belltown, Seattle, Washington. It also had the same kind of microwave built directly into the cabinetry. Unlike my previous microwave, this one would do its job: channel heat energy directly to the molecules inside my food. It could cook stuff.

Oh, joy! Now I could make my first OMM!

I don't know that I'd even unpacked before I was whisking together milled nuts, egg, and sweetener. I plopped my goo blob of batter into the microwave and anxiously watched the greased mug spin in circles. The microwave politely hummed along.

MMMMMmmmmmmmmmmmmmmmmmmmmm mmmmmm......

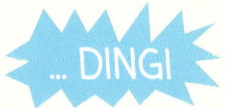

Out popped a fluffy, squat, cylindrical sponge; hot, steaming, flat-topped, and aromatic. DELICIOUS!

I was so excited by it that I *had* to blog about it. By this point, I'd already posted a good hundred or so recipes on the Internet, each with varying degrees of popularity, but... *this* was a clear runaway smash! It was little more than a basic vanilla OMM, but the powers behind social media grabbed onto it and championed it to all ends of the Internet.

Holy frijole! Lightening in a coffee mug! I had to try it again. The people had spoken!

I next tried a chocolate one. BOOM! These little 60-second sodium-bicarbonate-leavened pucks were undeniably popular with those following my shenanigans on Facebook. I was on to something...

I tried something a little more complex. Say... Carrot cake? HOME RUN!

An ex-professional baker, now *microwaving* grain-free, sugar-free batter in coffee mugs, several YEARS after discovering the concept... was now spreading this information virally...

Wacky, huh? Whodathunkit?! Never me!

Over the next few months, I created even more tasty treats. Each time, without fail, each recipe was more popular than the last!

While I never really meant to, I became known as the King of the OMM!

I didn't just limit myself to the coffee mug. I branched out into other shapes. I'd cut them up and use the chunks in other ways. I'd infuse the OMMs with liquids and fry them. I'd suspend them in gelatin. I'd split them and use them for sandwiches, hamburgers, and hot dogs. I made them both sweet or savory; occasionally BOTH!

I also stopped microwaving them. As quick and easy as nuking is, it robbed me of my personal desire to *cook*. Nuking isn't cooking. It's *nuking*!

I come from the restaurant world where microwaves are evil and taboo. They're okay for defrosting *in an emergency*. Otherwise, microwaves have no place in a professional kitchen. I don't necessarily feel *that* strongly about it. I certainly don't begrudge others who love theirs, but those thoughts and memories are always lurking whenever I push the wide, white, spring-loaded button opening the microwave door.

And honestly? I just like them better when they come out of the oven.

Also, as popular and as loved as they are, I often collect comments from naysayers proclaiming, "That nuked puck looks like a sponge!" They're not wrong, either. They *do* look like sponge-pucks.

A microwave cooks by rapidly vibrating all the food's molecules evenly. The *micro*waves drift like a frenetically dancing ghost, through a solid wall of muffin batter. The mixture cooks and rises uniformly, all at once, and all in one consistent level. Therefore, true OMMs have flat tops. Because there is no direct surface heat, there is no roasty-toasty browning of the top.

I personally prefer my muffins to have a golden caramel-flavored crown. A microwaved OMM is often a pale, colorless puck, without that magically burgeoned muffin top. While quick, delicious, and spot-hitting, they simply lack that little bit of specialness. I'm a gigantic fan of that specialness and am willing to wait for it.

See, an oven cooks from the outside in. Heat has no way to frenetically drift through the center of the muffin. The outside surface is cooked first, as the heat slowly seeps through the muffin, cooking and heating, cooking the center last. As the leavener does its job and molecules expand, the outside cooks and hardens, and the still-wet batter in the center feels pressure and rises up, trying to find a way to escape as the edges continue to heat and harden. The batter continues to seek escape.

This often results in a magnificent rounded top. Other times the top hardens, cracks and splits, releasing a fresh flow of raw, lukewarm batter, which pushes above the crest, cooking, browning and solidifying into tantalizingly petrified lava spills.

I love this natural and organic look. I also love the extra boost in flavor that comes from caramelizing the crown, as well as the little bit of browning that occurs around the rim of the muffin.

None of this happens with a microwave.

So, while none of the primary recipes in this book will be nuked, just know that this book was *born* in a microwave and that any of these batters can be poured into a greased, non-porous, microwave-safe container. Said shmoo will quickly turn into a tasty and thoroughly cooked-through little morsel. Just don't fill your cup too high, for fear it shall runneth over.

OK, SO WHY " THE FAKERY "?

Traditional baking is grain-based, is typically starchy, and almost always contains at least a little sugar or honey, and is baked in an oven. A book based on grain-free, sugar-free baked items, with a genesis in a microwave? What is it, if not faking? I mean...

... right?!

I know a lot of people from my past that would slap me silly if I were to call it *baking*. "That's not baking!"

Keep in mind, the term "faking" is *firmly* tongue-in-cheek. It's a loving sarcastic term of endearment. If there's anything I should say about my passion for food and these dietary philosophies, it's that I approach them from a heavily playful place. So many of these ideas and concepts don't register *fun* on the surface. I imbue a good time whenever I can. So, I fake!

For me, faking *is* baking. My wish for the future is that this is what all baking should eventually aspire to. However, any casual muggle glancing in, without our frames of reference, would only see our healthy alternative fakestuffs as nothing more than bizarrely odd fake fakery.

My aim with this book is to hand the keys of faking to those who read it. While the book contains only 30-ish primary recipes, the goal is to give all y'all the skills to locate, tweak, or even create your own tantalizing fakestuffs from scratch.

I aim to give you the skills to convert a recipe into a grain-free (gluten-free), nut-free, egg-free, dairy-free, and sugar-free goodie, all without sacrificing flavor. I also aim to showcase how to take a basic recipe and layer in your own ideas. The included recipes are there simply to illustrate flexibility and provide starting points. Use these lessons, then envision the millions of possible combinations!

Read this book from cover to cover. With a little practice, you should become a top-notch, grade-A, master-faker in no time!

WHAT IS A "QUICK" BREAD, ANYWAY?

A quick bread is typically viewed as a bread leavened (gas forced into the dough/batter) with baking soda and some form of acid, like lemon juice or a tart buttermilk. It isn't clear to me that there is any one definition of a quick bread, but I DO know that it's not bread leavened with yeast. It takes too long to be "quick." It's also unlikely to be a bread leavened by forcing air into eggs, without leavener.

A perfect example of a quick bread is a baking powder-leavened zucchini bread.

THE BLOB THAT ATE CINCINNATI

I've always been somewhat of a computer geek. My parents made video games in the '80s and '90s. I was raised in a computer household. I like to joke that I *typed* my first word, rather than speaking it. I programmed tedious "Choose Your Own Adventure" type, text-based adventure games in Basic, when I was 8 years old. I attended Computer Camp, alternating classes on robotics with horseback riding. I've always bridged the gap between kitchens and computers, loving both and eventually blending them into the same career path!

At one point, I was working for a new content management system company called TalkSpot. It's a company similar to Wordpress or Wix.com. I was trying to conjure up a new-fangled word for what is now more commonly known as a website widget, app, or applet (small application). I read and read and tried to think of a term that encapsulated the idea of having this one single thing that could morph and change into a variety of different things. It also needed to be technically relevant. During all that pondering and researching, I stumbled upon the acronym BLOB (Binary Large OBject).

A BLOB is a large piece of data stored in a database, but can be anything from an image, to a song or a video. Then I read about a database architect named Jim Starkey who lovingly referred to BLOBs as "The Thing that ate Cincinnati, Cleveland, or whatever," in reference to the 1958 movie *The Blob* with Steve McQueen.

The tagline for *that* famous movie? "Indescribable… Indestructible. Nothing can stop it!"

That was it. I now knew the name for the little gizmos we'd drop into our webpages. If you wanted to drop a "text thingie" or a "video thingie" into your webpage, you'd be dropping blobs!

Dropping blobs became my career for a good few years after that. I was a professional blob dropper by day and a caterer at night. All documentation written at the time described blobs. A wide variety of blobs were made.

Years later, blobs have managed to stay on the forefront of my mind. As I sat and tried to think about the title for *this* book, I kept wanting to call it "The Blob that Ate Cincinnati." But that would only make sense to *me*, my past coworkers, and some guy named Jim Starkey. Also, all of this is tech-speak nonsense, which has exactly zero to do with grain-free quick breads.

This book is focused completely on quick breads. More than that, it's about teaching you to build your own quick breads. First, we'll cover the ingredients used. Then we'll make a batter. It is this batter that I view as the new blob.

A quick-bread batter is little more than an amorphous blob. It can be cooked as is (pancakes) or it can be poured into any number of different forms and molds from waffles to muffins to doughnut pans.

From a purely conceptual standpoint, it really helps me to picture the batter as a big blob that can be formed and baked. Too much reliance is often placed on a specific pan or cooking method, when the reality is, a blob will bake or cook and be tasty no matter if you do it in a mug in a microwave or in a cake pan or a series of silicone mini-loaves. Sure, maybe you may have a little extra blob here and there, but that's okay. Just put it in a mug and nuke it up as a snack. The rest will turn out exactly as desired.

RATIOS

I attended cooking school in New York about 25 years ago, in what can only be described as the late 1800s. I remember the classes all focusing on techniques, like peeling and sautéing. Techniques seemed to be all you needed to know in order to *cook*.

The baking courses all relied on a far more standardized form of *ratios*, combined with techniques. Cooking is all about technique and creativity. Baking is about technique and creativity, built around a backbone of ratios.

What do I mean by a *ratio*?

If a recipe for salt water lists 1 cup of salt and 8 cups of water, then it's reasonable to assume that that you could double the recipe and use 2 cups salt and 16 cups of water and arrive at twice the original amount of perfect salt water.

This suggests that the *ratio* for salt water is 1 to 8 (1:8) salt to water. Provided the ratio is maintained, you can make as much or as little as you'd like, and the taste and texture of the salt water will not change one iota. 1 teaspoon of salt and 8 teaspoons of water to create just a little, or 2 liters of salt and 16 liters of water if you'd like a lot!

One incredibly famous and historic recipe, one that predates the idea of a "quick" bread is Pound Cake.

Pound cake, based on a famous ratio of flour, butter, eggs, and sugar, with a 1:1:1:1 ratio (by weight, usually a pound [.45^{kg}] of each), is not a quick bread and it has no leavening agents at all. So what gives it its lift?

Here is where technique comes into play. If one were to simply toss a pound of each of those ingredients into a blender and blend them for 5 minutes... they'd end up as some kind of gluey glop that would probably bake and probably even rise. However, it would be a tough, unrefined, unsophisticated random lump of browned wonkiness.

When making a traditional pound cake, one would cream the sugar and butter until smooth, light in color, and aerated. That's right... *aerated*! By beating the dickens out of the butter and sugar for a good 6 to 8 minutes, you're incorporating millions of tiny little pockets of air, all trapped in itsy-bitsy little bubbles, evenly dispersed throughout the soft, sweetened butter.

From here most people just slowly add their pound of eggs to the butter and continue the aeration process, as they add an egg, mix, add an egg, mix, etc., until all the eggs are added and the batter is even more nicely aerated.

There are a variety of different pound cake methods. Some, just after the creaming, call for the eggs to be separated into whites and yolks; the whites are whisked to frothy meringue-y peaks and the yolks whisked to the softest and lightest lemony yellow. The eggs are then gently folded, bit by bit, into the creamed butter. This act introduces even *more* air and will result in an even LIGHTER pound cake (**Warning:** this approach can also fall flat, without the right touch and experience. This is why I believe adding the eggs directly to the butter is the more desirable approach).

Finally, slowly add *sifted* flour (sifted will have more air in it), about 1/2 cup (120^{mL}) at a time and gently incorporate it into the sweetened egg and butter batter.

Once smooth, place this blob into two greased loaf pans and set into a cold oven. Turn the oven to about 325° F (165° C) and let the cakes bake until a toothpick comes out clean. Set aside on a cooling rack and enjoy. Pound cake!

So what's really happening here? What's the story with the air? Why does that matter?

The method and order of mixing incorporates and traps little tiny air bubbles. The mixing method is designed to maintain as many of those little bubbles as possible and not to overwork the gluten in the flour, which would result in tough cake, because the gluten strands were over-elasticized.

Once the batter is placed into an oven, the entire sum of the batter is heated. Heat expands, so the air trapped inside the little bubbles also expands inside the expanding batter. Eventually, the proteins in the eggs and flour all cook and become solid, trapping the expanded air inside slightly enlarged little pockets all throughout the batter. Additionally, a good portion of water that may have been introduced into the batter evaporates and escapes, further adding to the empty pockets and firm protein matrix left behind.

Now, as much as I love a good pound cake (not that I'm advocating pound cake, mind you), I personally feel the real thing could use a touch of salt. A little salt enhances the flavors of the exquisite farm-fresh butter and farm-fresh eggs you potentially used. What about a little vanilla? Maybe... fold some pecans into the mix and substitute 10% of the sugar with brown sugar?

Now we're combining *creativity* with technique and ratios. Oh, we're baking now!

Without dramatically altering the ratio or the method, we've just gone from a tasty and very traditional 300-year-old recipe to one which has a bit more flavor, a bit more textural nutty crunch and a new layer of charisma and complexity from the addition of the brown sugar. YUM!
NOW let's take 1/4 pound (113^g) of that butter out of the equation and replace it with sour cream. Sour cream has acid in it. NOW let's add 1/4 tsp (1^{mL}) of baking soda to the flour and whisk it together.

BOOM! With the addition of sodium bicarbonate (baking soda) and acid, we've just turned this recipe into a QUICK bread and introduced a chemical reaction that results in pockets of carbon dioxide being formed in our batter. Combined with the existing trapped air, we'll get even MORE lift!

Armed with a little bit of information, one can nudge a very basic simple ratio one direction or another without *dramatically* altering the recipe, yet creating very different variations on the original.

WELCOME TO THE FAKERY!

Buried within these pages are tips and techniques that should help release the creative inner faker within us all!

I've said it before and I'll say it again... My aim is to teach people how to cook and take their lives and health back into kitchens. This is the primary goal of anything I write. I just happen to also strongly believe in going without grains and refined sugars. As a result, these cooking lessons are intertwined with my culinary, philosophical, and physiological beliefs.

My hope is that by focusing on simple ratios, but twisting them with a variety of angles, that each angle can bring its own new life in your repertoire, making you a stronger, more confident cook.

I aim to release you, free, into your own kitchen.

Here are the two primary ratios and methods this book follows:

SWEET QUICK-BREAD RATIO

3 tbsp (45 mL)	nut flour (ex: almond, hazelnut, pecan, walnut [or sunflower seed])
1 tbsp (15 mL)	coconut flour
1 tbsp (15 mL)	sugar replacement (if no other sweetener exists, such as a flavored syrup)
1/2 tsp (3 mL)	baking powder
1/8 tsp (.5 mL)	salt
1 large	egg
1 tbsp (15 mL)	water-based liquid (ex: water, almond milk, flavored syrup)
1 1/2 tsp (8 mL)	fat (ex: melted butter, ghee, or coconut oil)

- In a bowl, combine and mix the dry ingredients: nut flour, coconut flour, sweetener, baking powder, and salt.
- In a separate bowl, combine the wet ingredients: egg, liquid, and fat.
- Whisk wet ingredients into dry ingredients.

SAVORY QUICK-BREAD RATIO

2 tbsp (30 mL)	nut flour (ex: almond, hazelnut, pecan, walnut [or sunflower seed])
2 tbsp (30 mL)	chia seed flour or flaxseed meal
Heaping 1/2 tsp (3 mL)	baking powder
1/8 tsp (.5 mL)	salt
1 large	egg
1 tbsp (15 mL)	water-based liquid (ex: water, almond milk, hemp milk)
1 1/2 tsp (8 mL)	fat (ex: melted butter, ghee, or olive oil)

- In a bowl, combine and mix the dry ingredients: nut flour, seed flour, baking powder, and salt.
- In a separate bowl, combine the wet ingredients: egg, liquid, and fat.
- Whisk wet ingredients into dry ingredients.

Everyone knows Pound Cake. Everyone knows flour and sugar. It's a known and historical way to establish some context. Take the known and establish a bit of a parallel to help explain the unknown. Let's see how we can apply these lessons to grain-free, sugar-free, sodium bicarbonate–leavened blobs of batter!

These ratios, poured into small greased containers and baked, will result in a very simple and very solid pound-cake-like, muffin-y quick bread.

WHAT ABOUT BLOB?

A blob will essentially form and mold into any shape you give it. If you add a touch more liquid, the blob will thin out and make great pancakes! Want to bake a blob as three 9-inch-round (23^{cm}) cakes and layer them with whipped cream? Yep! You can do that. Doughnuts? Check. Pizza? Check! Loaves, even?! CHECK!

Blob is there for you. Pour and bake. Enjoy!

Just double, triple, quadruple the ratio to make more and larger blobs. Adjust the consistency a little bit and pour into your mold, whatever it may be. As long as your mold will withstand sustained heat (without releasing any chemical nasties), you'll end up with a tasty baked treat!

These two ratios create highly versatile and durable blobs. It's been my experience that "precision" is not precisely required. *Baking* is often a precise science, where ratios, techniques, heat, and time must be carefully and dutifully controlled. With *these* ratios, this is not exactly the case. It can help to tune your favorite recipes to your specific tastes over time. However, provided you're approximating *these* ratios, you're going to get something worth eating. With time, tweaks, and modifications, you'll drill your ideas into your specific and unique view of perfect, but... *do not fear* experimentation. Short of an all-out bad idea, small scale fire, or the inclusion of a bad egg... even your worst creations are still likely to bring a subtle smile.

SHORT AND SWEET

There is one area where a clear and obvious problem exists.

Most baking is done with wheat-based flour. Wheat-based flour has gluten. Imagine a tangled knot of rubber bands. As you massage and stretch the knot, the bands increase in length, straighten, and become more and more taut. Now imagine baking the stretched bands inside a wad of starch and fiber. It'll harden, forming a firm structure that holds the cooked starch and fiber in place. This is roughly how gluten functions in baked goods.

Gluten in standard wheat-based flour is a protein and a surprisingly tough cookie. As it is mixed, massaged, and exercised, it gets even stronger and tougher, allowing for some pretty large and substantial loaves of bread. As the gluten cooks, it hardens and forms a large portion of the internal structure of the bread. Its strength prevents the loaves from collapsing in upon themselves. Gluten is load-bearing stuff!

Grain-free breads do not have gluten, which means that they're structurally weaker. A large grain-free blob poured into a deep loaf pan may collapse without some gluten replacers (rubber band alternatives).

Because there is no structure-giving gluten to hold the bread together, it can buckle and fall under its own weight, resulting in a dense, rectangular pancake, of sorts. It'll still probably taste good, but it's not what you want. Large loaves are often tough with grain-free quick breads. Keep your blobs short in stature. I typically try not to ever pour my blobs into anything much over an inch (2.5^{cm}) in depth.

However, if we're discussing something like a muffin, meaning it's an individual, self-contained morsel with a narrow diameter and steep walls, you can go upwards of two inches (5^{cm}). It's the wider cake, loaf, and casserole pans where height really begins to be a problem. On the individually baked portions, the hardened walls of the treat help hold it up.

With these ideas in mind, you should be free to form your own shapes to suit your own goals and needs from here!

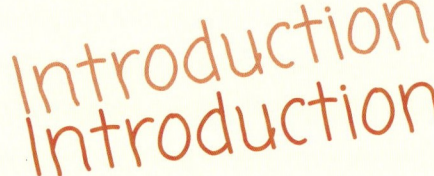

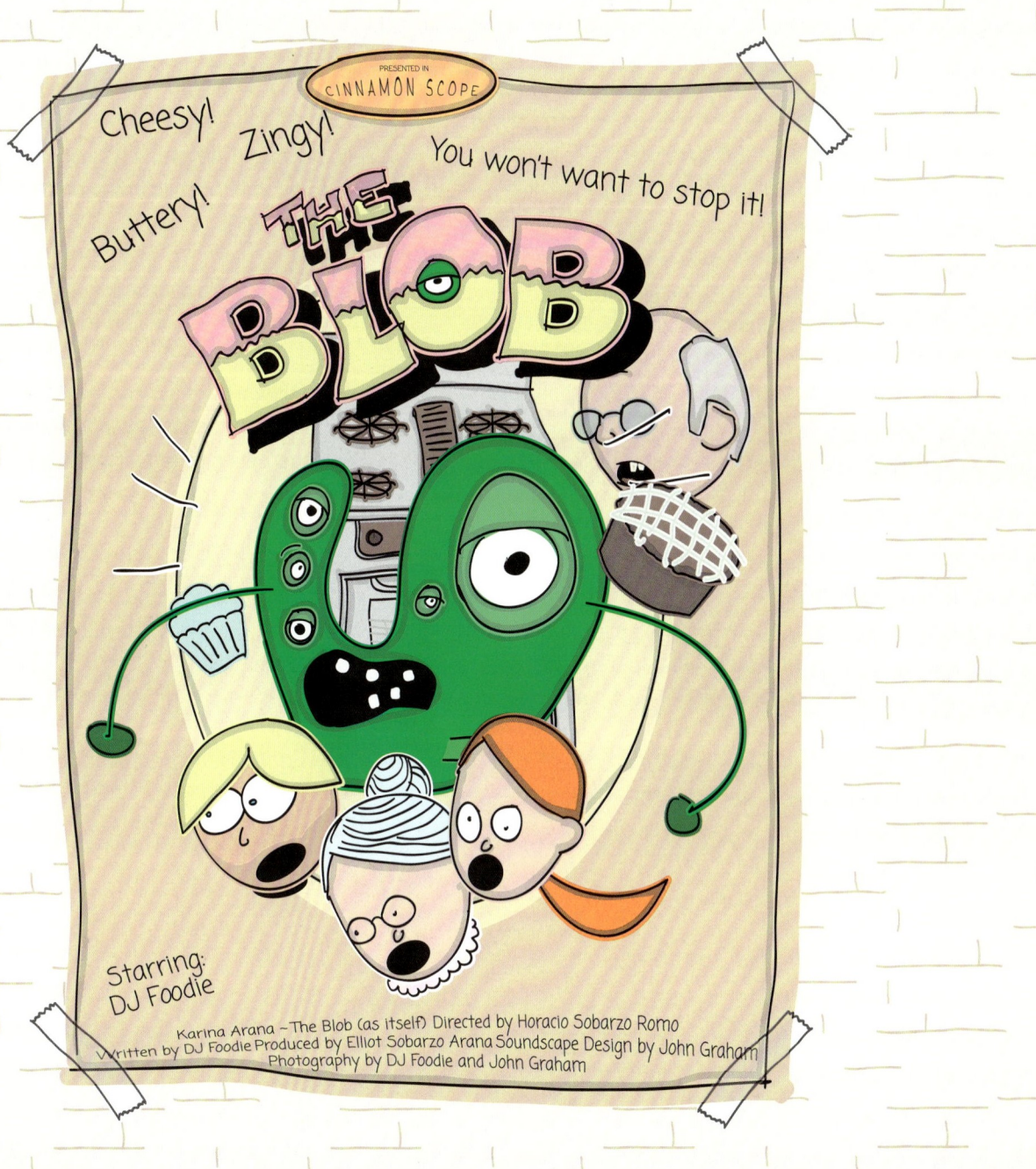

STUFF YOU'LL NEED

As of this writing, I've been blogging for several years, I've worked on 3 cookbook projects other than my own, and have also released my own 6½-pound behemoth of a cookbook, all based around a philosophy I call Low-Primal. The idea is to enjoy the lower glycemic ingredients stemming from the *Primal* philosophy: a modern whole-foods spin on the diet of 10,000-year-old ancestors. It's based on a lot of nuts, seeds, meats, fruits, quality fats, veggies, and some dairy. Everything is minimally processed. No grains, no legumes.

Now, it's silly to think our ancestors were using spice grinders to pulverize their nuts. It's even more silly to think of Grok whipping cream or making eggnog. It's in this vein that I refer to my approach as a modern rationalization.

Realistically, a whole almond will be chewed, digested, and processed in a body differently than a ground one. The ground one, in many ways, enters the body somewhat *pre*digested. Some of the effort of breaking it apart has already been done. Even though we're still just discussing a single almond, it's reasonable to assume that the body will work harder and get fewer nutrients from a whole almond than a ground one. This has both good and bad ramifications. Ultimately, the point is that 10,000 years ago, our ancestors didn't eat ground almonds. Today... we do!

I try and use ingredients that I know how to make in my own kitchen. If there is a level of processing that is impossible for me to do at home... that falls outside the scope of what I see as low-primal (with periodic thoughtful micro-cheats), I will typically avoid it. That's my personal line in the sand.

COUGH COUGH xanthan gum

In all my experiences with blogging, writing and sharing, I've had hundreds of thousands of people engage me in all manner of discussion. It's my belief that most unhealthy people understand that they'll need to change *something*. While they may be prepared for change, a lot don't know what to change or how to begin. They can often get upset or critical when hearing something they weren't prepared to hear.

The everlasting grumble I get from people typically sounds like this: "I can't find that!" or its cousin, "I can only get that at the *health* food store!"

This approach to eating is often seen as riddled with hard-to-find, expensive, and exotic ingredients; things like hazelnut flour, erythritol, and arrowroot. Some people get outright mad at me, like "How will I ever be able to afford this?!" or "Can't you just use *regular* ingredients?!"

Seeing as I have financial problems of my own, it's often difficult for me to tell others how they should prioritize their money. I'm simply not equipped to comment on this.

However, on the use of *regular* ingredients, the regular ingredients *are* the problem! So, no. I can't use those in my recipes. Especially in faking. I wish I could!

Here's the problem: If you want to bake a goodie, most all baked goodies are made from 4 ingredients: Flour, sugar, eggs, and butter. Beyond those ingredients it's a whole host of flavorings, toppings, fillings, colors, textures and hoo-has, but those 4 form the overwhelming bulk of any baked item. *Half* of the ingredients that go into baked goodies are terrible for us in excessive quantities (*far* worse than the eggs and butter). Flour and sugar are likely *the* heart of the matter for most of us. Unfortunately, they're simply not easy to replace.

There is no simple, common, and affordable "Flour II: Electric Boogaloo" that I'm aware of. There is no magical alternative to bleached, all-purpose flour, made from potentially addictive, terminally delicious, and heavily modified modern-day wheat.

Sure, there are "low-carb" flours out there, but they're often HIGHLY processed, full of ingredients I can't pronounce, and (at least in my opinion) taste twangy and bizarre. They're also expensive and hard to find.

There are also organic gluten-free flour blends made from *far* more natural sources, high in ingredients like rice and potatoes. These are tasty, largely functional and a step in the right direction, but still chock-full of starch. Better, to be sure, but we're already standing in the exotic ingredients aisle, pouting at our empty coin purses and we're *still* facing a blast of blood sugar.

In lieu of any other affordable, tasty, and easy-to-find flour... we have a difficult choice.

We can avoid baking and all forms of bread, cakes, cookies, muffins, waffles, and pancakes, *or* accept that there are no simple and direct substitutions for flour. Then do our best to mix and match low-glycemic (low impact on blood sugars) nuts, seeds, drupes, and the various sweeteners at our disposal. I COMPLETELY understand how the question arises.

I get it. I asked it myself at one time. I mean, it's a simple one, right?

Moving deeper into the conversation, I'll hear, "Okay, I get it. Flour is bad. You've convinced me. Now, I want a *good* all-purpose flour. The best. Which one is that?"

To my knowledge, there simply *isn't* a simple answer. Not all simple questions have simple answers. I can't just say, "Almond flour is the answer." It's not. It's a far more complex subject... At this point, peoples' eyes start to glaze over and they take a defensive stance. I persist and hope they're continuing to listen, despite their new posture. Different goals require a different blend of a variety of flours. Like you, I wish it weren't so complicated, but we live in a world where cuisine has evolved with flour and sugar for hundreds of years. *Faking* is a new concept and hasn't yet been streamlined or embraced by the populace.

As much as I love cooking, I loathe dirty dishes. Some of the time I just want an effortless Twinkie. I'd *LOVE* it if there were an affordable and healthy Ding-Dong. I'd do backflips for an easy to find, affordable, comforting and delicious Entenmann's cake; one that which helps tone my abs, increases my lifespan, and slides easily down the back of my tongue.

These things simply don't exist. Sorry. Don't shoot the messenger!

What I've done is to *try* and distill this all down into the bare minimums, while keeping ease of access and affordability in mind. I've read and read, having committed my own health and profession to all of this. I've got serious skin in this game. You can trust that this is the best I've been able to come up with.

If you are aware of better alternatives... by all means, please let me know!

> In order to bake the goodies in this book, at minimum, you'll need the following:
>
> - One nut flour (probably almond, as it's the easiest to find)
> - Coconut flour
> - Chia seed flour
> - A powdered or granular sugar replacement
>
> With *just* those 4 ingredients, you can MOSTLY replace flour and sugar in most quick breads.

I use a far wider range of different ingredients because I think they lend diversity, nutritional variety, and a bit of razzle-dazzle. The synergy can also heighten the quality of these quick breads, but they're not required. Most nut flours are interchangeable with one another. Flaxseed is interchangeable with chia. Most of the other starches, fibers, and proteins just give a nice positive, but optional, nudge.

If you skip to the recipes and see a wide range of things you've never heard of, read on to learn to simplify (or complicate, depending on your desired outcome!).

> I may also suggest for those carefully attending to their budgets that they seek out the following two items, be it new or from garage sales, friends, thrift stores, Craigslist, etc.
>
> - A hand-held spice/coffee grinder or nut grinder.
> - A fine-meshed sieve or flour sifter.

I typically buy almond and hazelnut flours, then grind the rest of my nuts and seeds. Grinding my own almonds from the hulled almonds in bulk bins would likely save me some money, but I usually don't for reasons of ease (*laziness*).

All the rest except coconut are ground fresh, as I need them. The few dollars spent on the above items will save oodles on nut and seed flours in the future, quickly paying for themselves, while also decreasing the likelihood of rancid nut flours.

Let's start talking some more depth!

FLOURS

ALMOND AND OTHER NUT FLOURS

Almond flour seems to be the supreme leader of the nut flours. It can often make up the bulk of the volume in fakery items. I'm a fan of Honeyville's Blanched Almond Flour (Super Fine Grind). That said, I personally prefer *hazelnut* flour/meal (Bob's Red Mill) and use it interchangeably with the almond flour. I find the taste is just a shade cleaner and it's got a few less carbs. However, it's more expensive and results in treats that appear a bit speckled and dirty in appearance. *Almond* flour, when blanched, peeled, and finely milled, results in delightfully clean and consistent-looking treats!

There isn't much *to* nut flours. They are little more than ground nuts. Some are hulled/peeled, some aren't. Some are ground more finely than others, but they're all just nuts. Nothing is added to them and there are no additional bizarre processing techniques applied to them. There is no bleaching, refining, or isolating. They're nuts, plain and simple.

If you purchase almond flour, you're buying precisely ground almonds. Companies like Honeyville and Bob's Red Mill have well-defined methods that give them precision and a very consistent nut granule. We must take a few extra precautions when we grind our own (see tips on *p. 82*), but nothing dramatic and nothing that isn't worth the money saved.

Other notable tidbits...

Nut flours are full of fat. Depending on your view of the world, this can be seen as a good thing or a bad thing. One truth, however, is that it creates baked goods that are decidedly "heavier" than their grain-based counterparts. While you may be able to put away six standard doughnuts in one sitting... one or two nut-flour based doughnuts will likely do the trick. They're just far more action packed in the fat and satiety department.

Nut flours are expensive! Pound-for-pound, yes, nut flours are quite a bit more expensive than wheat flour, but it's not a fair comparison. You'll eat a lot less of the nut flours. Smaller amounts will go further and bring greater satiety. They are far more nutrient dense, so your body is gaining more than it would from the wheaty stuff. Even mathematically, a carb has 4 calories per gram, whereas a fat has 9 stuffed into the same gram. This suggests you're getting more than 2 times the food! Finally, a *substantial* percentage of people are discovering nut flours because, frankly, the cheap wheaty stuff did them no favors. The potential medical and medicinal expenses down the line, don't help either!

A quote I like to bandy about when I'm feeling preachy: "Pay now. If you don't, you're *certainly* going to pay later!"

You get what you pay for.

Ground sunflower seeds (sunflour) works as a fantastic alternative to nut flours, for those with nut allergies. It's just a 1:1 ratio and can be easily substituted.

Powdered nuts, nut meal, nut flour, blanched or not? What's the deal?

There is not one clear standard consensus on all of this. I often read that people are trying to standardize the terms, but as of this writing, I use (and refer to) them all interchangeably and don't notice drastic changes.

Because of these inconsistencies between products, I've had varying degrees of success using the same ingredients made by other manufacturers. Therefore, each recipe suggests the potential for adding liquid. I hate to do it, but short of requiring people stick to my favorite brands, there's no alternative but to suggest people adjust the batter consistency on their own.

That said, typically the finer the grind, the better. Blanched, peeled, or hulled nut-flours typically have a lighter flavor and a more consistent appearance. If the goal is a clean off-white vanilla muffin, a finely ground blanched almond flour is the way to go. If the goal is a more rustic, rough and tumble hazelnut streusel topping for your next cattle ranch picnic amongst the dairy cows, then... of course, untoasted hazelnuts with the lightly bitter skins might give you the dirty appearance and earthy contrast you're seeking.

Sure! Let the *setting* guide your creativity.

You'd think a product labeled "flour" is going to be more finely ground than one that says "meal," and it does typically *seem* to work out that way, but not always. I also often see meal as being unpeeled, whereas flour is often peeled. Again, it doesn't *always* work out that way, though. Just... *mostly*.

These inconsistences often burn my biscuits, but none of them really end in a complete disaster. It can just result in lighter/heavier/darker/dirtier end results, which we enjoy and learn from!

Too much of a good thing?

It takes A LOT of nuts to make nut flour. Sitting around eating a cup (240^{mL}) of nuts (about 90 almonds) sounds unfathomable to some. Yet eating a large piece of coffee cake made from the very same cup of nuts somehow seems okay. You're *still* eating A LOT of nuts. They're just taking a different form. The good news is, your body will likely be happy halfway through that slice of coffee cake.

Eat knowingly and thoughtfully.

Ultimately, the goal with any good dietary philosophy is a healthy mix of varied foodstuffs and nutrients. Vegetables, meats, nuts, seeds, fruits, etc. At no point would I suggest eating massive quantities of pork belly, nor would I suggest downing daily giant bowls of kale. Nut flours largely fall even further from this tree, sliding into the "treat" camp.

Here falls the obligatory: Treats are wonderful, inviting, comforting, and pleasant, but... *not too much*.

COCONUT FLOUR - LESS IS MORE

Coconut flour is a *wonderful* product. I personally opt for the Organic Coconut Flour from Nutiva. While it's a fantastic ingredient, it's a wildly different beast than the nut flours discussed in the previous section.

While nut flours are easy to grind in the home, coconut flour presents challenges. It's *possible* to make at home, but it doesn't come easily and is unlikely to function as well as a bag of the store-bought stuff. Whereas nut flours are little more than ground nuts, coconut flour is a byproduct of coconut milk. In short, coconut meat is pressed, so that a substantial portion of the fats and waters are removed (coconut milk), leaving behind a fiber-rich mulch of coconut flesh. This is dried, powdered, and packaged as coconut flour!

Coconut flour is an off-white, slightly sweet powder. Like a sponge, it's *hungry* in that it absorbs and holds a ridiculous amount of moisture. This unique behavior of coconut flour puts it in a class of its very own. I know of no other direct substitute.

Very early on in my experience developing low-primal, I purchased a bag of coconut flour. Without doing much reading, I relied on what I felt I knew of regular flour. I tried to use it liberally, like I would regular flour. I don't recall what I was trying to make, but I know what I made. I made dry, crumbly lumpules which unquestionably offended my tongue.

I decided, right then, that coconut flour was just the worst, closed the bag and hid it in the back of my pantry, behind the bag of Werther's Originals that I'd been hiding.

A good year or two later, after repeatedly seeing references to the *hungry* coconut flour, I finally dug my heels in and did a little reading on the subject.

General Rule of Thumb: Use 25% coconut flour to replace another flour.

So, if you wanted 1/4 cup (60^{mL}) of a nut flour, you'll theoretically get the same bang, with just 1 tablespoon (15^{mL}) of coconut flour.

The processing method largely explains the hunger of the flour. It's basically de-fatted/de-hydrated ground coconut. Picture a raisin. A raisin is a dried grape. Picture a grape next to a raisin and you'll quickly understand the difference in size, volume, and shape. If you were to soak a small pebble of a raisin in warm water for a while, it would slowly absorb that liquid and eventually grow in size back to roughly the size of a frumpy ol' grape.

Its *hunger*, when quenched, leads to weight gain. Its volume and weight increase.

A single tablespoon (15^{mL}) of coconut flour with all of its water and fat added back to it, each little grain, will swell to about 4 times its size. The grand total would be roughly the same weight and volume of 1/4 cup (60^{mL}) of another type of flour. From a cost perspective, this also suggests each bag of coconut flour actually represents something 4 times bigger. Bang. *Buck!*

Further, it seems that most coconut flour recipes also use a good deal of eggs. This is likely an effort to replace the fat removed during the making of the coconut flour. This is likely why it's not a suitable direct alternative to nut flours, even if less is used.

It's very common to see a ratio of 1 egg to 1 tablespoon (15^{mL}) of coconut flour. Add a touch of sweetener and a bit of baking powder, possibly a small toot of liquid like cream or almond milk and *bake*. Baking this rough ratio will result in a golden-crowned little muffin-y thing!

Once I dug the dusty old bag out from behind the nearly empty bag of Werther's Originals and retinkered with it, I started to realize the coconut mantra "less is more" is true. I started to form a little crush on coconut flour.

Nut flours form a fantastic bulk in faked goods. Fine nut flours, baked, can form a bready-like texture when combined with eggs and a leavener, but I often view nut flours as merely the *bulk* in a recipe.

Depending on your goal, straight nut flours are the way to go. Tougher, crumblier varieties of faked goodies do well with pure nut flours. *Coconut* flour, on the other hand, tends to create a lighter/cakier fakestuff.

However! Coconut flour has a taste not entirely unlike coconut!

That isn't phrased sarcastically, either. I am often asked by the persnickety if coconut flour tastes like coconut. However, that's a lot like asking if flour tastes like wheat. I mean, *sure* it tastes like wheat, but it's not the *same*. Not at all, really. The tastes, textures, mouth feels, etc. are all quite a bit different.

Coconut flour is a bit sweet and definitely aromatic, almost *floral*. It's got a very unique taste, not entirely unlike coconut (but not exactly). I happen to really enjoy it in a wide range of recipes.

I've found that using it in a recipe is wonderful if my goal is something sweet and/or tropical. However, it can be a bit unusual in something like a bacon-cheddar waffle. To my mind, the tastes of cheddar cheese and coconut just don't mesh well. The coconut flour taste is on the persistent side. It stands out above other savory flavors in faked treats. This, of course, is my humble opinion, mind you. Some people LOVE IT!

Because of its mellow, floral, pleasant, but oddly prominent taste, I almost always dilute it by blending it with other flours. Blending a variety of nut, drupe (coconuts are *drupes*), and seed flours can result in some of the best textures in the long run, while also smoothing out and balancing any of the stronger tastes that may come from any *one* flour. It harmonizes and neutralizes. *Synergy*, my friends...

In my experience, blending a small amount of coconut flour, like 1 tablespoon (15_{mL}) and meshing it with roughly 3 tablespoons (45_{mL}) of almond flour results in a very nice little blend, suitable for a wide array of sweet treats. It's got the coconut flour taste, but it's not at the forefront of the flavor because it's counterbalanced by the almond meal.

I also find ground chia seeds make an *incredible* flour, exhibiting some of the lighter/cakier aspects of coconut flour, but without that lightly dominant coconut flour taste (however it does bring a subtle *buckwheat* vibe). I typically use this in blends for savory treats, but more about that later.

CHIA SEED FLOUR

Chia is *incredible*! If you haven't started using it, *start using it*. I usually buy mine from a vendor at the local farmers' market. I have no idea where they get it from, but I enjoy it. I've also had great experiences with Nutiva's range of chia products.

Spending as much time in Mexico as I do, I've been very aware of chia seeds for a very long time. I've always avoided them, believing them to be a *health* food (Yuck! Right?!). I simply assumed chia would taste like dirty chlorophyll and have no redeeming flavors or qualities, short of being spectacularly excellent for my body, and who really wants that?!

I *wish* I could remember what it was that finally got me to open that dusty old bag of whole chia seeds bouncing around my pantry. I just know that once I opened it and used it, I was *forever* smitten. My new crush!

I originally used it for a type of pudding or porridge, but later discovered it's also an *exceptional* tool in the faker's arsenal.

Chia, as many of you may recall, was made famous by the *Chia Pet*, a little terracotta figure used to sprout chia, popular in the early '80s. While you can still purchase hippo- and SpongeBob-shaped Chia Pets around the holidays, I suggest skipping the middle figurine and just go for the seeds.

The *seeds* are indigenous to Guatemala and South/Central Mexico. Chia is in the mint family and may have been as important as corn to the pre-Columbian Aztecs. Ground or whole, the seeds are still commonly used for food and drinks all around Mexico, Guatemala, Paraguay, Bolivia, and Argentina. Oh yeah, in the USA, too!

Chia, like flaxseed, can be found in a darker shade or a more golden-white color. I've noticed less difference in behavior between the colors than I have the producers. Some produce larger, heartier seeds and others produce lighter seeds. The *color* seems to have little impact, short of being a different color. It's the size of the seed that seems to make the biggest functional impact; smaller grains absorb liquid more slowly.

Chia can be found in both seed and ground versions. However, I have found that it's somewhat of a challenge to find preground. Chia grinds *very* quickly, easily, and incredibly fine, without any additional squeezing, isolating or sifting. I prefer to grind my own, anyway.

I'm going to throw an *AMAZING* chia seed recipe right here. It's a porridge and not a fakery item. However, it makes for an outstanding snack, dessert, or breakfast food, while also illustrating the gelling aspects of chia, similar to flax in the next section. I think it's important to understand the behavior of this seed and see the gelling occur. It's good to see how much it swells and increases in volume, but also to see what it does to the viscosity.

Try it! Chances are high that you'll love it!

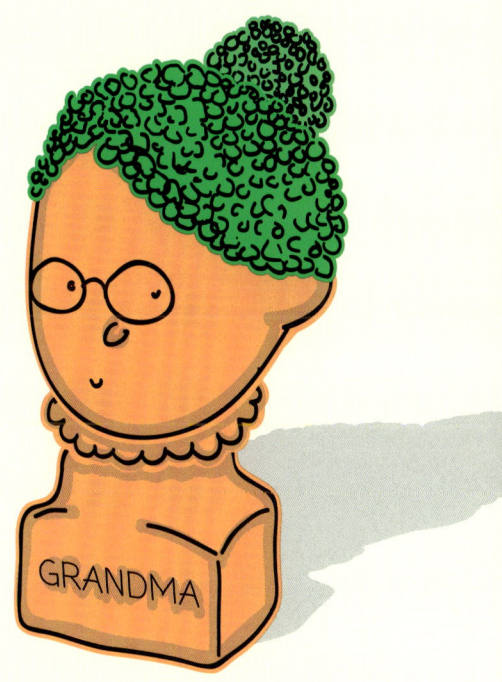

Orange-Blueberry Chia Pudding

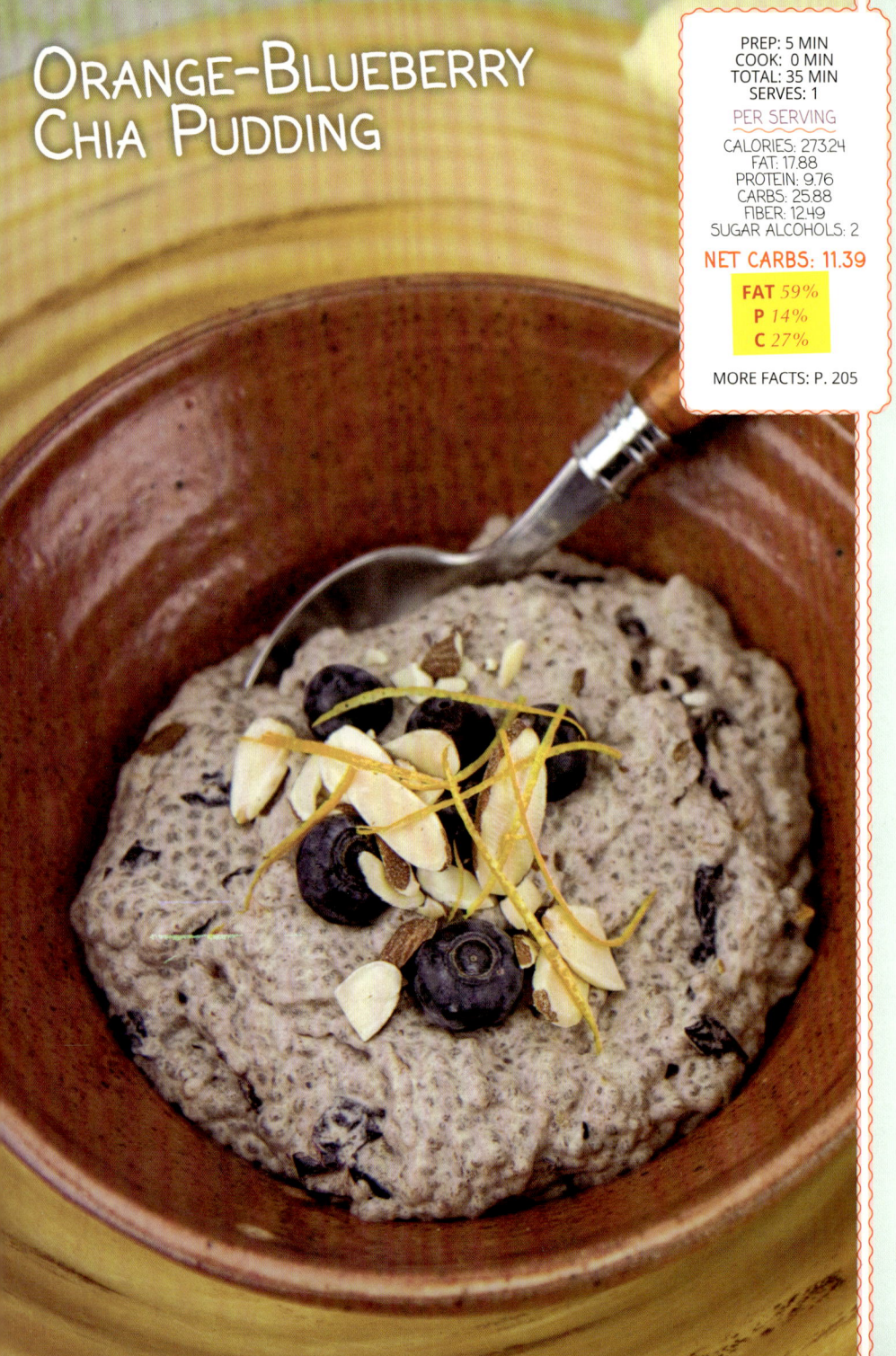

PREP: 5 MIN
COOK: 0 MIN
TOTAL: 35 MIN
SERVES: 1

PER SERVING

CALORIES: 273.24
FAT: 17.88
PROTEIN: 9.76
CARBS: 25.88
FIBER: 12.49
SUGAR ALCOHOLS: 2

NET CARBS: 11.39

FAT 59%
P 14%
C 27%

MORE FACTS: P. 205

Rather than using a fresh orange, I often put a few drops of orange oil into this. This drops the carbs by about 3 or 4, while still contributing a very similar taste sensation. Just add a touch more almond milk and sweetener to make up the lost volume and sweetness. I didn't want to add it to the recipe, as it might be viewed as a strange, exotic ingredient (even though it's one I love!).

3 tbsp (45mL)	chia seeds
1/4 cup (60mL)	fresh or frozen unsweetened blueberries
1/2 cup (120mL)	unsweetened almond milk
2 tbsp (30mL)	sugar replacement
2 tbsp (30mL)	fresh orange juice
1/2 tsp (2mL)	vanilla extract
1/2 tsp (2mL)	fresh orange zest (peel)
2 tbsp (30mL)	blanched and slivered almonds, toasted
Dash	salt

- In a cereal bowl, mix together chia, blueberries, almond milk, sweetener, orange juice, vanilla, orange zest, slivered almonds, and salt. I like to mush my berries a little bit, but you can leave them whole. Stir, then set aside.
- Mix again, about 2 minutes later, to break up lumps that can form.
- Mix again, about 5 minutes later, breaking up any lumps.
- Mix again about 15 minutes later.
- After a total of about 30 minutes, the seeds will fully plump, creating a flavorful and thick pudding-like mixture. Eat!

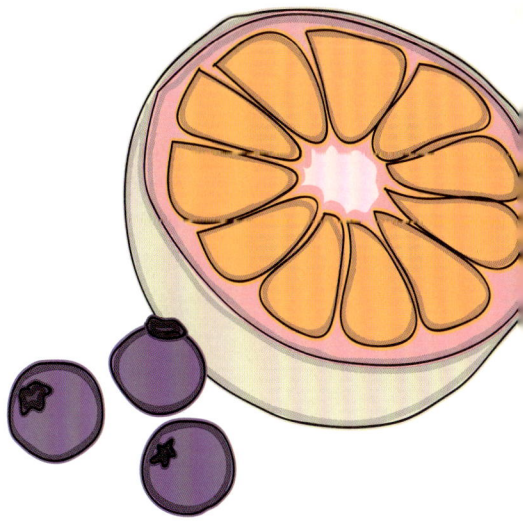

See? Chia is outstanding! I told you!

Chia and flaxseed are almost interchangeable as flours. I find chia to have an overall softer flavor and texture. Even more cakey and a touch lighter. You also need just a little bit less, but mostly, the two can be used interchangeably in quick breads. I am a fan of blending them for a nice synergy.

I typically use chia and flax in stronger tasting sweet treats and savory breads. I'd use them in a chocolate muffin, for example, but not a vanilla one. For the vanilla, I'd likely use the coconut flour (although I might throw a smidge of ground white chia seed in, for good measure). I also find that ground chia is fantastic mixed with chocolate. The tastes really complement one another. Interesting that they both come from the same place!

Chia seems to be a relatively new addition to the modern culinary scene. As such, the jury is still out on any meaningful health claims. Generally speaking, it's seen as positive and healthy, with no known adverse reactions. It's high in thiamine and niacin. Like flaxseed, it's also high in omega-3 fatty acids. Unlike flax, chia does have a long and sustained history as a food for humans. So, I believe it's a very good and healthy food, while ADDITIONALLY being just straight up tasty!

As a porridge, it's got little to no flavor of its own. It's more about the gelatinous gelling that occurs. It's perhaps a distant spiritual cousin of tapioca pudding. As a flour, it's very slightly earthy, but much cleaner in taste than the murkier and muddier flaxseed.

Let's not overlook the chia egg.

Like the trick of substituting sunflower seed flour for nut flour, for those with allergies, it's also good to know how to substitute eggs, for those seeking to avoid eggs.

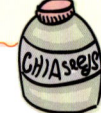

1 CHIA EGG

1 tbsp (15mL) chia seed flour
3 tbsp (45mL) water

- For any egg in any quick-bread recipe, substitute 1 tbsp (15mL) chia seed flour (or flax, but I use chia) and 3 tbsp (45mL) water (or a fuller flavored water-based liquid, like almond milk, fruit juice, chocolate milk, wine, etc.).
- Mix together and let sit for about 15 minutes. This will thicken and gel.
- Use in place of 1 egg. For 2 eggs, double the ratio!

Chia eggs are a very solid alternative to eggs. Yes, it changes the texture and taste, but it's just a lateral move.

I often use chia eggs in place of eggs, simply to switch it up! I find the final product to be a little wetter and a little more texturally delicate, but in a good way! In much the same way a really moist brownie can be delightful, a good chia egg can bring some moisture. I may occasionally do half and half, as well. Hey, some of the time I only have 1 egg, but need two! *SQWINK*

Ultimately, I've seen whole and ground chia seeds used in all manner of smoothies, beverages, puddings, granolas, baked goods, faked goods, and more!

Good stuff. Find some!

FLAXSEED MEAL

When I first began low-carbing, I found a lot of recipes that used flaxseed meal (ground flaxseed). I've only ever used Bob's Red Mill (whole or milled). Way back in 2010, flaxseed was one of the many high-fiber super foods being bandied about as a magical ingredient, perfect for baking and amazing for the body. Volatile flaxseed oil was making the rounds, etc. I think 2010 must have been a great year for the flaxseed industry. I used loads!

Flax, also called *linseed* is a food and fiber crop, mostly known for making the textiles known as *linen*. Yep! Flax makes a good fauxcaccia (*p. 106*), just as well as a nice bed sheet! It's also grown for its oil, which is high in omega-3 fatty acids and makes a spectacular wood finisher.

Much like soy was once (and still is in some circles) a popular health food, the decline began as people learned of the health issues. Most soy is genetically modified, the crops are heavily sprayed with chemical herbicides and the unfermented products (soy milk, tofu, TVP, etc.) contain loads of antinutrients. This has led to a whole slew of issues from infertility to cancer.

Like soy, flaxseed *also* mimics estrogen, which can lead to serious issues, in excess. Flax contains phytoestrogens called *lignons*. Thus, flax can increase estrogen levels and have a blood-thinning effect, lengthening one's menstrual cycle or causing midcycle bleeding. Flax has hundreds of times more estrogenic properties than soy; more than any other plant food, in fact. Clearly, this isn't great for men, either.

On the other hand, it reduces total and LDL-cholesterol in the blood. Flaxseed is a fantastic seed when used as a substitute for eggs in faked goods. However, flax is also quite volatile and can go rancid easily. It's best kept, whole, in the fridge or freezer and then ground when needed. Ground flaxseed can go rancid in less than a week.

So what does this all mean, as I weave in and out of positives and negatives and discuss things like linen and wood finish? Where does this leave *us*?

Eat *sparingly*. Like nuts, go easy! Don't inhale mass quantities of flaxseed. The stuff tastes great and is wonderful as a flour, but *too much* is a problem.

Small amounts, however, have some positives. A bit here and a little there is just fine. I don't consciously shy away from it, but I'm also still working on my same frozen bag of seeds that I have, for a good year or two. I enjoy it, *sparingly*; never more than about 2 tablespoons (30^{mL}) per day.

In terms of faking and flavor, it brings a decidedly earthy taste to foods. There are golden and brown flaxseeds, both of which function in the same manner. I used to use golden simply because of the consistent color, but it was preground and would go rancid quickly. I later purchased a bag of organic brown flaxseeds. It lives in the freezer and is ground fresh, as needed.

It creates a great cakey texture, but can also be a bit on the heavy side. Like within chia seeds, the fiber absorbs liquid and swells, creating a gel. This gel helps form a mild gluten-like structure in faked items. Typically, I'll use this and/or chia seed flour in place of coconut flour for savory treats.

It's a great tool to have, but is optional. Chia is likely a better way to go... (though, I like the synergy of the two, combined).

PROTEIN POWDER

I see protein powder in a lot of low-carb and gluten-free baking recipes. I theorize this is born from the bulking and cutting weight-lifting community. It's used in an effort to bolster protein intake.

I personally use protein powder in baking because I like the flavor and texture, but I also try not to use too much. I get *more* than enough protein in my diet from other sources (bacon). My personal pick is Jay Robb's Whey Protein Isolate (normally vanilla). As with my other favorites, there is no affiliation, mind you. I just get asked a lot, so I'm sharing. On this particular one, I've tried many types. Over the years I've just gravitated towards this product. It's all natural and quite tasty, even with a modicum of stevia!

I have found different protein powders to behave *quite* differently in recipes. I don't know why this one is such a wild card, but it tends to be. Tread carefully.

For one, be sure you're using an "isolate;" by definition, it has no meaningful fat or carbohydrates. It's *just* protein; protein *isolate*. Even here, most issues I've experienced seem related to moisture content. Protein powder, like coconut flour, tends to be a bit "hungry." It likes moisture; some brands more than others. Some of the time, a little extra moisture may be needed, depending on which type you're using (be it another brand, egg, rice, casein, hemp, etc. [don't use pea... it's too different]). It *also* couldn't hurt to sprinkle in a small, mild-mannered dab of fat, as well. Coconut milk and heavy cream are both good combinations of water *and* fat.

The recipes in this book were built using Jay Robb's Whey Protein Isolate, but most protein isolate (again, except *pea*) should work with some tweaking, and ALL are optional. Keep in mind that I never bake with it as the primary bulk. It's always a small part of a blend. Any recipe that uses it, uses it for a tasty nudge and/or a little extra lift. I simply like the flavor and the extra little bit of sponge-like strength I get from it.

Don't sweat it if you don't got it. Just add the equivalent of nut flour, a skosh extra sweetener and you'll be *just* fine.

In terms of the *lift*, or that "protein matrix" in breads, protein powder can somewhat mimic gluten in faked recipes. Many brands also include xanthan gum, which is *also* a common addition to gluten-free baking. If you're looking for something with a bit more rise and a little extra height, protein isolate can be a nice addition. Keep in mind, however, that too high a protein isolate content will render your food dry and rubbery; a rubber biscuit for your wish sandwich. In quick breads, never more than about 25% of your mix should be whey protein isolate.

GLUTEN REPLACERS

GELATIN, XANTHAN GUM, GUAR GUM, GLUCOMANNAN & AGAR-AGAR

Huh? Gesundheit!

Welcome to the gluten alternatives, replacers, and substitutes.

Flour and floury treats have evolved over thousands of years, with the most significant evolutionary changes occurring within the past 60 years.

Wheat flour has *very* specific properties that allow it to stretch, brown, hold liquid, taste great, etc. There are different kinds of flours (high-gluten, bakers, cake, etc.) that are specific to different types of baked goods. As these are being developed, we're all enjoying our pizza crusts and croissants, while the manufactures find ways to cut costs, make a chewier pizza crust and a flakier croissant. These characteristics have become the defining hallmarks of our treats. If a pizza crust isn't chewy, it's not a proper crust. If a croissant isn't light and flakey, it's not a proper croissant.

Remove the flour and you remove the one ingredient that brings *all* of those characteristics to the table!

It would be absolutely fantastic if ground macadamia nuts functioned in exactly the same way as wheat flour, but with an added healthy dose of good fats, no gluten to gum up the works, and no starch to blast the blood sugars. Sadly, this is not the case.

The above list of fibers, gums, and protein-based riddles and games help nudge our baked, moistened blend of nuts and seeds a step closer to the characteristics we seek. Yes, like you, I wish these were easy to find, easy to understand, and offered for free at the grocery store check-out. Alas, that just isn't the world we live in. The best we can do is learn and strive to come *close*, in hopes that prices drop and cultures change.

For now, until then... *wonkiness*.

Before we delve into the following fantasy land of exotics, I feel I need to *strongly* state that none of these are required at all. I've tried to build this book in a way that shows why and when you would use these, but also how to avoid them entirely, should that be your aim.

In fact, I considered omitting them entirely. However, I find them to be fascinating ingredients and worth knowing about. I also think it's fun to see the roles these ingredients play in our food chain. It lends perspective to the various oddities we enjoy and lends some logic to support what may seem like an otherwise daffy choice.

I *also* know that for every person that sneers about the use of synthetic, processed, expensive, exotic, and/or strange ingredients, there is another equally passionate person who is happy to purchase batwings and eye of newt, just to tinker, play, and endlessly refine and perfect their grandmother's pudding-stuffed Bundt cake.

Colors of a rainbow. Choose your own adventure.

XANTHAN GUM

Xanthan gum is the heavy lifter in the gluten-free replacement category. I personally use Now Foods Xanthan Gum Powder. Because xanthan is such a heavy hitter as a gluten replacer, any writeup on gluten-free baking will likely address it the most.

> **Rule of Thumb:** Use about 1/4 tsp (1^{mL}) per cup (240^{mL}) of a gluten-free flour blend, and upwards to 2 tsp (10^{mL}) (or a *smidge* more if really needed) per cup (240^{mL}), for bigger yeast-leavened treats.
>
> Careful, though. Too much xanthan gum makes the final product feel undercooked and gummy. I try to never go over much more than 1 tsp (5^{mL}) per cup (240^{mL}).

Interestingly, xanthan falls outside the scope of my low-primal ideology. I can't make it in my kitchen (not without some of the bacteria *Xanthomonas campestris*, anyway). It's overly technical to create in a home environment. I mean, I suppose it's *possible*, but well outside anything I'd ever actually do.

Like erythritol (smappy), bread and beer, xanthan gum is a product of fermentation.

Baker's and brewer's yeasts are both strains of the *Saccharomyces cerevisiae* species of yeast, a kind of fungi. During fermentation, this strain of yeast converts carbohydrates into alcohol and carbon dioxide. This is how bread and beer are made.

Whereas *those* yeasts turn carbohydrates into alcohol and carbon dioxide during fermentation, the *Xanthomonas campestris* bacteria converts carbohydrates into a gelled form of xanthan gum. This is further solidified by isopropyl alcohol (rubbing alcohol is mostly isopropyl alcohol mixed with about 35% water). It is then dried, powdered and added to products like yogurt to give it a more pleasant mouthfeel.

Ultimately, xanthan gum is a powdered complex exopolysaccharide (a string of multiple sugars) and a polymer. So… yeah, totally wacky stuff. It's used in cosmetics, faked goods, jellies, lotions, medicine, pudding, toothpaste, and more. I personally love it in ice cream!

So, while I could make the argument that it's all natural and that I understand the process, given that it's both fermented *then* precipitated by the stuff that aids my swimmer's ear (isopropyl alcohol), I feel this one stepped over the line into *processed* ingredient territory.

However, to frame the issue in a different light, it takes really just two steps to get from bacteria to a thickening agent and gluten replacer. The most mass-produced form of stevia is known as *Rebaudioside* A. The trade name is "Rebiana." It takes a *42-step* (forty-two!) procedure to derive Rebiana. This process of extraction is chemically driven, using acetone, acetonitrile, methanol, ethanol, and isopropanol for extraction and likely starts with genetically modified stevia leaves.

Compared to the most mass-produced form of stevia, xanthan gum is *wildly* natural and unprocessed.

Sometimes, ignorance is bliss, ya know? Poor Smappy Goodness… *sigh*

The options, as I rationalize them:

1. Skip anything sweet tasting and/or without the textures brought on by gluten.

2. Pursue and enjoy low-glycemic alternatives that have no meaningfully known health issues associated with them.

3. Enjoy treats loaded with wheat and sugar, with loads of known health issues related to them.

I vote for a balance, the middle ground. I typically choose to enjoy periodic treats made with harmless and essentially inert processed ingredients, from natural sources (#2).

Yep. A *total* rationalization, with a side of wiggle room. I've said it before and I'll say it again. It's how I get my cake *and* eat it, too!

These rationalizations *do* tend to keep me on track, though. That's what really matters, no matter the logic to support it. For me, *it works*. It allows me freedoms and variety, without illness and weight gain. Purists will argue, but they can be a grumpy lot, can't they?

wink

Xanthan gum is kind of a thickener and emulsifier, a *texturizer* of sorts. I use it a lot in ice cream, where I find it helps to keep sugar-free ice creams "scoopable," as opposed to the hard rocks they can freeze into. It helps maintain some of the behavior that sugar lends to ice cream. I also find it to be a decent thickener for sauces and salad dressings. Be warned, though, too much and things become *slimy*, quickly.

While xanthan gum is very common as a gluten replacer, some people still have issues with it. It is ultimately a protein, like gluten. Some people experience headaches and varying degrees of digestive issues. Xanthan gum has been found to be an excellent laxative. Upwards of 15 grams per day is fine. Too much or too high a percentage can cause issues with texture and taste in baked goods and can additionally result in tummy trouble. Finally, xanthan gum loses its potency and function over time. I buy the smallest amount possible, once a year. It noticeably loses its powers after that. I probably shouldn't store it next to my powdered kryptonite, though.

Benefits: A great thickener, emulsifier, and gluten replacer. It has some cancer fighting properties. It tends to lower the glycemic index of foods, as it increases the overall viscosity. Some also claim it's good for the skin and hair.

Lots to think about, huh?

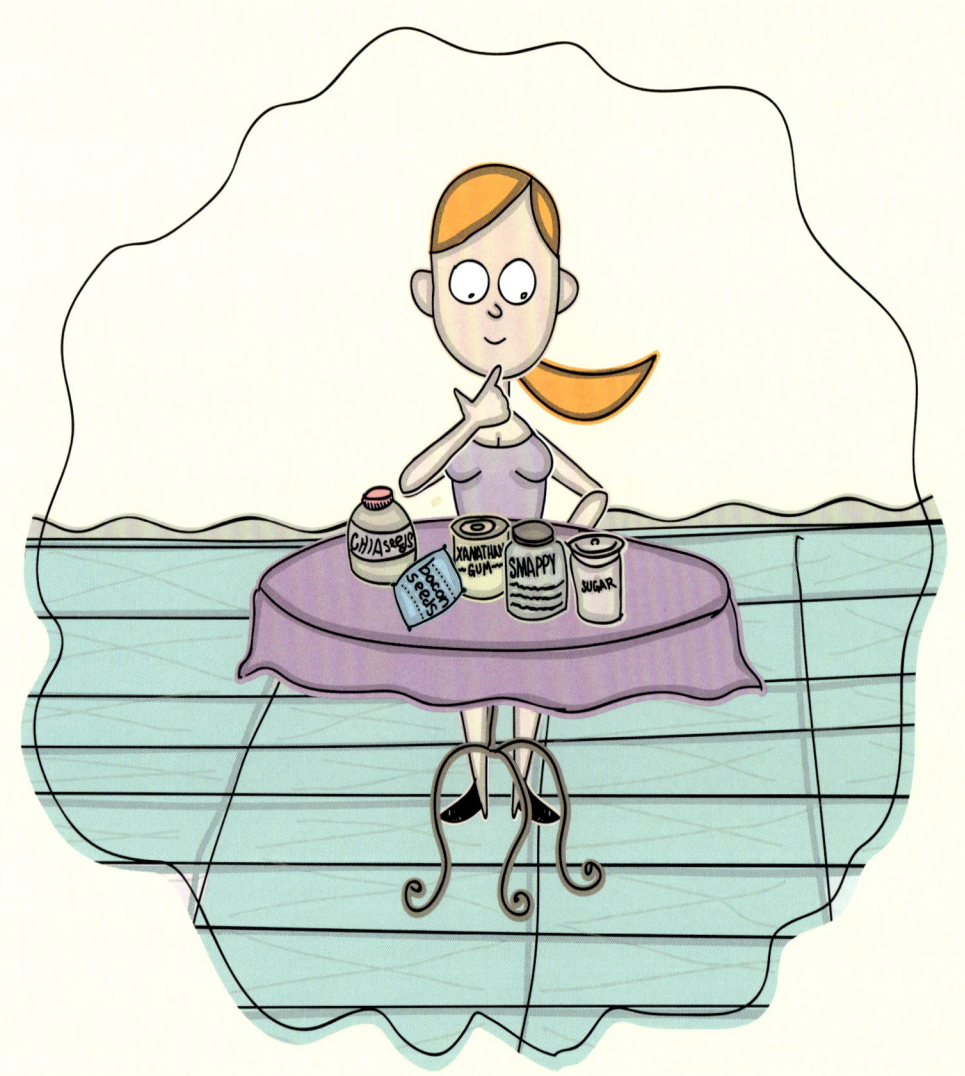

Eat Thoughtfully

GUAR GUM

Guar gum is often used instead of xanthan gum, or in a blend mixed with xanthan gum. I also tend to buy Now Foods Guar Gum. While the two gums *do* share a lot of similar properties, they are not the same.

Guar gum (guaran) is a gummy substance made from guar beans (or cluster beans), a legume (uh oh, Paleo people!). This product is less processed than xanthan gum. As a simplified overview, the guar seeds are husked, milled, and sifted. That's about it! It's mostly used in food as a thickener, texturizer, and stabilizer, but is also apparently used in fracking (to thicken water, helping to carry away sand).

Both xanthan and guar are used as thickeners, but guar doesn't need to be heated to thicken and it's also a great emulsifier. It's used in a lot of cold foods, like ice creams and pastry fillings.

In faking, guar improves overall texture and can help with crisping, something difficult to achieve in low-glycemic, gluten-free baking.

Guar gum will not work as well as xanthan gum as a gluten replacer, but it's close. It should also be noted that acid reduces its thickening powers. So, recipes high in acidity will weaken it. For these, use xanthan gum or a bit more guar.

> **Rule of Thumb:** 1/4 to 1/2 tsp (1 to 2.5^{mL}) of guar gum, up to 1 tbsp (15^{mL}) per cup (240^{mL}) of flour.

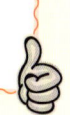

GELATIN

Now for those of you already flabbergasted at the difficulties of replacing flour with blends of other things, it doesn't help to know that within the universe of grain-free faking, there is a further series of potential issues. Some simply can't do nuts due to allergies. Others won't do legumes. Further still, some can't digest eggs.

Another issue is related to xanthan gum. Again, it's the heavy lifter in the gluten-free department, but some experience issues with it. Gelatin often becomes the xanthan replacer (although it's not anywhere near as good... and is clearly not vegetarian).

Gelatin or gelatine (from Latin *gelatus* meaning stiff or frozen) is a translucent, colorless, brittle (when dry), flavorless food derived from collagen obtained from various animal body parts.

Yum, right? I wonder what this would taste like if I added strawberries?! *yummy!*

Yes, gelatin is what gives Jell-O its shape and jiggle. I typically buy Great Lakes unflavored gelatin (red can), but Knox works just as well. Gelatin is definitely an odd foodstuff, but because it's been a part of modern culture for about 100 years, it has crossed over from the weird ingredient it truly is, *into dessert*! And, actually there is a lot to love about gelatin. It's a fantastic source of important nutrients.

Gelatin is great for the gut and digestion. It's wonderful for joints and joint pains. It's helpful for growing strong hair and nails. It's great for the skin and heart. It improves sleep, mood, and thought. It's great for bone density. It aids regulation of the body's metabolism. It helps satiety, too! Low-primalists love Jell-O. You can find sugar-free iterations at pretty much any grocery store. They're fun, colorful, and tasty, while also having virtually no carbs and containing the wonderful gelatin. I usually prepare my own gelatin treats and am a huge fan of using it with chocolate or to make panna cottas.

Currently gelatin is breaking out so much so that fancy powdered supplements are being sold and added to smoothies, coffees, puddings, teas, and more. In fact, there are even little shops opening that serve bone broth, much in the same way cafés serve coffee. What is bone broth full of? Gelatin!

Gelatin isn't a great gluten replacer, but if you can't use gluten and you can't use xanthan, then you're out there slumming a little bit. You must work with what you've got or go without.

Rule of Thumb: 1/2 tsp (2.5 mL) of hot soluble (standard Knox powder or "the red can") powdered gelatin, up to a heaping tbsp (15 mL+) per cup (240 mL) of flour.

GLUCOMANNAN

Glucomannan is a dietary fiber made from the konjac plant. Like guar and xanthan gums, it's used as a thickener and emulsifier. It's also sold as a supplement for constipation, obesity, cholesterol, acne, and diabetes II.

There are a lot of positives to glucomannan. I use Now Foods. Where we're most likely to have heard about glucomannan is as the ingredient *shirataki* noodles are made from. For anyone who's tried these rubbery, zero-net-carb noodles, you'll understand the texture. Now, imagine infusing those noodles with a myriad of small air pockets, which expand as the noodles firm up around them and trap the air.

Glucomannan can be difficult to work with and a bit hard to find. However, it's an interesting substance and fun to play with! Like most of my pantry items, I order mine from netrition.com. You'll find it in capsules, bags, or little plastic jars. If you have the capsules, you can simply separate them and use the powder inside. Otherwise the bags and jars should be what you're looking for.

> **Rule of Thumb:** a dash of glucomannan powder or up to a 1/2 tsp (2.5mL) per cup (240mL) of flour.
>
> **Caution:** Go lightly on this one, or else you'll wind up with bricks. Less is more.

AGAR-AGAR

Agar-agar is essentially the vegan gelatin from the sea. In fact, it's an extract from seaweed and can turn liquids into solids, similar to gelatin, but with a very different texture.

Agar-agar was discovered about 350 years ago, in Japan. You may also find it under its Japanese name, *kanten*. Like most of these wackadoodle ingredients, this one is not just used as a food. It is also used as a laxative, an appetite suppressant, a clarifying agent in brewing, and for sizing paper and fabrics. Mostly, though, we're just focused on its gelling properties as it relates to gluten-free baking. It is used as a gelatin alternative.

Agar-agar is for use by those who can't use anything else. It's vegan, natural, and potentially better than nothing.

> **Rule of Thumb:** 1/2 tsp (2.5mL) of agar-agar, or up to a tbsp (15mL) per cup (240mL) of flour.

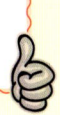

PSYLLIUM SEED HUSK FIBER

Psyllium fiber is the bulk ingredient in Metamucil and Colon Cleanse. I buy mine from GNC. I used a lot of psyllium seed husk fiber early in my adventure, *well* before I discovered all these other ingredients. I mostly used it for rubbery pancakes.

If I had to be point-blank honest, even though it's a fantastic ingredient, I no longer use it simply because of its association to laxatives. It's illogical and ludicrous, I know, but... it's the gosh-to-honest truth.

Psyllium powder is a rough beige powder. It's basically flavorless. It's hygroscopic (it loves to absorb and hold moisture, like other similar gelling fibers [chia and flax, for example]).

A little bit of psyllium goes a long way. Unless you're accustomed to eating a lot of fiber, don't jump off the diving board into a pool of psyllium husks. There are choking hazards: it can swell in the throat without enough water to dilute it.

Then, the other obvious issue is a clear lack of constipation.

Psyllium is completely natural.

Rule of Thumb: Upwards of 1/4 cup (60^{mL}) of psyllium per cup (240^{mL}) of grain-free flour blend to gain some gluten-like benefits (a firmer structure and more height).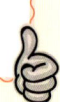

STARCHES

Starch is another oddity in a low-glycemic book about faking. Starch will convert to glucose quickly in the bloodstream, raising blood sugars and bringing out the insulin, the primary thing we're trying to avoid. However, it's such a big part of the gluten-free baking world it seems irresponsible not to cover it on some level.

Further, some starch is fine in the diet, in my opinion. Some people can enjoy more of it than others. There are also those in the Paleo and Primal communities who don't really pay much attention to their carbohydrate intake, focusing more on nutrient density.

Starch is the main component in grain-based flour. In wheat, it can consist of as high as 75% of the flour. Losing it and replacing it with nuts and seeds is also complicated. Starch is key in absorbing and holding water in baked goods, while also influencing appearance, texture, taste, and shelf life. This is why most gluten-free flour blends are mostly starch. Even Paleo folks who eschew potatoes, rice, and corn still use other forms of starch in their treats. Namely...

TAPIOCA STARCH/FLOUR

Tapioca flour or starch (same product) is a very fine and lightweight flour made from the cassava/manioc root. It has a texture similar to that of cornstarch. It's mostly flavorless, but is *ever-so-lightly* pleasant and sweet. It's essentially a pure starch with no other meaningful nutrients. It has about 26 net carbs per 1/4 cup (30^g/60^{mL}), or about 2 net carbs per tsp (5^{mL}). As a comparison, standard bleached all-purpose flour actually has fewer net carbs, at about 23 net carbs per 1/4 cup.

Tapioca flour is *often* what provides the bulk in much of Paleo baking, but the Paleo ideology doesn't focus as heavily on carbohydrates as much as it does on nutrient density. In any event, tapioca starch is seen quite often in those circles. I personally have one foot firmly planted in those circles, but try and further cut out a lot of the unnecessary starch and sugars. Thus, tapioca starch rarely enters my cooking sessions. When it does, it does so in small amounts and is done thoughtfully.

One thing I can say for certain: *I* struggle with today's wheat.

I *love* it and find it terminally fulfilling and comforting, but I also experience shady and diabolical problems with it. Please keep in mind that this is *me*. You may be fine with it, but I know that if I even take so much as a corner off a Wheat Thin, I'll wake the next morning with ludicrous cravings. Wheat is an instantly triggering food for me. It releases my inner lunatic, regrettably and periodically resulting in less than stellar decision making. This tends to perpetuate itself until I wake with cinnamon roll in my eyebrows and on that hard-to-reach spot somewhere in the center of my back.

I personally avoid wheat as much and as often as possible, except for periodic planned events, where I go into it with an iron-clad resolve. I allow myself to eat as much "on plan" foods as I'd like for a few days afterward, allowing pain-free time for the wheat and cravings to clear my system.

Point being, *tapioca* flour doesn't do this to me. If I have a choice between the two flours, tapioca will always win.

Tapioca flour absorbs and retains water, suggesting it's great at binding, thickening, and moistening. While it's not a structure-giving protein (like gluten) and won't keep a bready baked good from falling, it *will* assist in keeping them from being too dry or crumbly. Tapioca flour will lend a lighter, more moistier, more delicate and cakier vibe. Because it doesn't help with holding structure, it's often used in flatbreads, tortillas, crusts, some low-lying cakes, and muffins.

It's not just great as a flour, though. It's a FANTASTIC thickener, which is where it *does* get some mileage in my kitchen.

I'm a big fan of "goo." I'll toss some fruit in a pan (berries, apples, peaches, etc.) and simmer them with some salt (to help remove the water, enhance flavor and speed up the cooking process). Once the water is starting to come out, I mix a small amount of sweetener with tapioca starch and glucomannan powder, then toss it into the simmering fruit. This will thicken it to something like a fruit suspended in syrup (compote), on up to something closer to fruit preserves for pie, depending on the amount used. I typically aim for the viscosity of *goo* and put it on my blob pancakes.

As a thickener, tapioca starch requires about double what would be needed to replace cornstarch. However, you'd need about one-third less than you'd need for the equivalent thickening power of flour. It is best to form a slurry (mix with a small amount of water [about 1 tsp {5^{mL}} tapioca starch to 2 tsp {10^{mL}} water], then pour the *slurry* in), but I often mix it in with other dry ingredients to help prevent lumping.

If thickening, add toward the end of the cooking process, as the thickening will lose its potency after too long in the heat. Keep in mind that a little goes a long way. Start with just a little bit and add more after about 1 minute, if you need it. As with many things, you can always add more, but once it's in there ... you can't take it out. Err on the side of caution.

Tapioca starch is a great product to have lying around, but a little bit goes a long way. Great in a blend, but we low-primalists should avoid using it as a heavy lifter. I typically use Bob's Red Mill.

Finally, there is another product found in some specialty markets called *cassava flour*. This is not the same thing. It's derived from the same root, but is far less processed and is not a pure starch. Don't confuse the two.

ARROWROOT STARCH/FLOUR

Arrowroot shares a lot of similarities with the aforementioned tapioca starch. It's also nut-free, grain-free (thus, *gluten*-free), dairy-free, egg-free, seed-free, GMO-free, and vegan. I also use Bob's Red Mill.

Arrowroot is a starch derived from the rhizome (that is, rootstock, an often-underground stem, like ginger, lotus, galangal, and turmeric) of the tropical perennial herb *Maranta arundinacea*. Arrowroot has a long history of cultivation, dating back over 10,000 years, in northern South America.

I personally first learned of arrowroot in cooking school, where it was touted as a better alternative to cornstarch. Cornstarch thickens with a cloudy opaqueness, while arrowroot thickens perfectly clear and shimmering.

Arrowroot has about 27 net carbs per 1/4 cup (32^g / 60^{mL}), just a shade more than tapioca starch.

Arrowroot has a long list of health benefits: everything from fighting foodborne pathogens and serving as a digestive aid to boosting immune system function and soothing mouth pain. It was even used to help pull poison from an injury caused by poison arrows!

In terms of faking, tapioca flour and arrowroot are largely interchangeable. Both are great in blends, but neither are particularly great on their own.

Nut- and seed-based baked goods are often considered quite heavy. Granted, this can be a good thing, in that you're likely to be satisfied with less. However, it's nice to know that there are options for removing some of that heavy density and providing a bit of levity. A wee little bit of arrowroot or tapioca will do the trick.

With nuts and seeds, the moisture is coming in the form of fat. By adding a starch, you're adding carbohydrates and can lose some of the fat. The starch holds water, which is also a moisturizer. Less fat means less calorie density and less "heft." Keto people are clearly of the fatty bandwagon, while Paleo people may thrive on arrowroot. Scales slide.

Colors of a rainbow.

Just remember that you're adding about 2 net carbs per teaspoon (5^{mL}). This can make it okay to throw 1 tablespoon (15^{mL}) into a 6-serving batch, as it only adds about 1 net carb per serving. It won't *dramatically* change the outcome, but even a subtle nudge or two may make something a nudge or two more enjoyable!

As a thickener, arrowroot also functions like cornstarch and tapioca flour. However, whereas you would multiply cornstarch times 2 to get the correct quantity for the tapioca, it's closer to 1.75 for arrowroot. It has slightly more potent thickening properties.

It should be said that this is just a quick overview of these products. I doubt most will even use them, but I have personally used both enough that owning small amounts has been worth it to me.

LEAVENING AGENTS

Leavening agents and leaveners may be combined with a range of techniques to add air and volume to doughs and batters.

AIR

It should be said that *air* is a leavening agent.

As illustrated near the beginning of the book, the original recipe for pound cake didn't include a leavening agent (the thing that puts bubbles into bread).

When butter is whipped, the volume increases because tiny little bits of air get trapped in the butter. This increases the overall size of the mass without increasing its weight. Further whipping of various ingredients, such as eggs, can trap even more air bubbles. Gently blending and folding these whipped and aerated ingredients together results in a light batter.

This mass of blob is then baked. During the baking process, the heat causes the air to expand, creating even bigger bubbles. As the blob bakes, the proteins coagulate and harden, trapping the air and forming a spongy skeletal structure that maintains its shape after the goodie is cooled.

Thus, it should be noted that *air* is its own leavening agent, but it should also be noted that working only with air is more time consuming, trickier, and will typically result in smaller/denser pockets of air than if a chemical or biological leavener is used.

WATER

Water functions similarly to air. At sea level, water freezes at 32° F (0° C) and turns to gas (water vapor) at 212° F (100° C). Only pressure (atmospheric, peer, or otherwise) can change these constants.

When a batter or dough is baking, it is heating up from the outside in. As the water rises in temperature, the water molecules increase in size. As they hit 212° F (100° C), they turn from liquid to gas, essentially leaving an empty water pocket in their wake, while increasing the overall size and volume of the baked goodie. The water *vapor* molecules continue to increase in size as they bake.

Eventually, the baked goodie will be removed from the oven, where some portion of the water has evaporated and filled the oven with water vapor, helping form the crust. The rest will stay trapped inside the treat, converting back to liquid when it's cooled, lending moisture (along with fat) to the whole affair as it's eaten.

Sometimes, however, water and air just aren't enough.

BAKING SODA

Baking soda is quite common and seems to be good for pretty much everything. If you're bored, try googling "uses for baking soda." It's good for cleaning, freshening your mouth, treating insect bites, soothing your feet, and so much more!

For our purposes, however, baking soda is a chemical leavener. Baking soda ($NaHCO_3$ or sodium bicarbonate) is a chemical compound that reacts with acid in a moist environment and liberates carbon dioxide. This carbon dioxide (CO_2) expands in the heat causing air pockets, which are trapped by the hardening batter or dough.

Everyone knows the science experiment where the kid has a volcano model topped with baking soda. Vinegar is added to the baking soda and the volcano erupts with white froth. *This* is the chemical reaction at work.

Baking soda without acid doesn't do anything, though. It just sits there, tasting a bit like my toothpaste. It doesn't convert to carbon dioxide. It sits, inert, and channel flips.

(Okay, that's not totally true. The truth undermines my point, but the reality is that heat—anything over 80° F [27° C]—also causes baking soda to release CO_2, but only half as much. Sodium carbonate is also produced, giving the food a soapy taste.)

Ever hear of the pH scale? It's a rating for the acidity or alkalinity of certain substances. The range is from 0 to 14, with *0* being highly acidic (battery acid) and *14* being highly alkali (liquid drain cleaner). In the center, at a cool neutral 7, sits pure water.

Acid is a substance that neutralizes alkalis, such as the weak alkali sodium bicarbonate. Acid turns litmus red, it dissolves some metal (try squeezing a lemon on aluminum foil), is corrosive, and has a sour taste in liquids.

For the purposes of our discussion, we're not talking about any bathtub-corroding acids, such as hydrochloric acid. We're talking about citrus juices (especially lemon and lime [pH of 2]), yogurt, buttermilk, vinegar, wine, and tomato juice (pH of 4), etc. Our range of acidy is between 2 and 4 on the pH scale, but even milk and rainwater are lightly acidic.

When faking, I personally try and match an acid to the taste of whatever I'm making. However, if I want something more neutral in taste, I use cream of tartar. Read on to learn how!

BAKING POWDER

Baking powder is not the same thing as baking *soda*. Baking powder *contains* baking soda, but it isn't baking soda.

Baking powder is a mixture of baking soda and a powdered form of weak acid (commonly cream of tartar [a derivative of tartaric acid]). Baking powder is also commonly mixed with other components to help with consistency, stability, anti-caking, helps absorb moisture, and to prevent a chemical reaction. It's this latter "filler" (commonly cornstarch [from grain]) that contains carbs.

Eliminating baking powder is a good way to eliminate a few carbs and enhance the likelihood that you're eating *clean*.

To skip baking powder, you can mix your own or follow some of the following general guidelines, keeping in mind that baking soda is about 4 times more potent than baking powder.

The following substitutions work quite well:

1 tsp (5^{mL}) baking powder = 1/4 tsp (1.25^{mL}) baking soda plus 1/2 tsp (2.5^{mL}) cream of tartar

1 tsp (5^{mL}) baking powder = 1/4 tsp (2.5^{mL}) baking soda plus 1/2 cup buttermilk, sour cream, or plain yogurt

1 tsp (5^{mL}) baking powder = 1/4 tsp (2.5^{mL}) baking soda plus 2 tsp (10^{mL}) lemon juice or vinegar

BAKER'S YEAST

Yeast plays no role in this book. I personally haven't used baker's yeast in years. For its tangential relevance, however, I feel I should still touch on it.

Baker's yeast (*Saccharomyces cerevisiae*) is a biological leavener. It's been used to leaven breads as far back as ancient Egypt. Yeast converts the fermentable sugars in doughs and batters into carbon dioxide and ethanol.

Random irrelevant trip down memory lane: I was a baker in San Francisco, which is famous for its sourdough breads (because of the wild yeasts that exist in that area).

I remember my first-day training with the head baker. She took me into a walk-in refrigerator and showed me to a shelf with a series of 5-gallon buckets, each containing a different starter (a prefermented mixture of flour, water, and various wild yeasts, microorganisms, and lactobacilli).

She asked me if I'd ever smelled a good San Francisco starter. I confessed that I hadn't. She told me a story about wild yeasts and explained the concept of starters and mothers and claimed that one of the mothers (just another name for starter) was well over 100 years old, and that she'd been feeding it daily for years. She said that the aroma was beyond anything I'd ever experienced or ever *would* experience.

She told me to get close to the bucket so that I could fully take in its fragrance.

"Closer," she said. "Get in really close and inhale *deeply*. You won't want to miss it!"

I leaned in and held my nose right against the lip of the bucket.

"Right as I remove the lid, inhale deeply and take it all in."

She removed the lid and as deeply as I could, I took in all the gases and vapors that had been collecting at the top of the bucket since its last feeding.

Oh, my dear friends, it was like doing 3 consecutive shots of gaseous tequila vapor... *through my nose*! All that ethanol had been collecting at the top of the bucket, waiting a hundred years for me to idiotically snort it all deep inside my head, frying my olfactory system.

It was like snorting an invisible cloud of mustard, crushed habanero seeds, and wasabi. Ever want to clear your sinuses? Inhale deeply over a 100-year-old sourdough starter!

Eventually, my tears ran dry and the head baker's laughter subsided.

Wow, that Hurt!

Needless to say, that was a quick lesson in yeast converting sugars to CO_2 and alcohol. Lesson learned!

Yeast is used in a wide range of foods, most notably bread. So why isn't it in use here? For the most part, even in the real world, quick breads are made without yeast (hence the term *quick*). Yeast requires time for the little single-celled fungi to do their work. Even quick-rise yeast takes a good while to get going. It's not in use here because it's not quick (and this is a quick-bread guide).

Secondly, yeast eats sugars and starch to create CO_2. As much as I personally enjoy my low-glycemic sweeteners, yeast *knows* something is up and won't convert it. Yeast thrives in honey, but gets grumpy in a wet, sandy pool of erythritol.

Finally, yeast is a fairly potent leavener, relative to the amount used. It's often used with heartier breads, higher in gluten. The gluten provides a tougher framework to hold the bread together as it fills with CO_2. Even the strongest gluten-free baking mixtures struggle to hold together in the same way many conventional breads do. We're limiting our gluten-free options to those without grain and low in starch and sugars. So, we're dealing with far weaker structures... perfect for cakes and muffins, but lousy for bagels or baguettes.

For the most part, when yeast is used in low-primal cookery, it's simply done for flavor.

That said, I should point out that there are many low-carb frankenfood recipes on the Internet that *do* use wheat gluten and are capable of holding together. In those instances, the yeast is fed sugar or honey. These carbohydrates are converted into CO_2 and ethanol (which evaporates). Do not count these sugars toward your total net-carb count. They're not there by the time the bread is eaten.

BRIEF MENTION OF SWEETENERS

Sweeteners are a big topic within the realm of baking and sweets. I wrote a substantial amount on this subject in my first book, Taking Out the Carbage. I hate to duplicate all of that and will provide only the bare essentials here. If you'd like more depth, you can grab a copy of my first book. Alternatively, I go into even MORE depth on my blog. Google "djfoodie Sweet Spot" to unearth loads of freely available information on my website, ranging from available sweeteners (natural, as well as synthetic), to recipes for your own blends and reviews of popular sweetener brands.

Like flour, sweeteners are also a bit of a challenge. Sugar is what all sweets have been built around. However, sugar has very specific properties that are hard to duplicate, right across the board. While some sweeteners are good at providing "sweet," they may not caramelize (brown) like sugar does. Or, another may taste great and brown, but will cause gastric distress. Another may have incredible flavor, but is concentrated and synthetic, lending no bulk to a recipe. Another may brown, measure like sugar and taste great, but ... has a high glycemic rating, causing elevated blood sugars.

So, what are we do to?!

Much like with flours, the key comes down to blending and mixing and matching. The goal is a delicious sweetener, with a taste, volume, and function as close to table sugar (sucrose) as is possible, but with as minimal a hit to blood sugar as possible.

I am personally a huge fan of the Swerve brand sweetener and believe it to be the best overall sweetener on the market, as of 2017. It's all natural, it's tasty, it measures like sugar and has a glycemic index of zero. The downside is that it can be on the expensive side and a bit hard to find (although their website will tell you where to find it). I typically order mine from netrition.com.

Beyond that, I encourage people to study sweeteners to learn what fits best into their lives. Because I know finances can often play a significant role in determining food choices, it stands to reason that homemade blends are the way to go.

A good homemade blend can be just as good (if not

better, in that it's both homemade AND built to your own tastes). It is also going to be more affordable, if the initial ingredients are purchased in bulk. And, like most pantry items, a powdered sweetener blend is not going to go rancid any time soon. Make a huge batch every few months and enjoy!

The average American enjoys roughly 160 lb (73^{kg}) of sugar per year. That's gosh-darned near 1/2 lb (227^g) a day! And, for some who only eat 10 lb (4.5^{kg}) a year (like me), there's another craving lunatic ingesting lethal amounts of sugar to the tune of 310 lb (141^{kg}) a year (like me, in 2010!)!

Granted, that's not all consumed through shovels full of crystalline saccharose. It's delivered through a wide variety of mechanisms, such as soda, doughnuts, breakfast cereal, and Weight Watchers Mint Chocolate Ice Cream Cups.

Assuming we're going to replace this sugar with 160 pounds of alternatives... it simply makes sense to invest in bulk ingredients for homemade sweeteners. Just make a huge batch every 6 months. It takes minutes to do and... you're all set!

TASTY VS. GOODNESS

I really see the sugar-free sweetener world as having two mainstream dominant super-potent sweeteners: sucralose and stevia. If I had to do a double-blind taste test, sucralose wins. I don't love it alone, but I prefer the taste to stevia. Stevia just has a bitter taste to me, which is less pleasant than the somewhat hollow or empty sweetness that I get from sucralose. However, stevia is going to win every argument put forth about health and nature, simply because it comes from a leaf (somewhere in there).

So, I'm going to create a split in my naming convention. Sucralose blends will be known as "Tasty," and stevia blends will be known as "Goodness," henceforth.

Tasty blends will often be less expensive than their Goodness counterparts. They're likely to be more synthetic in nature and are likely to be the better tasting of the blends. Goodness blends will be as close to nature as I can make them, without concern for costs.

Even though I personally believe that the Tasty ones are less expensive and taste better, I'm still likely to mix up a batch of Goodness for myself. I often call myself a "gateway cave hippy." It's the best way I can describe my desire to be open to all things, while trying to stay closer-ish to nature and eat like Grok.

"Smappy" is the term I concocted for erythritol, finding it to be a far more pleasant word for a sweet tasting natural sweetener, than the kerfugly multisyllabic erythritol. Because, all of my blends contain erythritol, they will all be Smappy blends.

Finally, all of these recipes are 1 to 1 (1:1) sugar replacement recipes, much like Swerve or Splenda.

BASIC TASTY SMAPPY

Basic Tasty Smappy is designed for simple applications. It's affordable, easy to make, and tastes great! It's good in most applications. This runs the risk of crystallizing in super-sweet recipes but is perfectly suited as a standard sweetener. This would be great for coffee or iced tea. This would be good to give a sweet kick to a pancake batter. It's great for adding a touch of sweetness to any savory dish.

1 cup (240 mL)	erythritol
14 drops	liquid sucralose

That's it! Put it in a bowl and stir it up! You can now use this mixture like you would for sugar, one cup to one cup.

BASIC SMAPPY GOODNESS

Like the Basic Tasty Smappy, this is good for simple applications. This is all-natural and basic. It's also good in most applications, but not in high concentration desserts. The erythritol will crystalize at too high a concentration. Good for mellow sweetening.

1 cup (240 mL)	erythritol
1/8 tsp (.5 mL)	powdered stevia concentrate

Mix it up! Powder it if you want to. That's it!

TASTY SMAPPY: BAKING BLEND

Now here's a sugar blend that's better for baking. Really, it's just as good as the Basic Tasty blend, but it's a bit more complex, a bit costlier, and certainly a bit stranger. *However*, it's also very tasty and will work fabulously in your muffins, cakes, and cookies. Again, the idea is to make a cup of sugar replacement.

1/2 cup (120 mL)	erythritol
1/2 cup (120 mL)	polydextrose
31 drops	liquid sucralose

Mix in a bowl, and/or powder in a Vitamix or coffee grinder. You may want to dry this in an oven if doing big batches, before giving a final mix in a Vitamix or coffee/spice grinder. The PolyD likes to absorb moisture and is quick to clump. Store in an airtight container.

SMAPPY GOODNESS: BAKING BLEND

This is the all-natural version of baking blends. The inulin helps bulk out this sweetener, to dramatically decrease the likelihood of the erythritol clumping in sweets. The stevia is increased to pick up the sweetness slack dropped by having less Smappy.

- 1/2 cup (120 mL)   erythritol
- 1/2 cup (120 mL)   inulin
- 1/4 scant tsp (1 mL)   powdered stevia concentrate

Mix it up! Powder it if you want to. That's it!

LIGHT BROWN SMAPPY: BAKING BLEND

- 1 cup (240 mL)   of either of the two Smappy Baking Blends
- 1 tsp (5 mL)   yacón syrup

In an electric mixer, mix the ingredients until well combined.

This will have a *slightly* muddy and wet texture. That's fine. I wouldn't make too much of it, and would just drizzle a bit of yacón into whatever it was that I might be making. You could also use one teaspoon (5 mL) of blackstrap molasses instead of yacón, but it adds about 5 net carbs to the whole recipe.

DARK BROWN SMAPPY: BAKING BLEND

- 1 cup (240 mL)   of either of the two Smappy Baking Blends
- 1 tbsp (15 mL)   yacón syrup

In an electric mixer, mix the ingredients until well combined.

Again, to learn more about these ingredients and the logic behind all of this, grab a copy of my first book, Taking Out the Carbage, from my website, or search for the "Sweet Spot" on my website. It's a series of 7 blog posts. If I do say so myself, it is as informative as it is fun to read!

VISUALIZE

As much fun as it is to write about and discuss different ingredients, a *picture* is worth a thousand words.

I created a small experiment designed to showcase the behavioral properties of each major ingredient. Each recipe is identical, with exception to the **one variable alternative**. The two tablespoons (30^{mL}) of water in each sample is a bit wet and loose for some ingredients and not quite wet enough for others. This bit of extra water helps to showcase the *thirst* of the ingredients.

As you peruse the photos, take notice of the size of the air bubbles, the shape of the crown, the color and more. Make note of the muffin size, as well as the snooks and craggles on the top. Imagine which ingredients absorb moisture and which don't. Imagine which hold their shape and which collapse. Creatively visualize what biting into it must be like. Imagine the texture and mouthfeel as you chew.

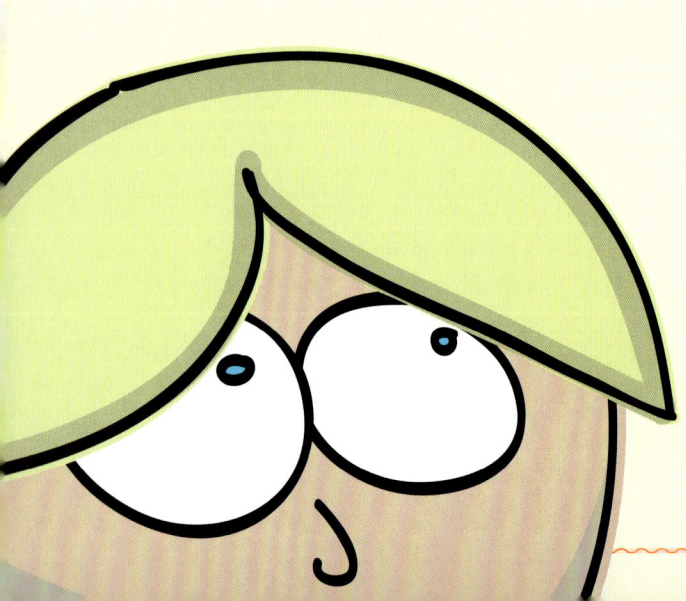

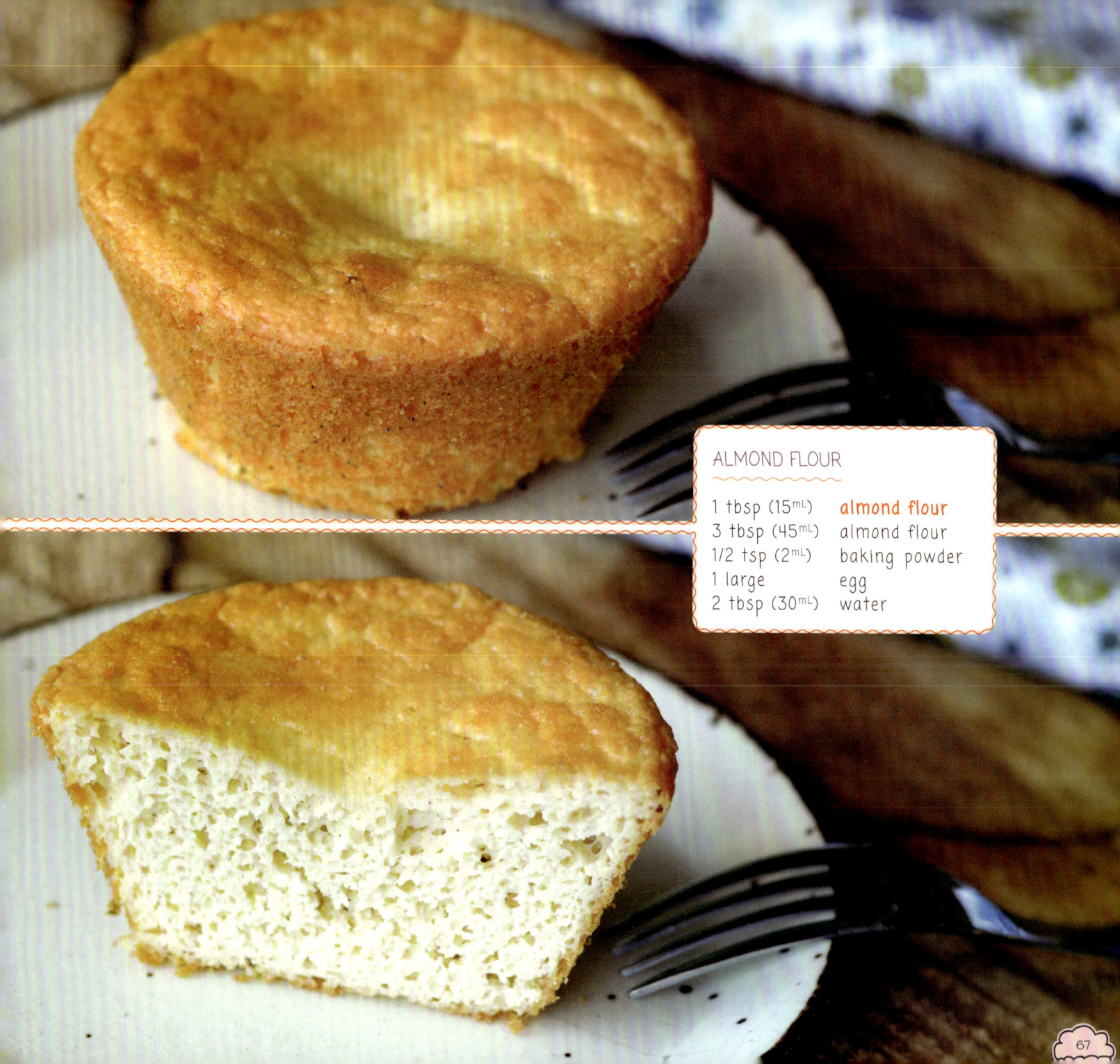

ALMOND FLOUR

1 tbsp (15 mL)	**almond flour**
3 tbsp (45 mL)	almond flour
1/2 tsp (2 mL)	baking powder
1 large	egg
2 tbsp (30 mL)	water

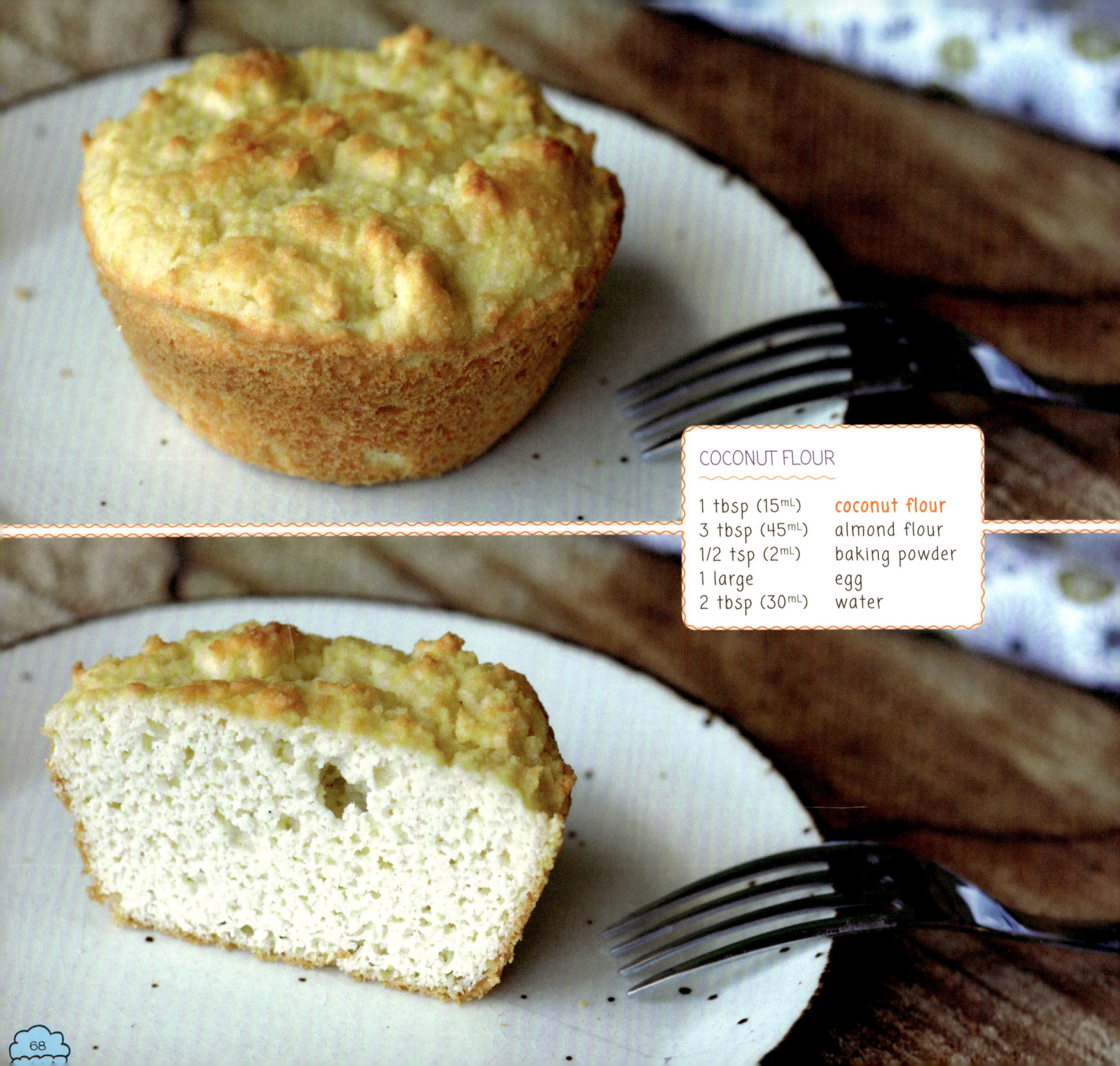

COCONUT FLOUR

1 tbsp (15 mL)	**coconut flour**
3 tbsp (45 mL)	almond flour
1/2 tsp (2 mL)	baking powder
1 large	egg
2 tbsp (30 mL)	water

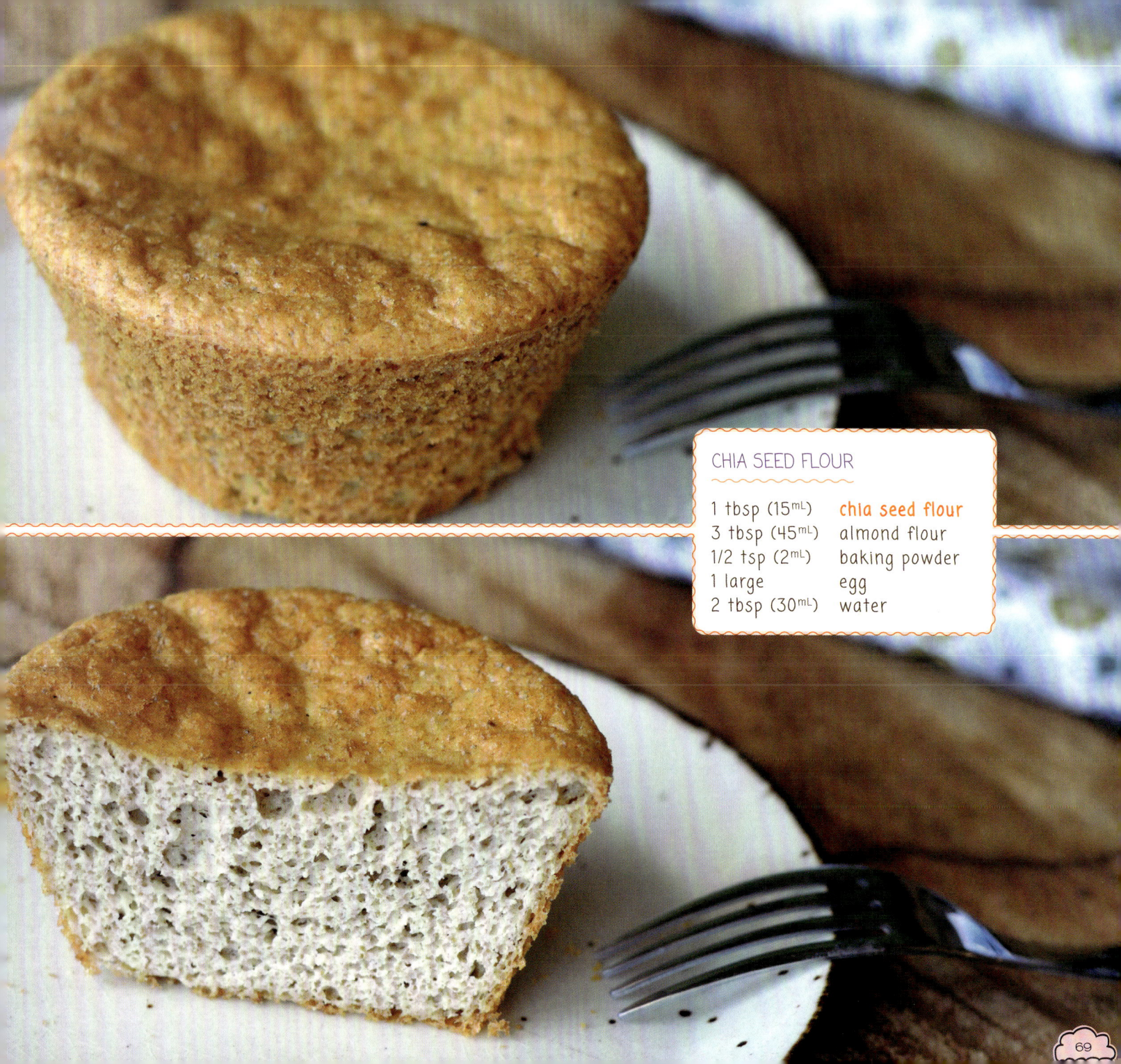

CHIA SEED FLOUR

1 tbsp (15 mL)	**chia seed flour**
3 tbsp (45 mL)	almond flour
1/2 tsp (2 mL)	baking powder
1 large	egg
2 tbsp (30 mL)	water

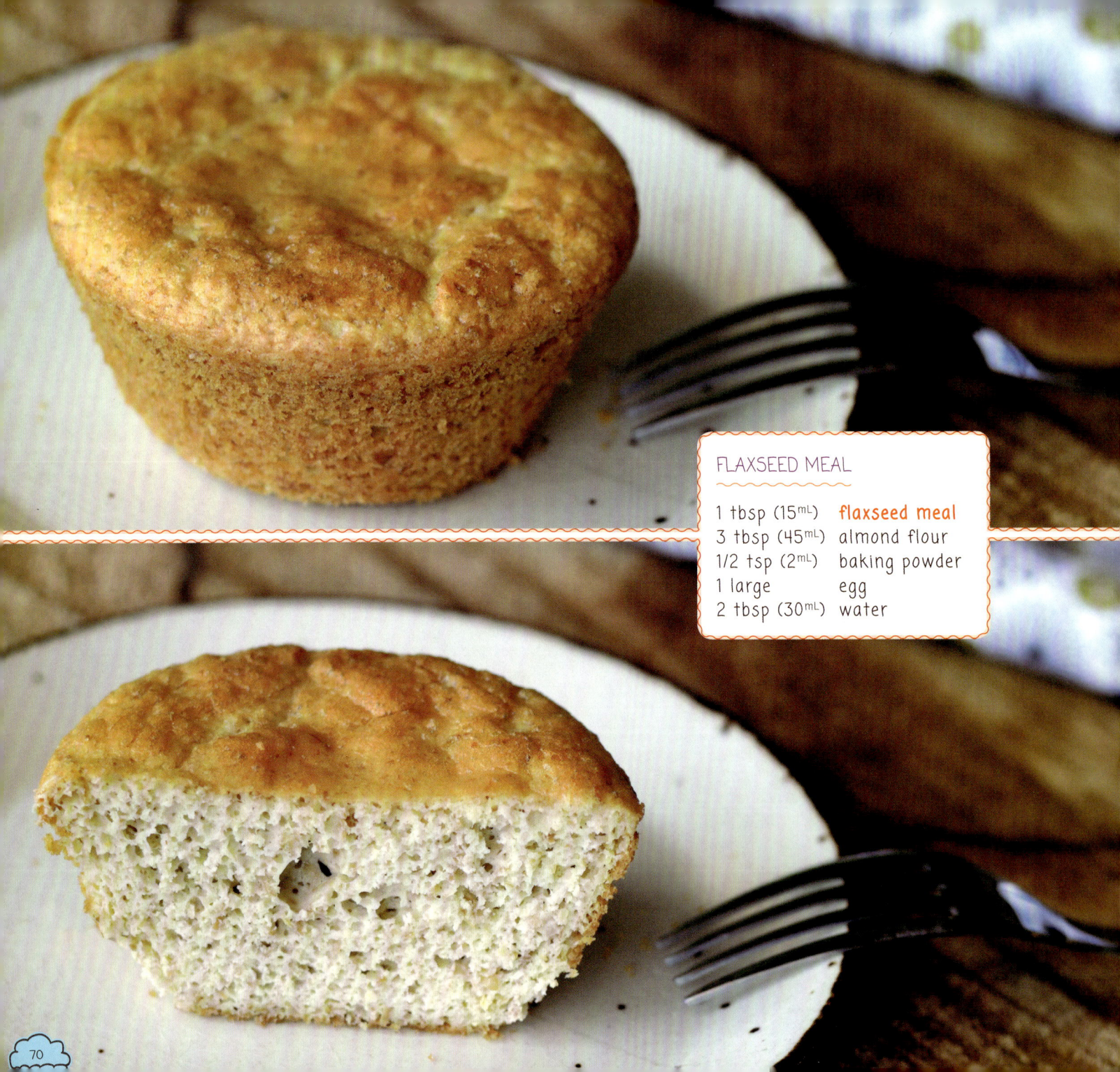

FLAXSEED MEAL

1 tbsp (15 mL)	**flaxseed meal**
3 tbsp (45 mL)	almond flour
1/2 tsp (2 mL)	baking powder
1 large	egg
2 tbsp (30 mL)	water

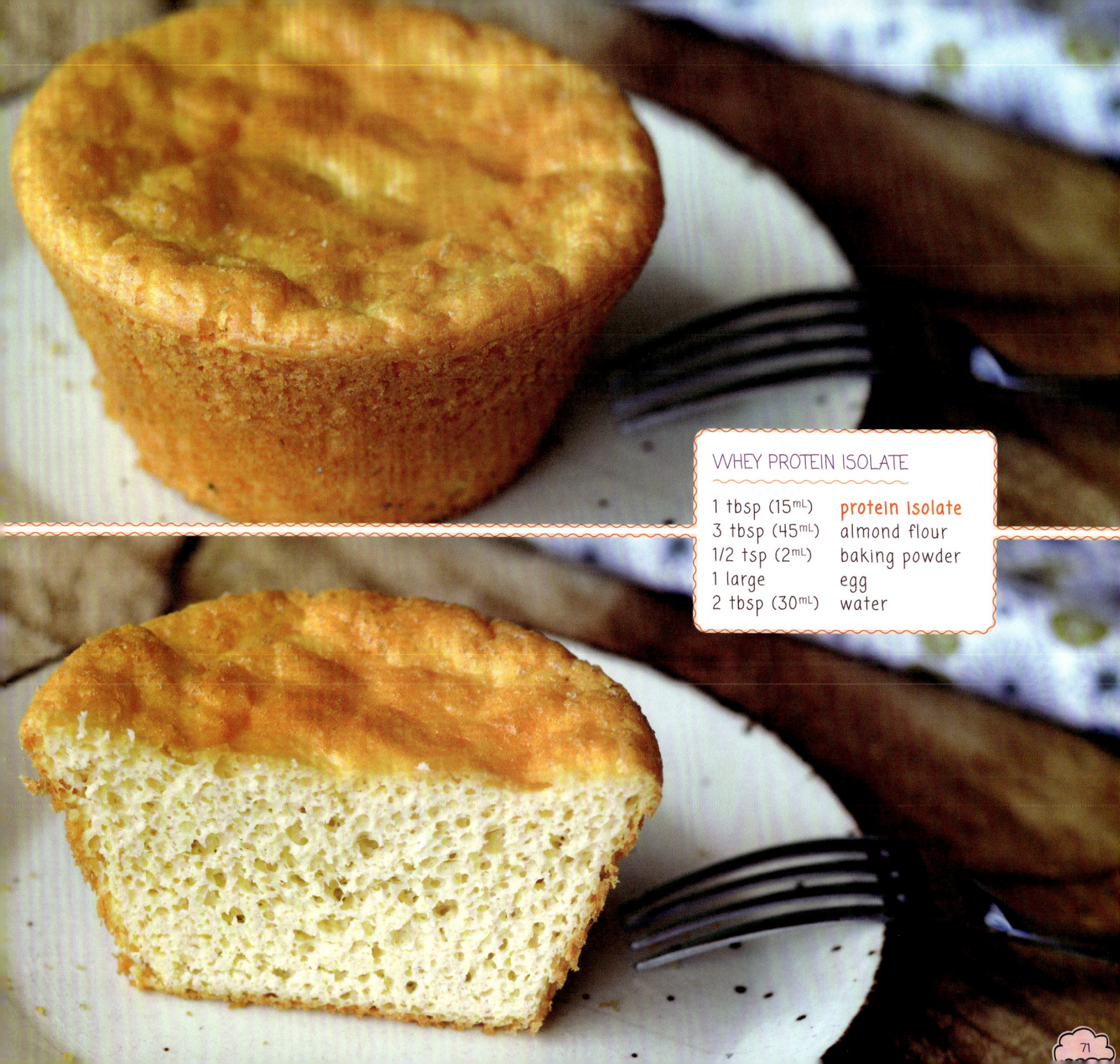

WHEY PROTEIN ISOLATE

1 tbsp (15 mL)	**protein isolate**
3 tbsp (45 mL)	almond flour
1/2 tsp (2 mL)	baking powder
1 large	egg
2 tbsp (30 mL)	water

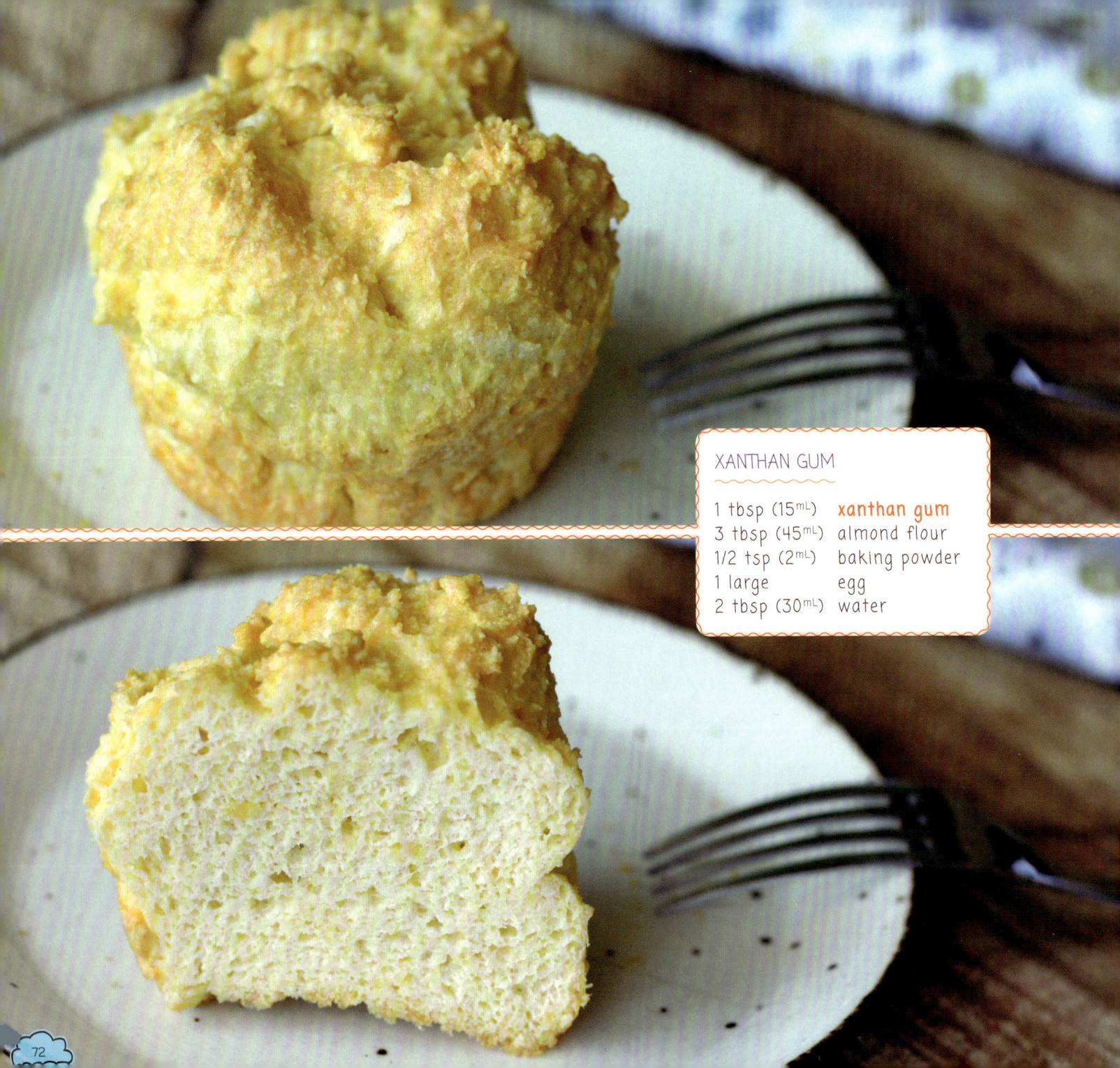

XANTHAN GUM

1 tbsp (15 mL)	xanthan gum
3 tbsp (45 mL)	almond flour
1/2 tsp (2 mL)	baking powder
1 large	egg
2 tbsp (30 mL)	water

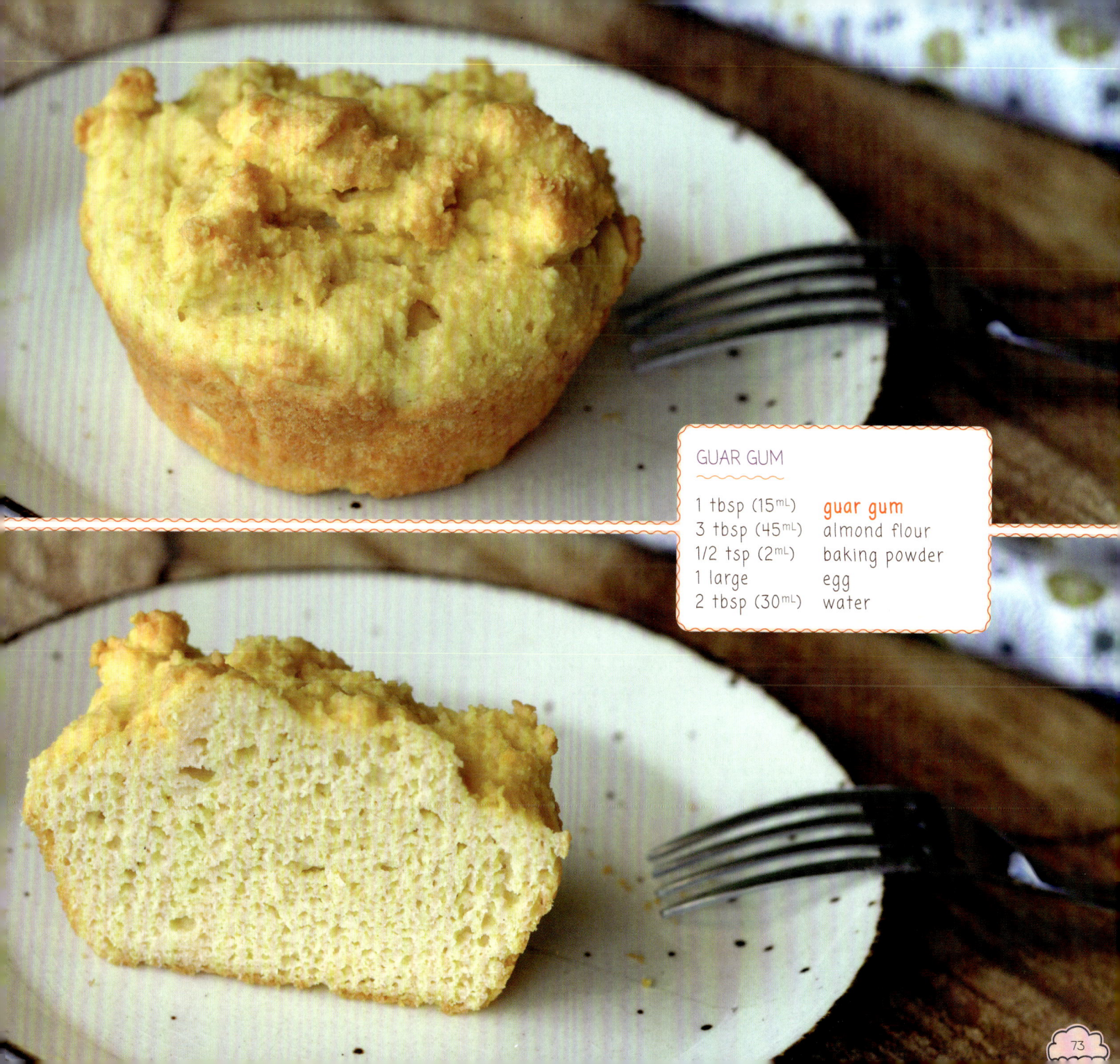

GUAR GUM

1 tbsp (15 mL)	**guar gum**
3 tbsp (45 mL)	almond flour
1/2 tsp (2 mL)	baking powder
1 large	egg
2 tbsp (30 mL)	water

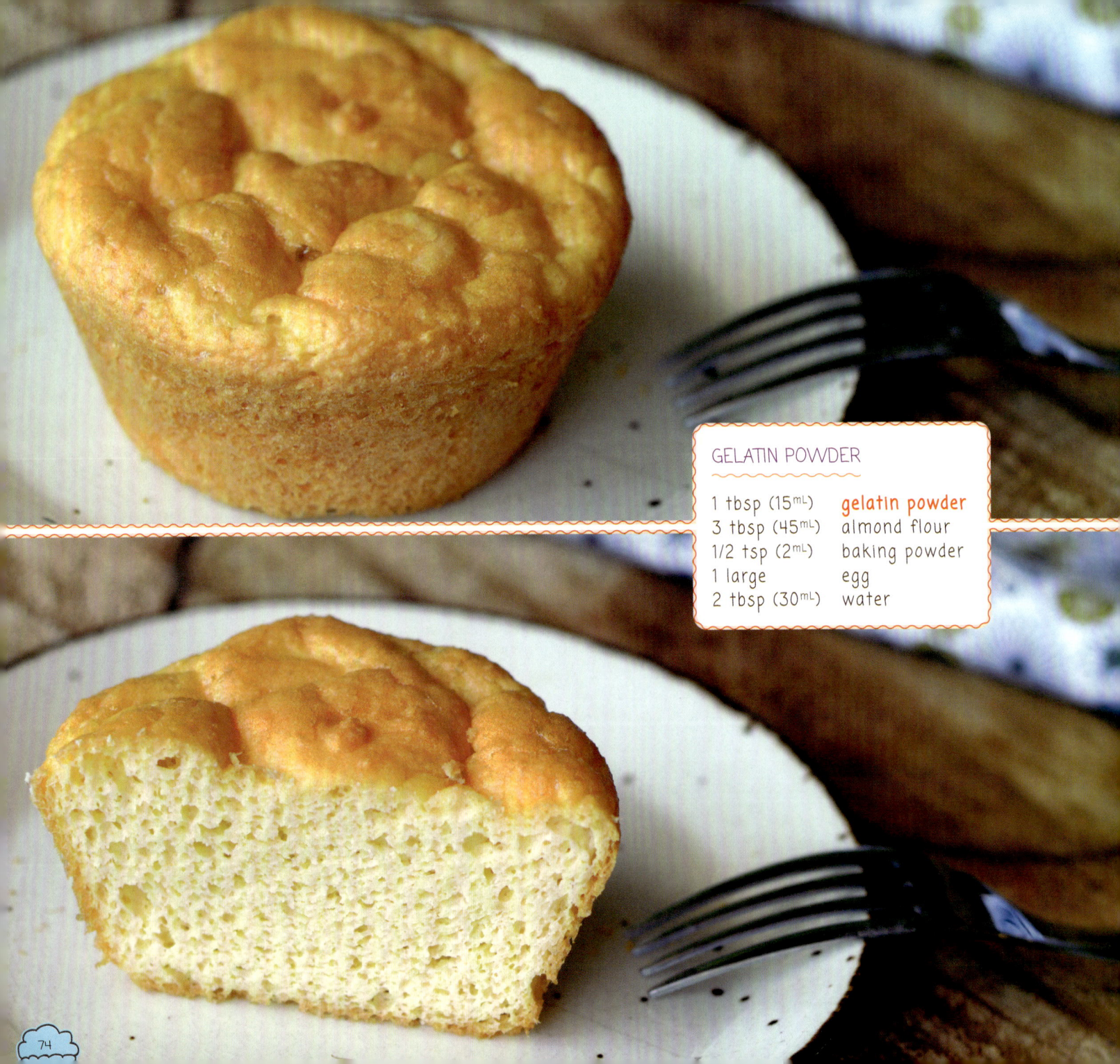

GELATIN POWDER

1 tbsp (15 mL)	**gelatin powder**
3 tbsp (45 mL)	almond flour
1/2 tsp (2 mL)	baking powder
1 large	egg
2 tbsp (30 mL)	water

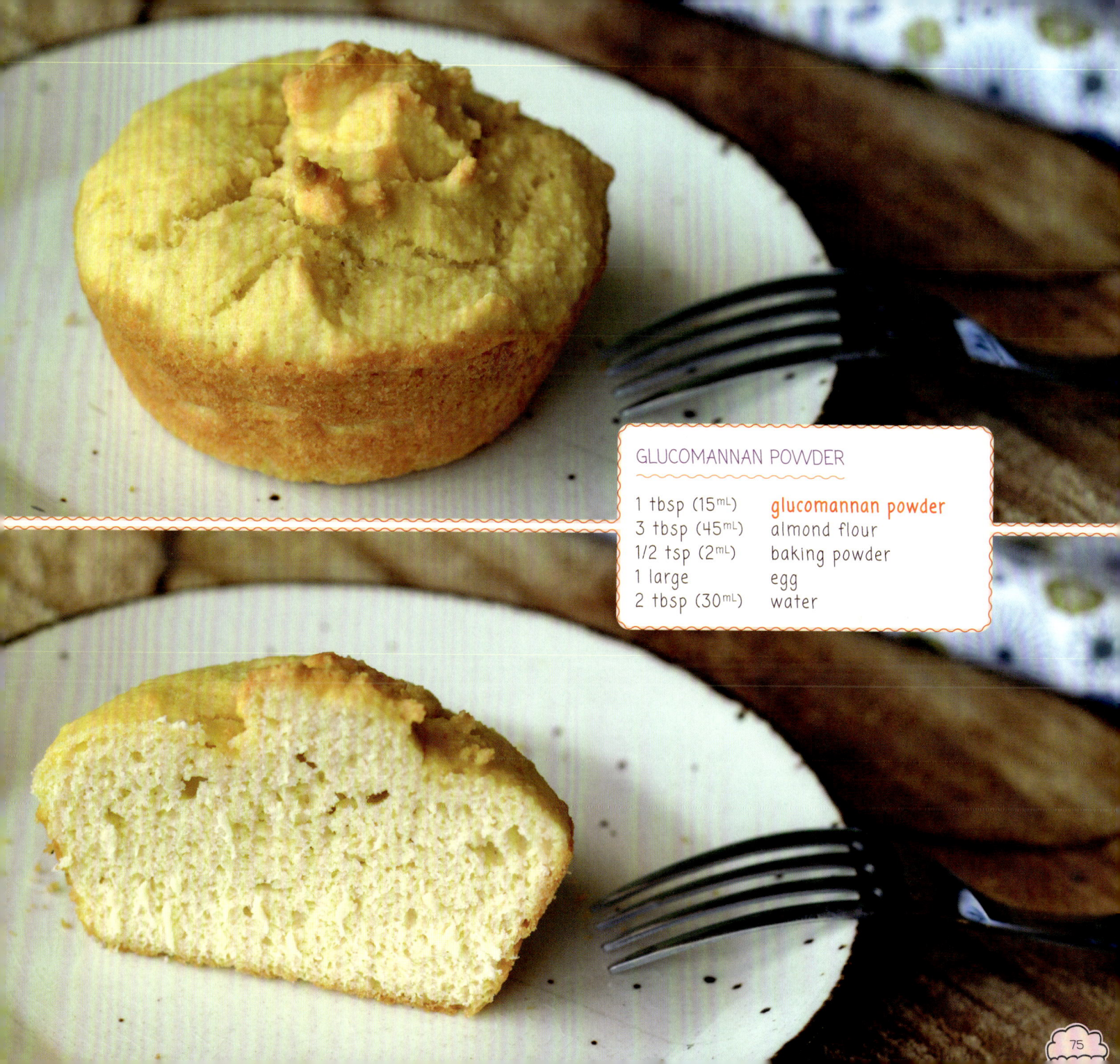

GLUCOMANNAN POWDER

1 tbsp (15 mL)	glucomannan powder
3 tbsp (45 mL)	almond flour
1/2 tsp (2 mL)	baking powder
1 large	egg
2 tbsp (30 mL)	water

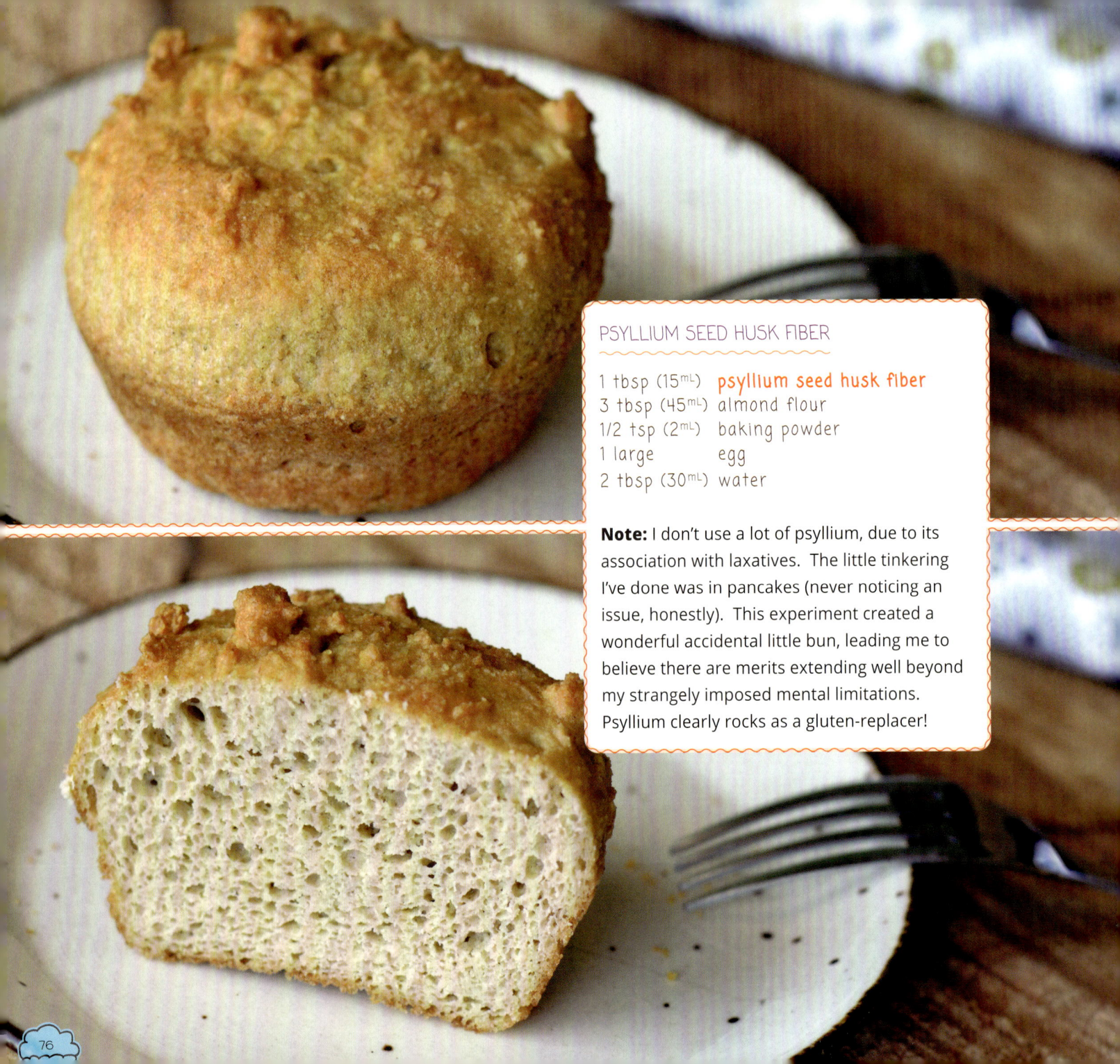

PSYLLIUM SEED HUSK FIBER

1 tbsp (15 mL)	psyllium seed husk fiber
3 tbsp (45 mL)	almond flour
1/2 tsp (2 mL)	baking powder
1 large	egg
2 tbsp (30 mL)	water

Note: I don't use a lot of psyllium, due to its association with laxatives. The little tinkering I've done was in pancakes (never noticing an issue, honestly). This experiment created a wonderful accidental little bun, leading me to believe there are merits extending well beyond my strangely imposed mental limitations. Psyllium clearly rocks as a gluten-replacer!

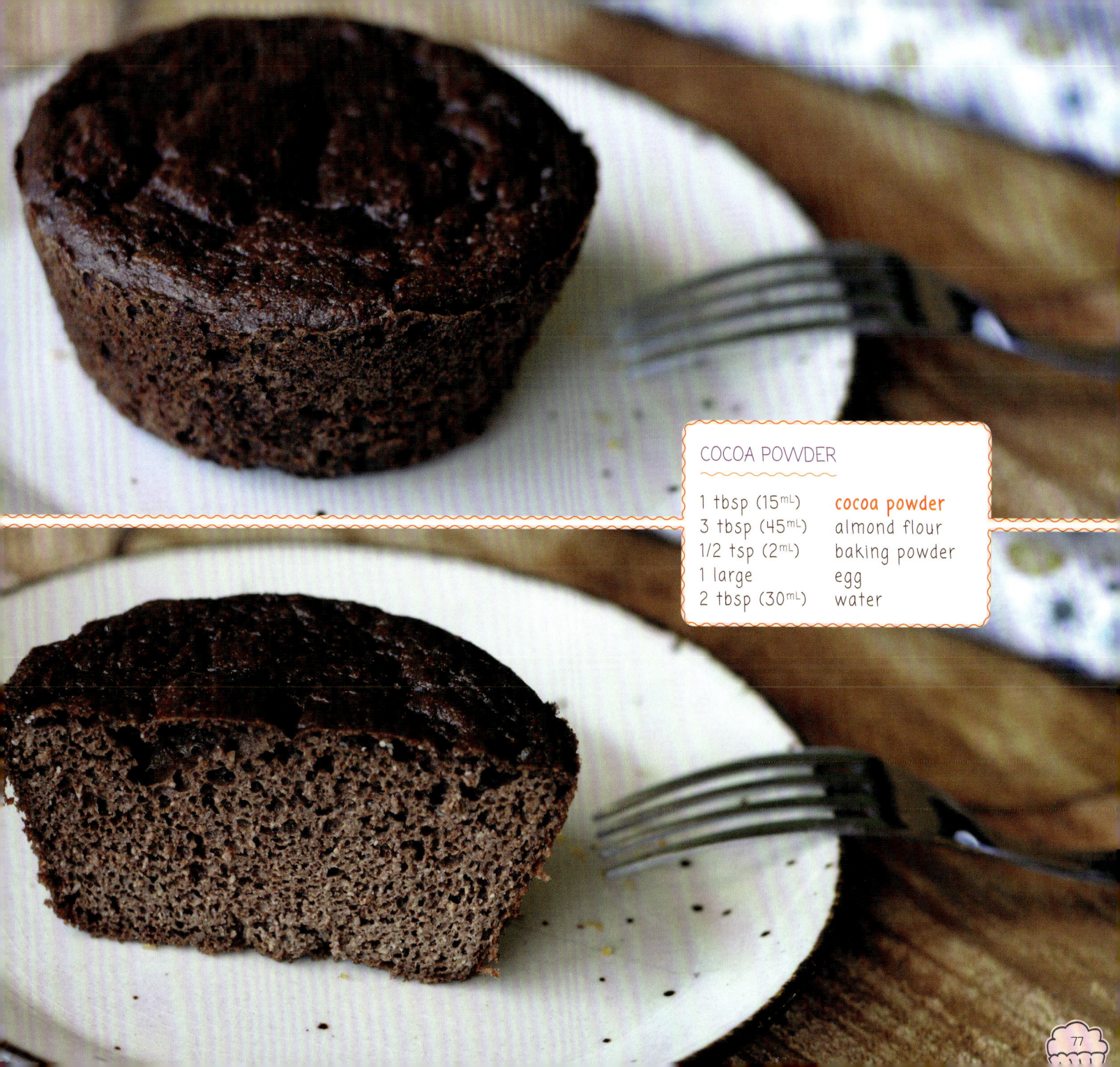

COCOA POWDER

1 tbsp (15 mL)	cocoa powder
3 tbsp (45 mL)	almond flour
1/2 tsp (2 mL)	baking powder
1 large	egg
2 tbsp (30 mL)	water

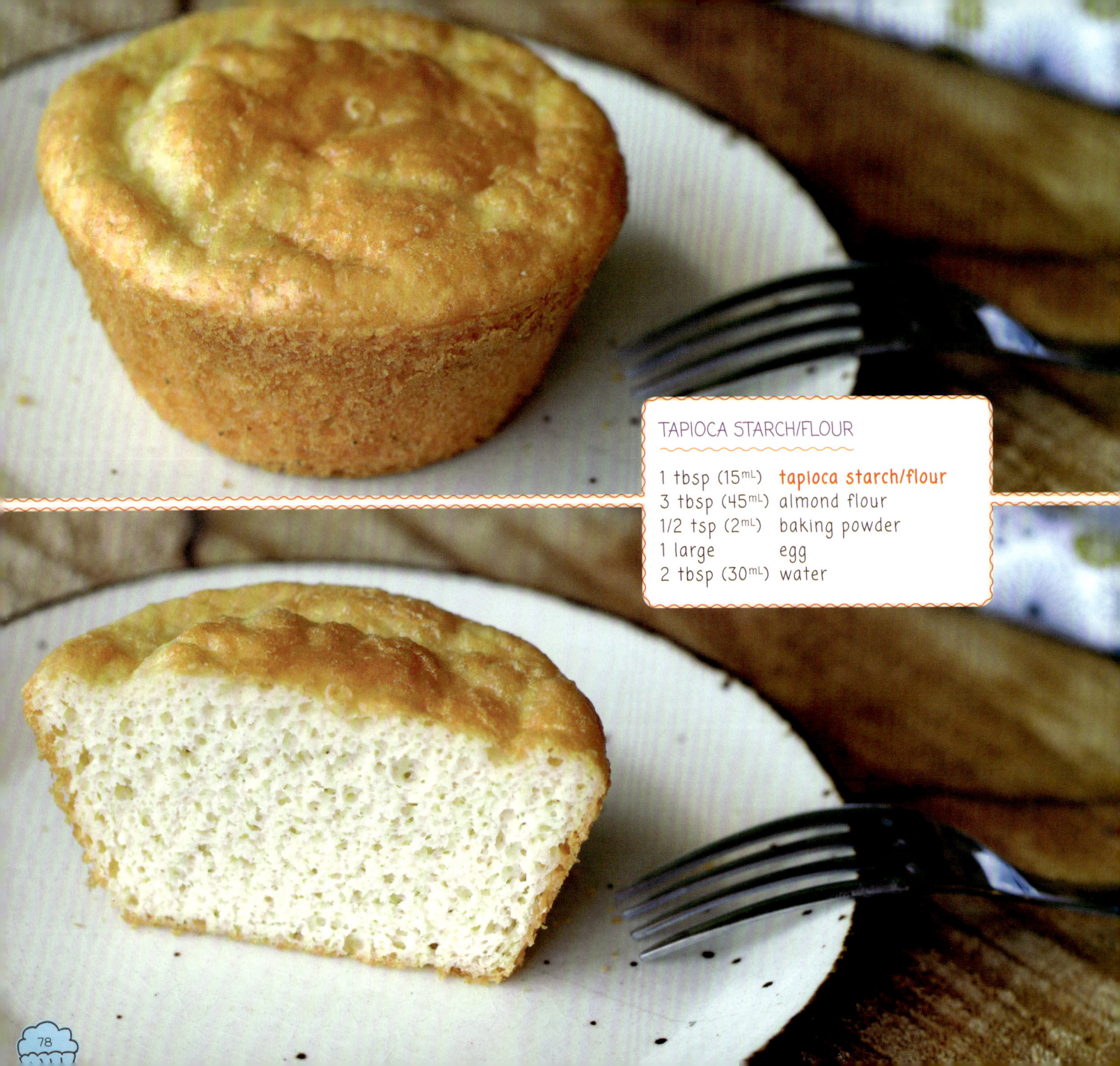

TAPIOCA STARCH/FLOUR

1 tbsp (15 mL)	**tapioca starch/flour**
3 tbsp (45 mL)	almond flour
1/2 tsp (2 mL)	baking powder
1 large	egg
2 tbsp (30 mL)	water

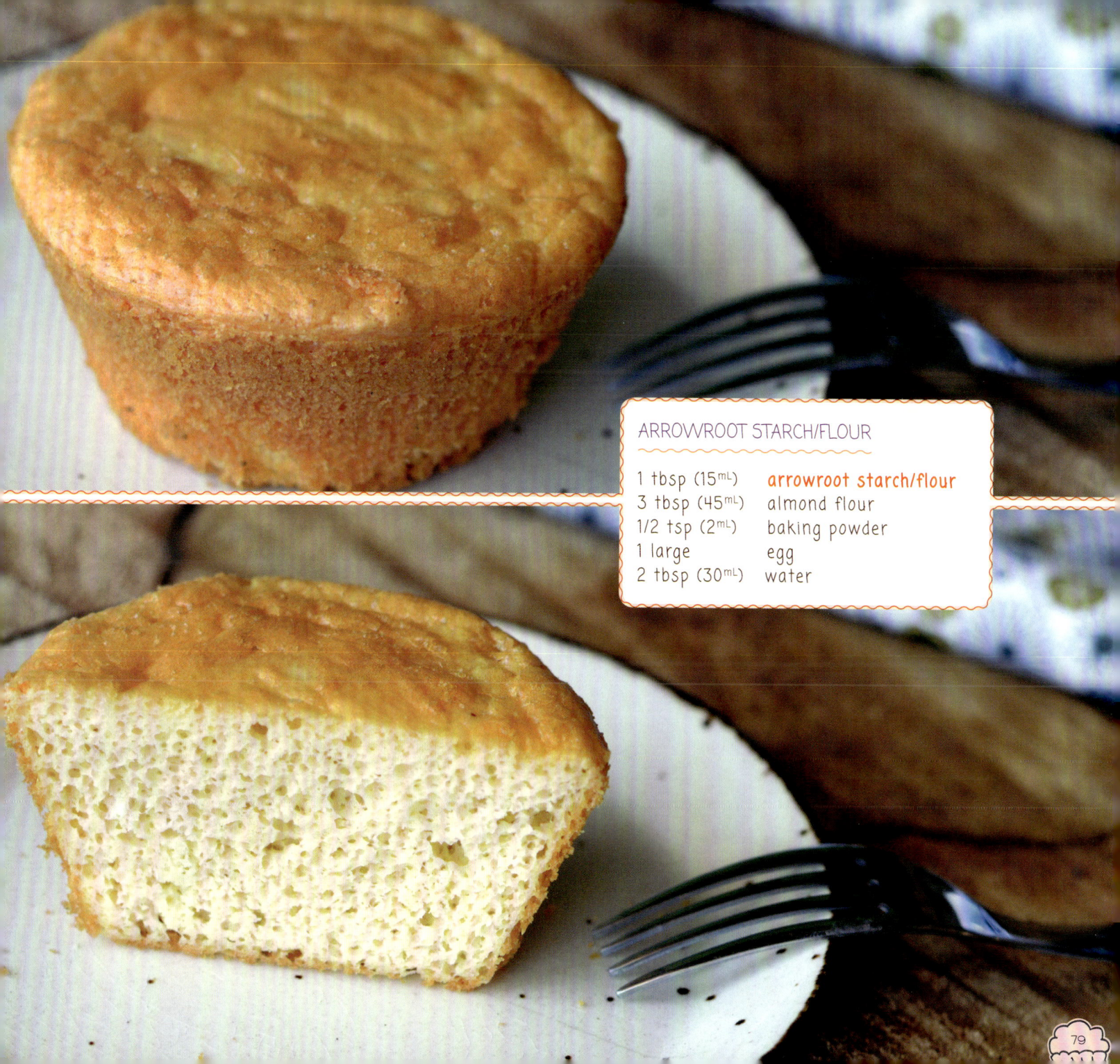

ARROWROOT STARCH/FLOUR

1 tbsp (15 mL)	arrowroot starch/flour
3 tbsp (45 mL)	almond flour
1/2 tsp (2 mL)	baking powder
1 large	egg
2 tbsp (30 mL)	water

SUBSTITUTIONS

For a wide variety of reasons, from allergies to dietary choices (and good old-fashioned pickiness), people do not eat certain ingredients. I'd like to point out basic alternatives for some of the more common ingredients.

Almond Milk:
Water, Milk, Hempseed Milk, Soy Milk

I use almond milk in a majority of my recipes. Within a standard American purview, I would use milk. However, due to the lactose (milk sugars), I opt for a nut-based milk. This is used for little more than adding water to a batter, most of which will evaporate during the baking process. I could just use water, but I like baking flavor into foods wherever I can. Water will add moisture, but will also literally water it down. Why not use something with a bit more character?

I tilt toward unsweetened almond milk largely out of habit, but also because it's only about 2 net carbs per cup. Hempseed milk is even lower in carbs, but is also more challenging to find. Soy milk would work, but I'd personally likely choose water over soy milk.

Nut Flours (like almond, pecan, hazelnut, walnut, etc.):
Sunflower Seed Flour

Nut allergies are quite common. I'm asked almost daily what can be used instead of the prevalent nut flours. Sunflower seed flour is a perfect 1 to 1 alternative. It's not a common ingredient, but is easily found online. You can also grind your own, if you can find raw, unseasoned sunflower seeds.

Melted Butter:
Coconut Oil, Olive Oil, Ghee, Bacon Fat

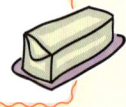

Within the scope of quick breads, fats are all interchangeable. Granted, butter has specific behaviors (stays solid at room temperature) that make it a wonderful spread. This makes it more challenging to replace with some of the other fats. However, within a batter and as a function within quick breads, the melted fats are all largely interchangeable.

I try to match tastes to the quick bread being made. It's less likely I'll use bacon fat in a chocolate muffcake, but... if it's all I have, it'll definitely work! And it might just be tasty. Chocolate-coated bacon strips, anyone?

There is one minor difference between melted butter and the other fats listed. Fresh butter is about 80% fat and 20% water. For smaller recipes it's not a big deal, but as more is used, it makes sense to decrease a fat substitution by about 20% and replace that lost volume with a little bit of liquid.

Let's say a muffin recipe asks for 1 tablespoon (15mL) melted butter, but the preference is coconut oil. Because the amounts are so small, I would use the equivalent 1 tablespoon (15mL) of coconut oil. However, if I were to make 16 muffins I would need 16 tablespoons (240mL) or 1 cup (240mL) melted butter. In this case I would use a little more than 3/4 cups (180mL) coconut oil and a little less than a 1/4 cup (60mL) liquid such as water, almond milk, coconut water, etc.

Again, this isn't a dramatic change. Being that these ratios are flexible and forgiving, I typically just eyeball it.

Eggs:
Chia Eggs

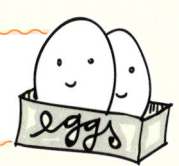

Chia eggs are a vegan substitution for those looking to avoid eggs. One chia egg will replace one egg in a quick bread. I personally like to use chia eggs from time to time, simply to change it up. Also, it's great to know about when I run out of eggs! Chia eggs are great in faking, but I wouldn't want to scramble one.

Chia egg recipe on *p. 40*.

Flaxseed Meal:
Chia Seed Flour

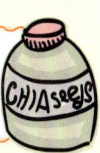

For those looking to avoid flaxseed, I find using chia seed is a great alternative. I *do* find that flaxseed bakes up a little stiffer and drier than chia does. They both behave quite well, but the end result is a twinge different. If you're looking to maintain a drier texture, but seek to use chia, use chia seed at a 1:1 ratio, but cut back the fat by about 50%. You may need to add a touch more almond milk or water.

GRIND YOUR OWN

I list powdered sugar replacement several times in this book, as well as in other books and on my website. I am *often* asked what that is, where to find it, or how to grind your own.

I'm also asked about grinding nuts and seeds, like pecan, sunflower, and chia, all of which can be hard to find in a preground form.

I personally own a KRUPS F203 spice and coffee grinder. It cost me less than $20.00 USD, gets used *a lot* and is showing no signs of slowing down. It's a small, handheld grinder that I grabbed from Amazon many years ago.

Read on for more info about grinding some of these valuable ingredients.

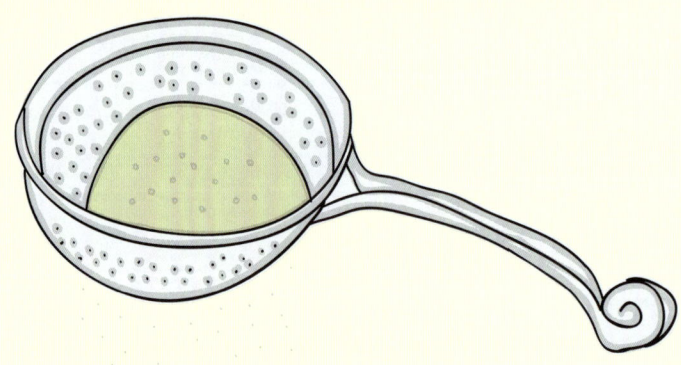

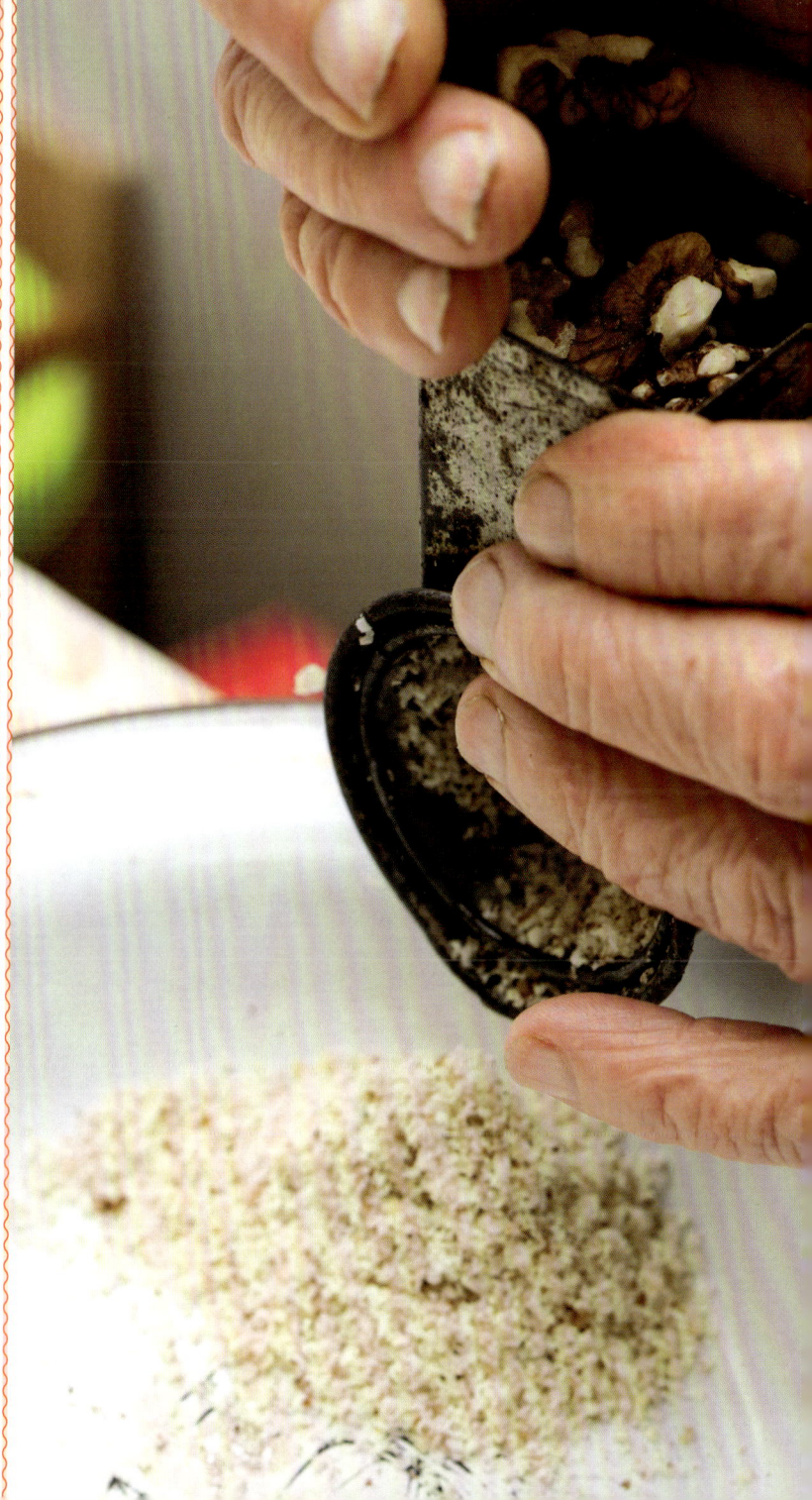

Sweeteners: For the most part, I purchase confectioner's Swerve. I use that as my primary sweetener. Generally, I don't need to powder my own. However, I HAVE used my spice grinder to powder my own sweetener blends. Neither home-powdered sweetener nor store-bought confectioner's Swerve will ever be as fine and delicate as standard powdered sugar. So don't feel like you're doing it wrong if it's not a luxurious pillow of clouds. Erythritol simply doesn't powder like that. The grains, however, can get much smaller, which goes a great distance toward helping them dissolve, as well as the mouthfeel (less intense sandy grit) in recipes where they don't dissolve.

Seeds: The only seeds I grind are chia and flax. I have ground sunflower, but the process is closer to that of nuts (see next section). Chia and flax powder up beautifully in a matter of seconds in the spice grinder. I buy both whole and grind my own. I store seeds in the freezer, then I just grind what I need for whatever I'm making. There's often a little left, but that gets stashed in the freezer. Later it is thrown into things like omelets or meatloaf, to help hold in moisture (great texture!). This is fast and painless. Just grind until fine and that's it. Use like flour!

Nuts: The nut category is the only one that really needs explaining.

I fill my spice grinder with a small amount of nuts (say walnuts). I then *pulse* (turn it on and off, in rapid succession) the grinder. I repeatedly turn the grinder on and off, while shaking its contents. Start small and pulse once or twice, to begin with. When a small portion of the nuts are finely ground, I pour the entire contents of the grinder into a sifting tool, resting on a plate, large sheet of parchment paper, or in a bowl. I sift the nuts. Some portion of them will sift into a lovely little hill. What doesn't fit through the holes goes back into the grinder, where I pulse the nuts for a few more seconds. When a bit more of the nuts are finely ground, I pour the contents back into the sifter. I sift the nuts once again. Whatever remains in the sifter goes back into the grinder, where it is pulsed again.

Be warned that you can *over*-process your nuts. Nuts have a high fat content. When ground in a food processor, the friction resulting from the consistent processing heats the fat, melting it and decreasing its viscosity. This can take a bowl full of nuts and quickly pulverize it into a nut butter which, while wonderfully delicious with jelly, it is not the goal.

The goal is to find a nice, finely grained nut flour without going so far as to create a nut *butter*. Walnuts and macadamia nuts are likely to turn to butter more quickly. Tread carefully.

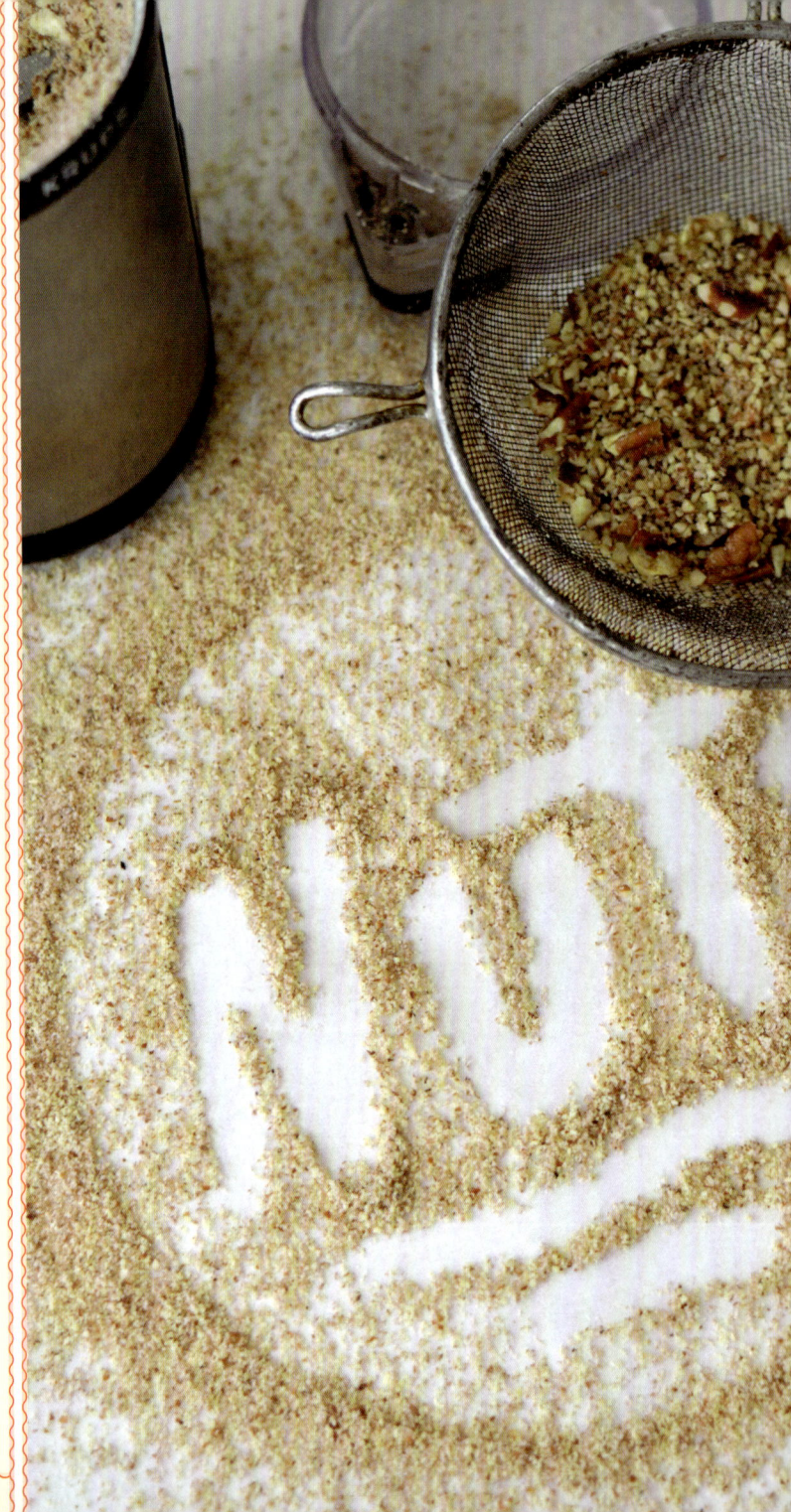

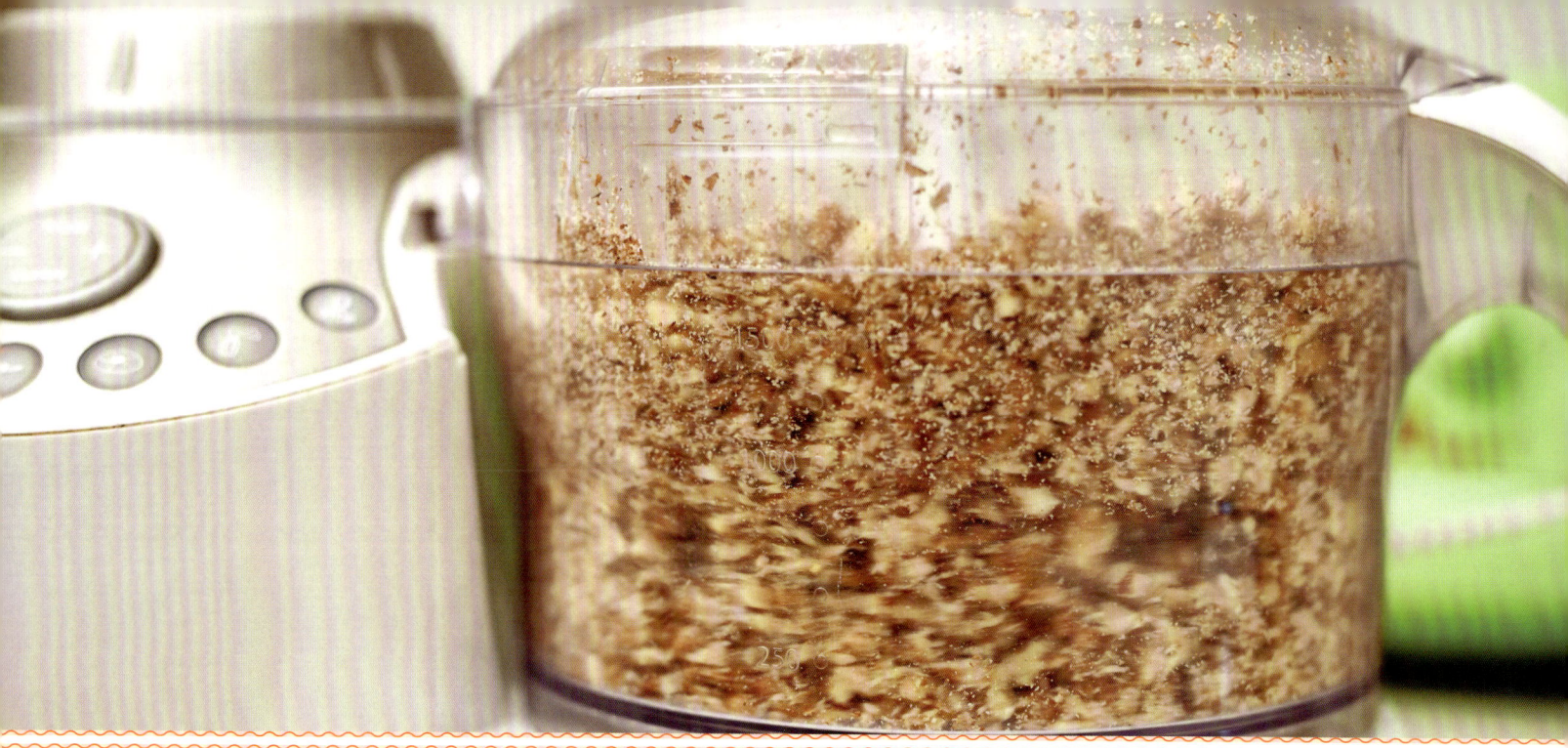

Pulsing is key, if using a spice grinder. Other forms of grinding are likely more straightforward (like a true nut grinder). I don't own a nut grinder simply because I'm in the habit of using my spice grinder. I don't do this so often to have felt the need to purchase one.

No matter how you grind the nuts, you should still sift them. Be aware that a very fine meshed strainer is good for a very fine grain, but it also takes a while longer and takes a little more patience as you go through the paces. A less fine strainer will yield a coarser grain, but will go more quickly. Remember, we are striving for a *flour*, so something like your pasta strainer is likely too large a hole. Strike a balance.

I have personally ground almonds, hazelnuts, walnuts, pecans, and macadamias (which can be a bit fickle because of the very high fat content... they want to turn to butter more quickly). Each of these functions interchangeably in recipes asking for nut flours. I have also ground sunflower seeds. They work as a wonderful replacement and are perfectly suited for those with nut allergies. Be warned, however, that sunflower seeds turn an alien gray/green color when heated or baked. Do not worry. It's completely harmless and barely noticeable (at least in my experience).

This may sound like a long, complicated process, but it goes much more quickly than you'd think. In the end, you wind up with a spectacular and airy little pile of home-ground nut flour.

It only takes a few moments to grind a cup of nuts, while saving money and boosting variety at the same time.

I personally store my nut flours in the freezer. Feel free to grind extra, if you have the time to grind and sift a lot of nuts. Try and store the flour in an airtight container in the freezer. I still don't suggest grinding more nuts than you can use in a week, if left on the countertop, or upwards of 3 months in the freezer. Nut oils are volatile and can spoil quickly, once the nuts are ground. Freezing slows the pace quite a bit, but it's still best not to grind more than you need.

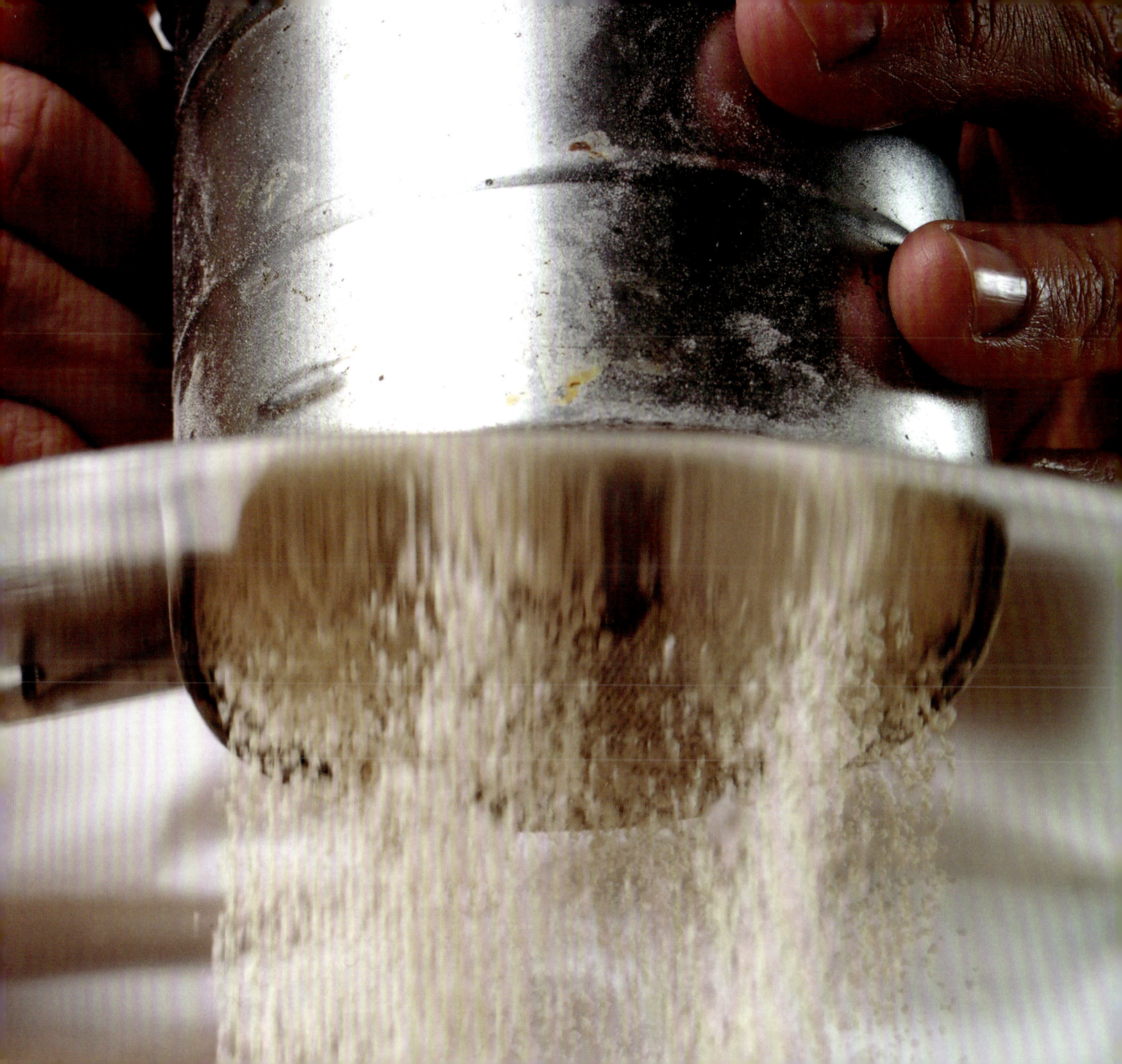

FURTHER TIPS

The following are tips and hints to help tweak and tune recipes to more closely suit your own tastes and dietary needs and goals. These can be applied to the recipes in this book, or used for recipes in other books or on the Internet.

In large part, the hope is that you can look for recipes like "Christmas Cakes" to locate loads of recipe ideas, then use the information learned from this book to convert those recipes into recipes that you can enjoy, without worry.

Increase leaveners by 25%.

Because these recipes have less structural integrity and tend to use heavier ingredients, it's a good idea to increase the leavener by about 25% over what seems necessary in a standard recipe.

Smaller is better.

Because these ingredients are less durable, smaller can yield a better product. Where something may not make sense "small," then keep it somewhat flat. Rather than a *loaf* of bread, consider something closer to a *flat* bread or focaccia. Rather than slices, split it in half to form sandwiches. If too large or too tall some recipes will fall and cave in upon themselves.

Blends, blends, blends...

Be it flours or sweeteners, the *blends* are the best. They typically combine well and form amazing synergies, far surpassing the qualities of any one solo ingredient.

I do *some* blending in this book, but nowhere near as much as I do in my personal life. One of my great fears of this subject is that people will see the seemingly long list of expensive, exotic, and hard-to-find ingredients and simply throw in the towel. The reality is, a muffin made with almond flour and coconut flour is going to be wonderful. The *same* muffin made with a blend of hazelnut, almond and sunflour, with a touch of tapioca, a pinch of xanthan gum and 1 chia egg is going to be even better!

Not only will it be better, but it will also give your body a wider range of nutrients. I often mix up my flours simply to give my body something new and not constantly give it almond flour.

Too much of any of these flours isn't good. Mix it up!

A little starch goes a long way.

Even a little tiny bit of starch helps lend a lighter and more familiar cakey texture and color. While *totally* optional, for many, this little blast of starch is worth the extra quality. Consider adding a tablespoon or two (15 to 30 mL) of arrowroot to your recipes. Granted, at 2 tbsp (30 mL) you're adding over 2 net carbs per serving, but for many with higher carb diets, 2 net carbs are no big deal and worth spending on a lighter muffin.

Use a gluten replacer to help with structure.

Use about 1 tsp (5 mL) or more xanthan gum per cup (240 mL) of flour for heavier things like bread and pizza crust. About 1/2 tsp (2 to 3 mL) for things like cakes and muffins.

Slower and lower.

Especially as your baked items grow in size, it becomes important to lower the baking temperature by about 25° F (14° C) degrees from the norm. Bake longer, by about 25%. I have also found that heavy reliance on gluten replacers can extend the baking time by even longer.

I have a habit of starting *hot* and lowering. I typically put my goodies in a 400° F (205° C) oven for 5 minutes (I always set a timer). Then I drop the temperature down to 325° F (163° C) for the remainder of their time in the oven. This tends to help give a quick OOMPH to the process, but then gives a mellower, consistent pace for the structure to stiffen.

Just keep an eye on things and you'll be fine. (Use the light in the oven, though. Constantly opening and closing the oven door causes dramatic increases and drops in temperature. Try and open the oven infrequently.)

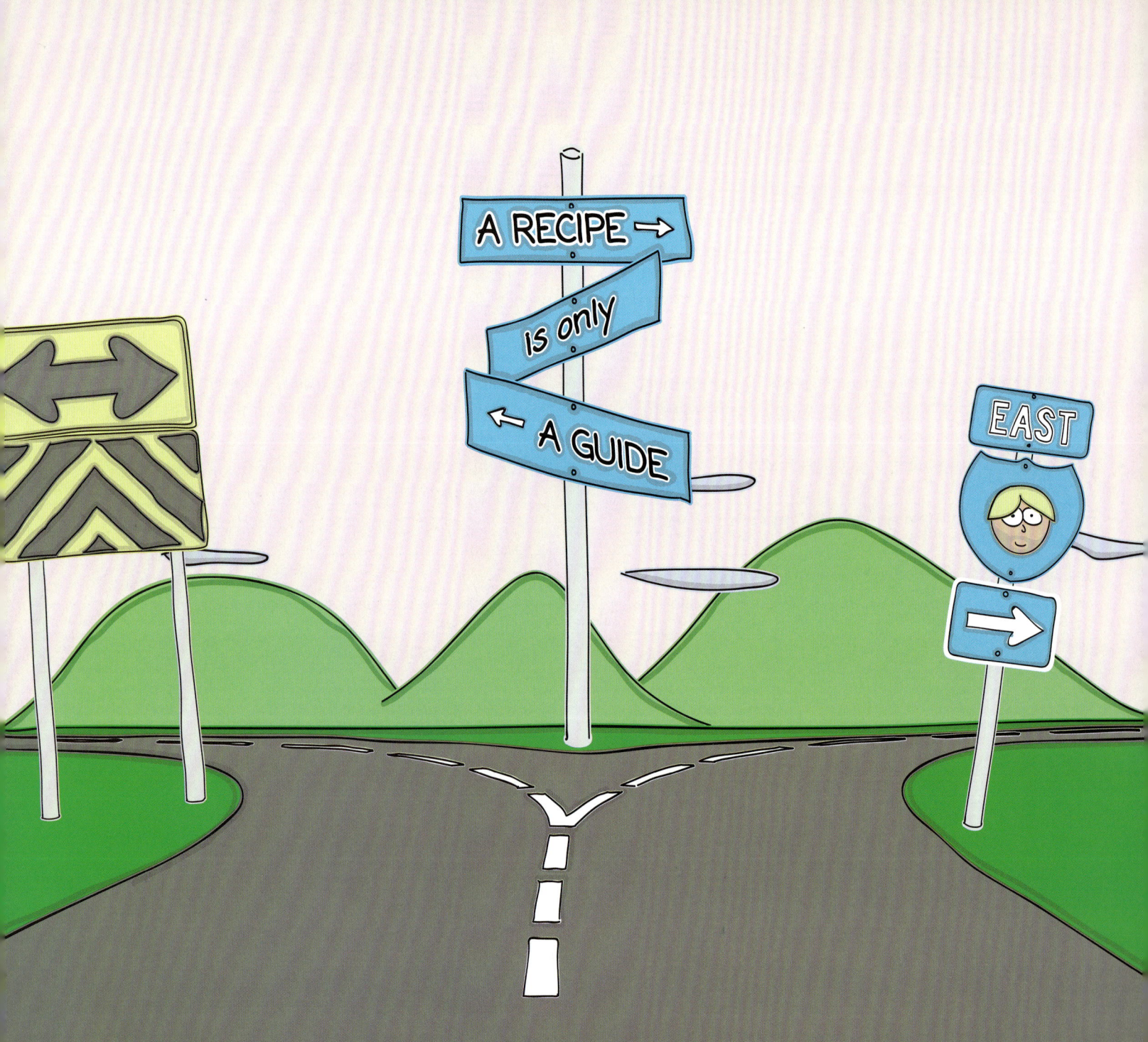

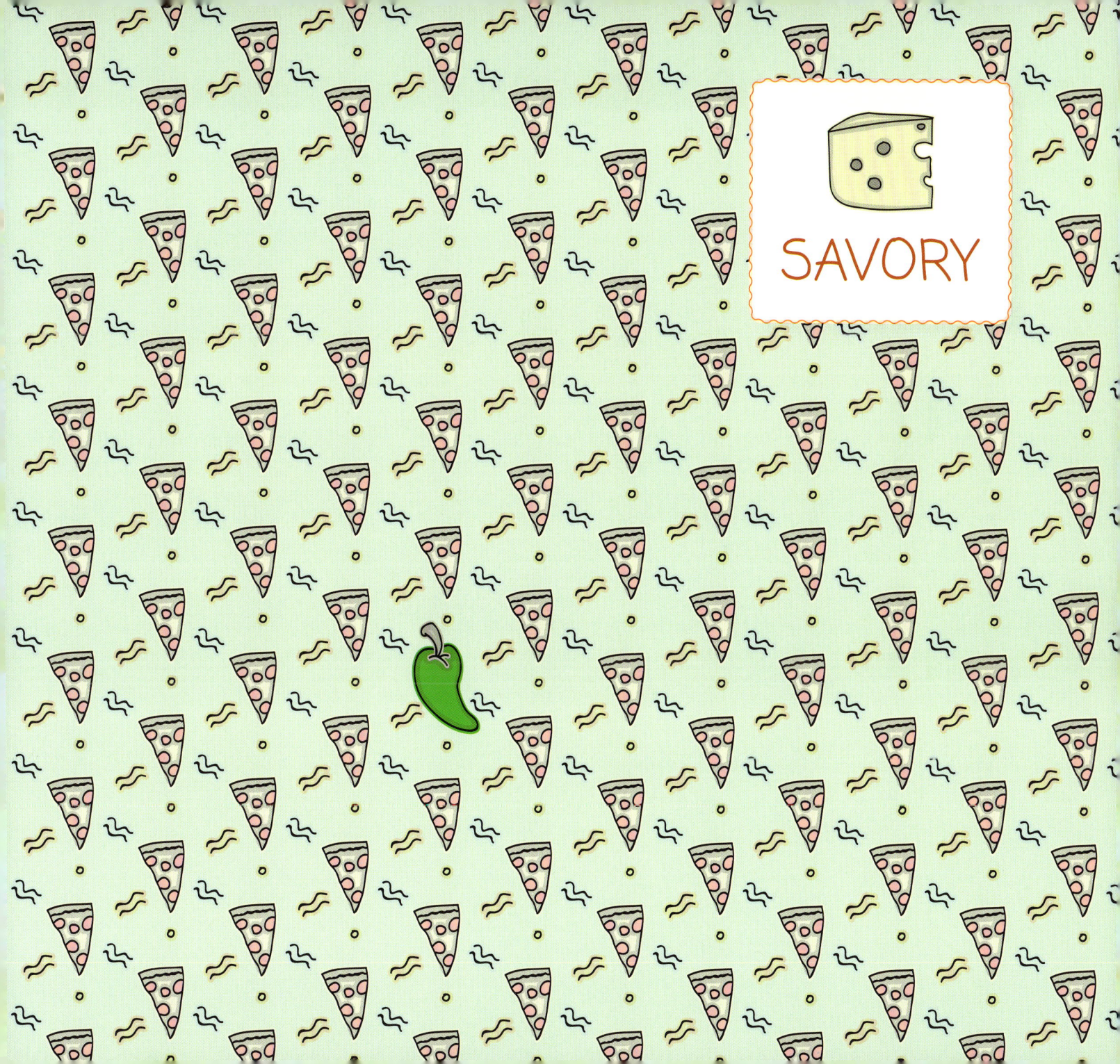

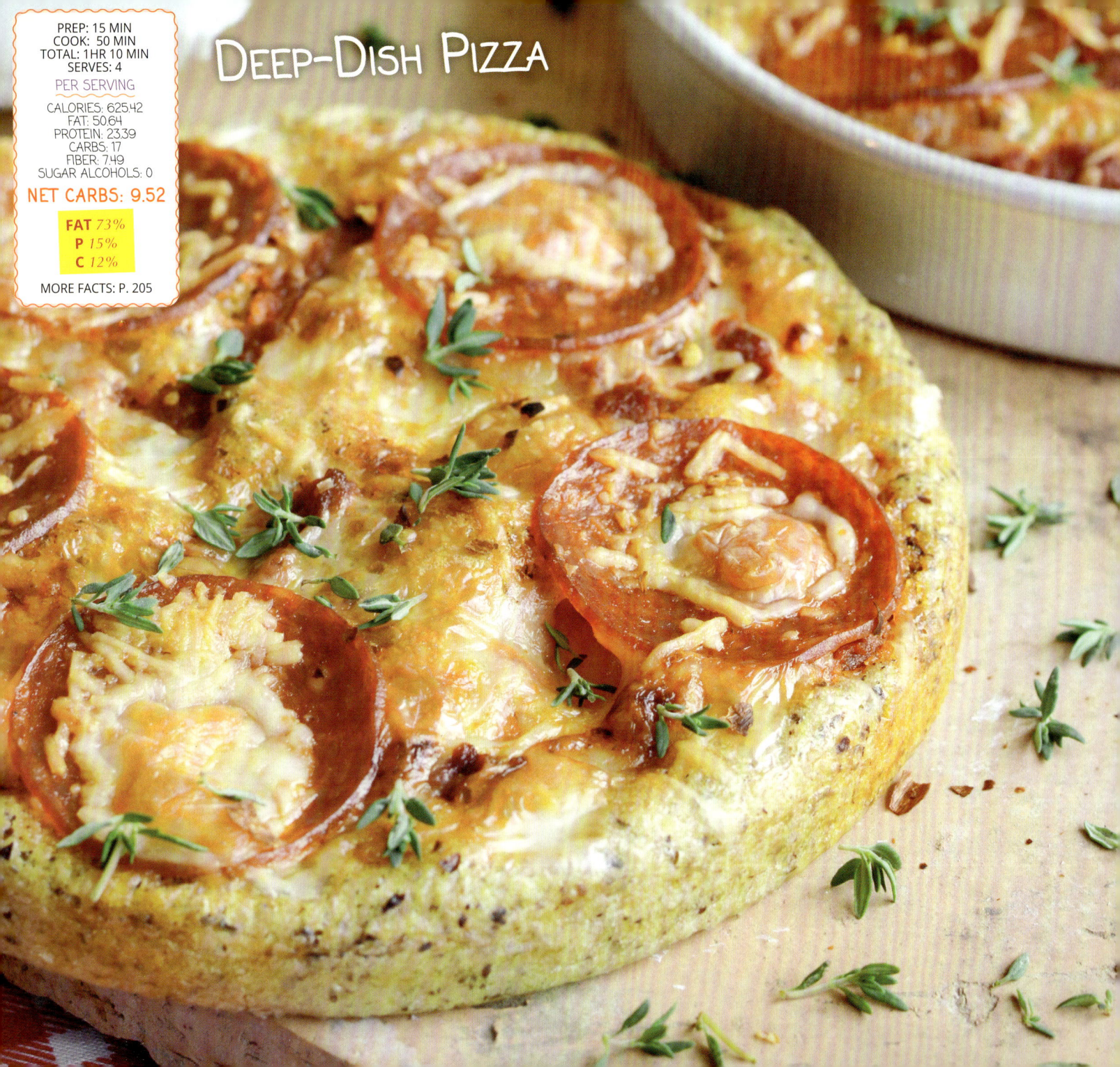

Deep-Dish Pizza

PREP: 15 MIN
COOK: 50 MIN
TOTAL: 1HR 10 MIN
SERVES: 4

PER SERVING
CALORIES: 625.42
FAT: 50.64
PROTEIN: 23.39
CARBS: 17
FIBER: 7.49
SUGAR ALCOHOLS: 0
NET CARBS: 9.52

FAT 73%
P 15%
C 12%

MORE FACTS: P. 205

For YEARS, I searched and searched for a solid pizza crust recipe that I could support. My blog is riddled with pizza-flavored treats and meals, but no actual *pizza*. Even my first book has pizza goodies, but no *pizza*. This isn't for lack of effort, mind you. I've tried store-bought crusts, store-bought crust *kits*, I've tried crusts made from zucchini, cauliflower, chicken, cheese, and meat. The Meatza was probably my favorite of these, but boy was it ever a mess!

I should make special mentions of Meatzas (I used raw bulk spicy Italian sausage as the crust), as well as the "Fat Head" pizza crust (Google it). Both are very good, but one was an absolute mess to eat and the other... wasn't mine!

I tried endlessly to make my own crusts from nut flours and seed flours and always found them to be too brittle, too soggy, too wonky, too messy, etc. They were all delicious, but none were fully worthy.

Finally, I came upon THIS combo! What's weird is, it's a very standard quick-bread recipe. I use variations of this recipe for sandwich bread, all the time. I used it for deep-dish pizza YEARS ago, but always felt it had a bit of a slimy texture, from the fibrous seed flours. I moved on.

On a lark, I decided to try a trick. I *reduced* the pizza sauce. I put the pizza sauce on the stove over a very low heat, until it was THICK. Tomato paste thick. *Toothpaste* thick.

By pouring a wet tomato sauce over a wet batter, then topping it with cheese, I found that the space between the crust and cheese stayed too wet, too gummy... too snoorky, for lack of a better word. It was enjoyable, easy to cut, eat, and handle. It very much looked the part, but the sensation and mouthfeel while masticating was *just* on the wrong side of pleasant.

However, by thoroughly removing most of the extra water from the sauce, the crust stayed firm and solid and maintained a very pleasant texture. Eureka! Yes, my friends, I'd finally found it!

The goal is to have a batter that is about 1/2-inch (1 1/4^{cm}) thick, and then splatter and spoon small consistent dollops of the thick sauce all around the batter. You can't "spread" it, as the batter is too viscous, but you can spoon it around, with the goal being "every bite will have a little." Then, top with cheese and your favorite toppings. Enjoy!

2 cups (480mL)	no-sugar-added pizza sauce
1/4 cup (60mL)	almond flour
1/4 cup (60mL)	hazelnut flour
1/4 cup (60mL)	ground chia
1/4 cup (60mL)	flaxseed meal
2 1/4 tsp (11mL)	baking powder
1 tbsp (15mL)	chopped herbs (oregano, thyme and/or rosemary), divided
1 tsp (5mL)	salt
Dash	chili flakes
4 large	eggs
1/4 cup (60mL)	unsweetened almond milk
3 tbsp (45mL)	extra-virgin olive oil, divided
2 cloves	garlic, chopped
1/2 cup (120mL)	grated whole milk, low-moisture mozzarella
1/2 cup (120mL)	grated parmesan cheese
4 oz (114g)	pepperoni slices

- Preheat the oven to 305 °F (177 °C).

- Over medium heat, place the pizza sauce on the stove in an uncovered small pot. Bring the sauce to a simmer, then turn the heat to low. Periodically stir and check the sauce. As the sauce simmers, water is evaporating, leaving the sauce behind. The goal is to reduce the sauce by more than half, so that it is very thick, almost like a paste. When done, you should have about 1/2 to 3/4 cup (120mL to 180mL) of sauce.

- While the sauce simmers, in a mixing bowl, combine almond, hazelnut, chia, flaxseed, baking powder, half of the chopped herbs (setting some aside for garnish), salt, and chili flakes. Mix these ingredients together.

- To the dried ingredients, add eggs, half of the almond milk (or water), 2 tbsp (30mL) of the olive oil, and garlic. Mix well. Allow the batter to sit for 5 minutes.

- Grease the inside of the pizza pans with the remaining olive oil. This recipe works well with four 6-inch (15cm) deep-dish pans (pictured), two standard 9-inch (23cm) cake pans, or one 9 x 13-inch (23cm x 33cm) casserole pan.

- While greasing the pans, the fiber in the seed flours will be absorbing the liquid, swelling and thickening the batter. After the 2- to 3-minute wait, the mixture should resemble a very thick pancake batter. Add more almond milk, if the batter is too thick.

- Evenly spread the batter along the base of your prepared pan(s).

- With a small spoon, spoon small dollops of the thickened pizza sauce evenly around the top of your batter. Do what you can to spread it around without breaking through the batter or touching the rim of the pan with the sauce.

- Evenly spread the grated mozzarella over the sauce.

- Evenly spread the pepperoni (and/or other favorite toppings) over the top of the mozzarella.

- Sprinkle with parmesan cheese.

- Bake in oven until cooked through and cheese is golden. Depending on the pan, it will take between 18 and 28 minutes. Just keep an eye on it.

- Remove from pans, cut (if necessary), garnish with remaining fresh herbs and enjoy!

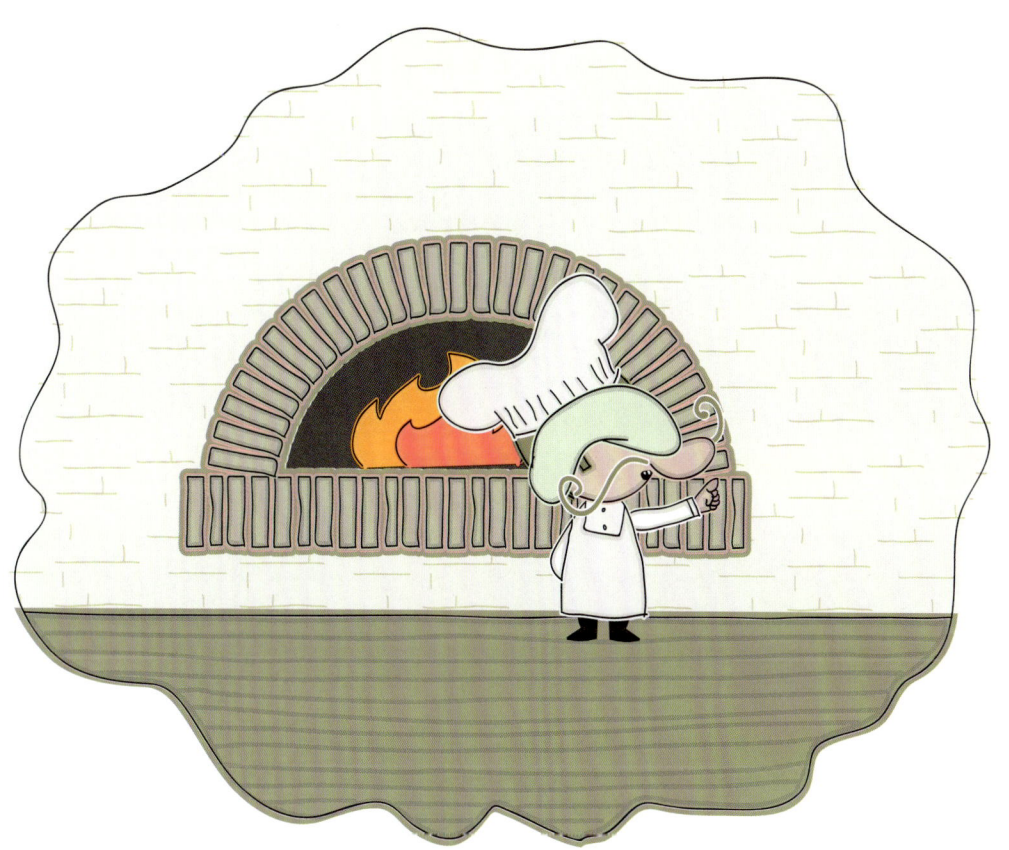

Cheesy Bacon-Chive Muffin

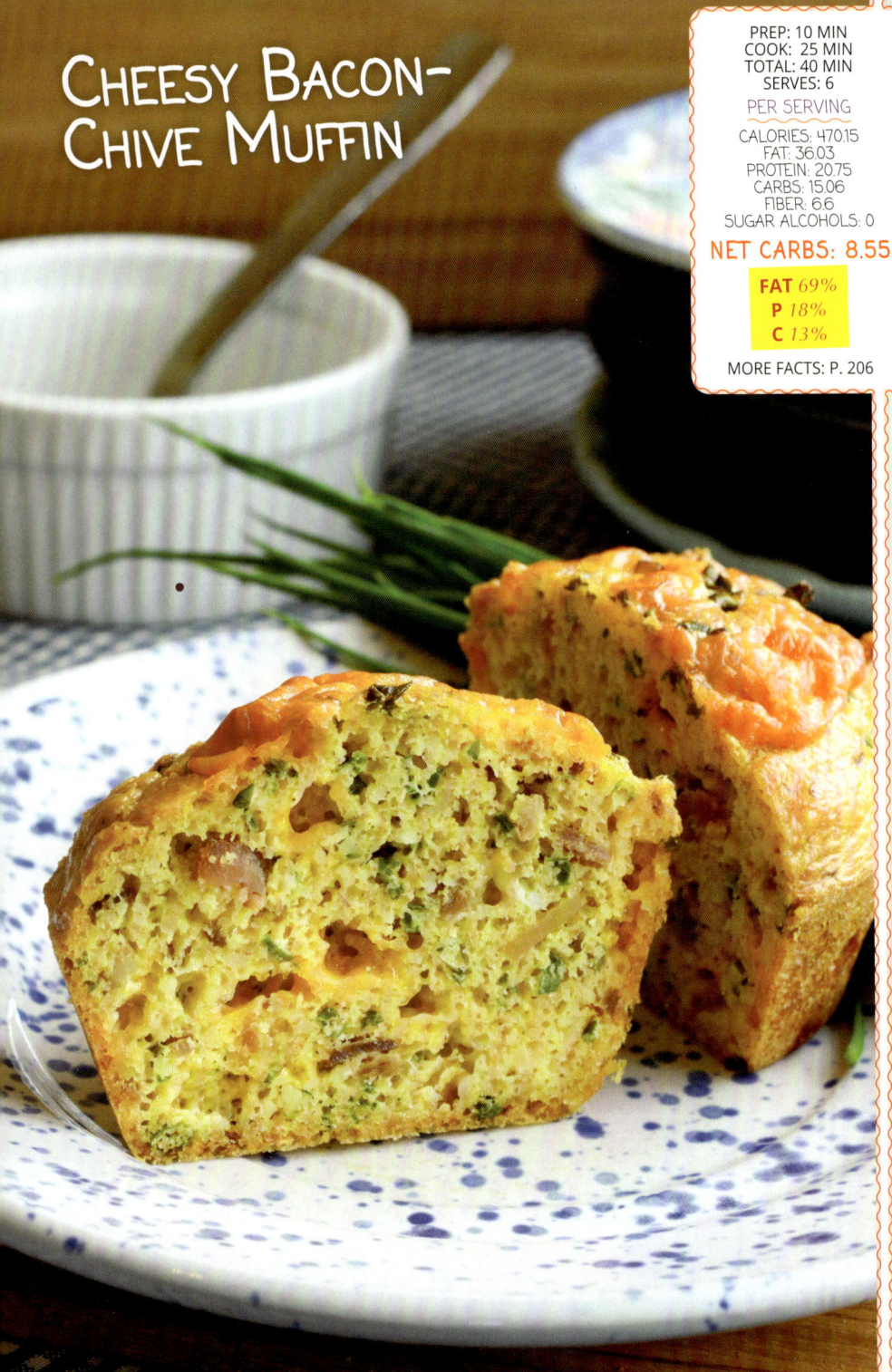

PREP: 10 MIN
COOK: 25 MIN
TOTAL: 40 MIN
SERVES: 6

PER SERVING

CALORIES: 470.15
FAT: 36.03
PROTEIN: 20.75
CARBS: 15.06
FIBER: 6.6
SUGAR ALCOHOLS: 0

NET CARBS: 8.55

FAT 69%
P 18%
C 13%

MORE FACTS: P. 206

I love the combination of bacon with, well, if I'm being totally honest... *everything*. A CLASSIC combination is bacon and cheddar cheese. I, like many, tend to like tying the two tastes together with a member of the onion family, be it through caramelized onions, sweet chopped garlic, or in this case, chives. My mind immediately jumps to the youthful memories of innocent potato skins at TGI Fridays. This makes me wonder how these full-flavored muffins would be slathered with sour cream. MMMmmmmm....

Flax and chia both come in light or dark colors. They are functionally interchangeable. If you have one, but I've listed the other, have no fear. Use what you have. Approach it color blind. The end result will still be excellent. In *this* case, I used white chia and golden flax because I'm looking for a lighter shade, so the yellow color of the cheese and the bright green of the chives would visually *POP*.

I also want to point out the addition of both tapioca flour and xanthan gum. These are optional additions, but they will help the muffin hold its shape. The cheese pockets may collapse under the weight of the batter. The gluten-like properties of the starch and fiber combo will help it stay puffed. If you opt not to use those two ingredients, I suggest making 12 smaller muffins, rather than the 6 Texas-sized muffins shown here. Alternatively, pour the batter into a small greased casserole pan and simply cut out squares. ALL delicious options that can help cut down on a few carbs, as well as the need for an exotic ingredient.

3/4 cup (180ᵐᴸ)	almond flour
1/2 cup (120ᵐᴸ)	ground white chia seed
1/4 cup (60ᵐᴸ)	golden flaxseed meal
1/4 cup (60ᵐᴸ)	tapioca flour (optional)
1 tbsp (15ᵐᴸ)	baking powder
1 tsp (5ᵐᴸ)	xanthan gum (optional)
3/4 tsp (4ᵐᴸ)	salt
Dash	pepper (or to taste)
Dash	chili flakes (or to taste)
6 large	eggs
1/4 cup + 2 tbsp (90ᵐᴸ)	unsweetened almond milk
3 tbsp (45ᵐᴸ)	melted butter
8 oz (227g)	cheddar cheese
1/2 cup (120ᵐᴸ)	real bacon bits
1/4 cup (60ᵐᴸ)	chopped fresh chives

- Preheat oven to 350° F (177° C).
- Grease a 6-cup large muffin pan. Set aside.
- In a large bowl, combine the almond, chia, flaxseed, optional tapioca flour, baking powder, optional xanthan gum, chili flakes, salt, and pepper. With a whisk or a fork, combine the dry ingredients so they are evenly mixed and distributed in and amongst one another.
- In a separate smaller bowl, whisk together eggs with the almond milk. Pour into the dry ingredients. Whisk together, while pouring in the warm melted butter. Set aside to allow your flax and chia to thicken and gel (about 2 to 3 minutes).
- Cut your cheese into cubes. Grated cheese would be quite tasty, but I like the small pockets of melted cheese globs. Cut the cheese into rough 1/4- to 1/3-inch cubes (just shy of a centimeter).
- Add the cubed cheese, bacon bits, and fresh chives to the batter. Whisk. The batter should be like a thick pancake batter. These ingredients tend to be a bit inconsistent from brand to brand and grind to grind. You may need to add a little more almond milk to thin it out (just not too much!).
- Once the batter is well mixed, pour even amounts between the 6 muffin cups.
- Bake for about 23 to 28 minutes, or until the muffins have crowned and the surface is dry, beginning to crisp, and has turned golden.
- Remove from the oven and let rest for 5 minutes before removing from the pan. Enjoy warm!
- Final thought: These reheat VERY well!

Chorizo, Cilantro and Cotija Muffins

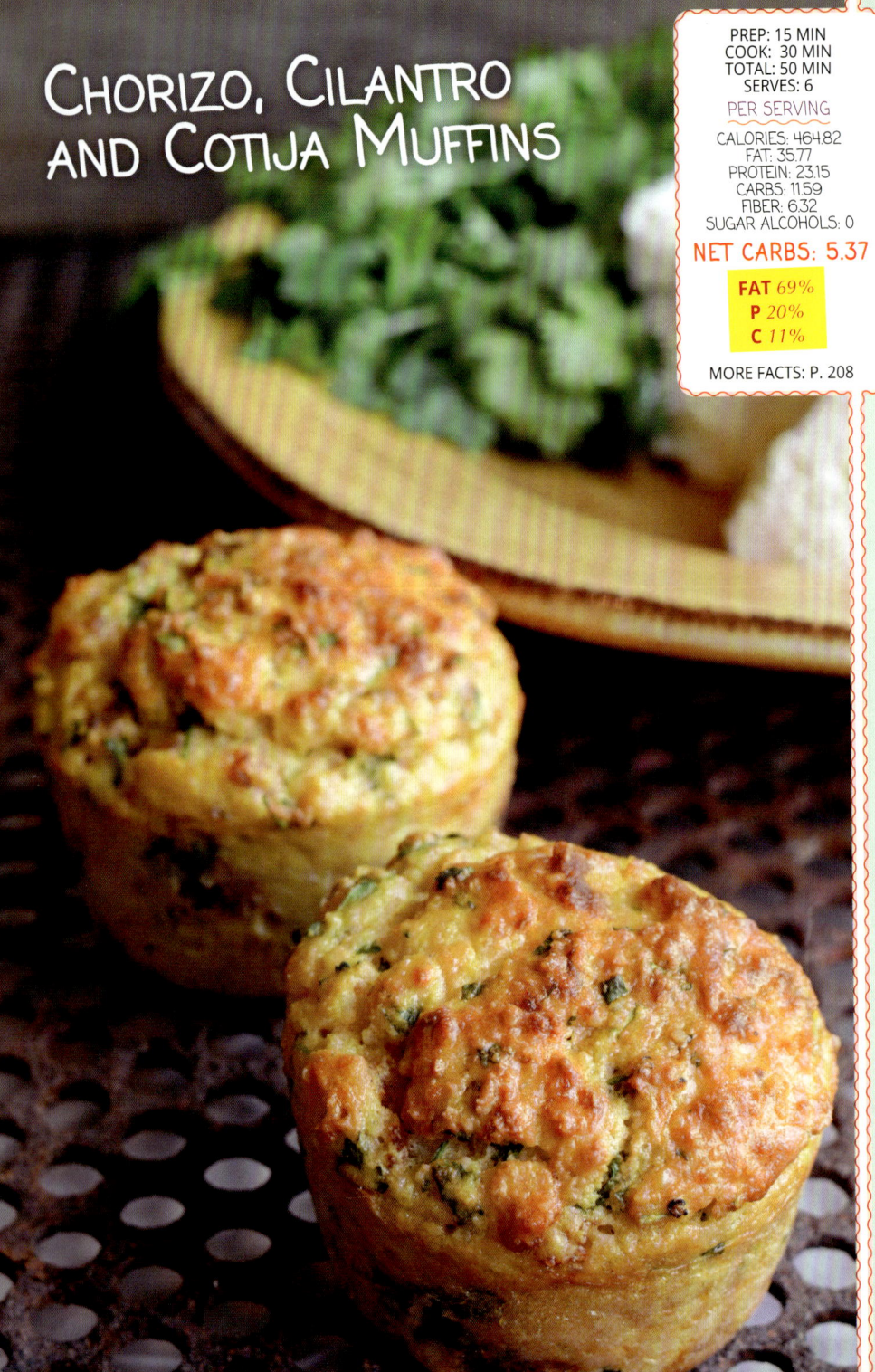

PREP: 15 MIN
COOK: 30 MIN
TOTAL: 50 MIN
SERVES: 6

PER SERVING

CALORIES: 464.82
FAT: 35.77
PROTEIN: 23.15
CARBS: 11.59
FIBER: 6.32
SUGAR ALCOHOLS: 0

NET CARBS: 5.37

FAT 69%
P 20%
C 11%

MORE FACTS: P. 208

My ultimate goal with this book is to teach people how to throw together their own fanciful blends, and do it with the confidence that the end result will be tasty. PERFECT may take a second attempt, but the first stab should still be highly enjoyable.

I personally spend a lot of time in Mexico. Chorizo, cilantro, and a cheese called *Cotija* are incredibly common ingredients in my neck of the woods. This could just as easily be Italian sausage, feta and oregano, but I opted to go for some local flavors. The result is a dozen firm, near-biscuit-like muffins, FULL of flavor. Take a look at my website and serve them with a big bowl of Sopa sin Tortilla.

Note: I cut back on the salt because of the use of salty ingredients.

8 oz (227g)	dry chorizo links (fresh bulk meat will work, too)
3/4 cup (180mL)	almond flour
1/2 cup (120mL)	ground white chia seed
1/4 cup (60mL)	golden flaxseed meal
1 tbsp (15mL)	baking powder
Dash	salt and pepper
6 large	eggs
1/4 cup + 2 tbsp (90mL)	unsweetened almond milk
2 tbsp (30mL)	melted butter or lard (as needed)
8 oz (227g)	crumbled Cotija cheese
1/4 cup (60mL)	chopped cilantro

- Preheat oven to 350° F (177° C).
- Grease a standard 12-cup muffin pan (or two standard sized 6-cup muffin pans [We're looking for 12 smallish muffins.]). Set aside.
- Place a sauté pan on the stove over high heat.
- While the pan is heating, cut your chorizo into cubes. Evenly spread the chorizo along the bottom of the pan and cook until the edges begin to crisp and color. Remove and strain off any fat or liquid that accumulates. Save that liquid and set the cooked sausage aside.
- **Note:** Many chorizos will yield a brilliant orange fat. You need 2 tbsp (30mL) of fat for this recipe. If there isn't enough, add a little melted butter to equal 2 tbsp (30mL) of warm liquid fat.
- In a large bowl, combine the almond, chia, flaxseed, baking powder, salt, and pepper. With a whisk or a fork, combine the dry ingredients so they are evenly mixed and distributed in and amongst one another.
- In a separate smaller bowl, whisk together eggs with the almond milk. Pour into the dry ingredients. Whisk together, while pouring in the warm melted fat (see note about fat, above). Set aside to allow your flax and chia to thicken and gel (about 2 to 3 minutes).
- Smoosh and crumble your cheese. It should look like a dry, salty pile of cottage cheese.
- Add the cooked chorizo, cheese, and fresh cilantro to the batter. Whisk. The batter should be like a thick pancake batter. These ingredients tend to be a bit inconsistent from brand to brand and grind to grind. You may need to add a little more almond milk to thin it out (just not too much!).
- Once the batter is well mixed, pour even amounts between the 12 muffin cups.
- Bake for about 18 to 21 minutes, or until the muffins have crowned and the surface is dry, beginning to crisp, and has turned golden.
- Remove from the oven and let rest for 5 minutes before removing from the pan. Enjoy warm!

Muffin aux Fines Herbes

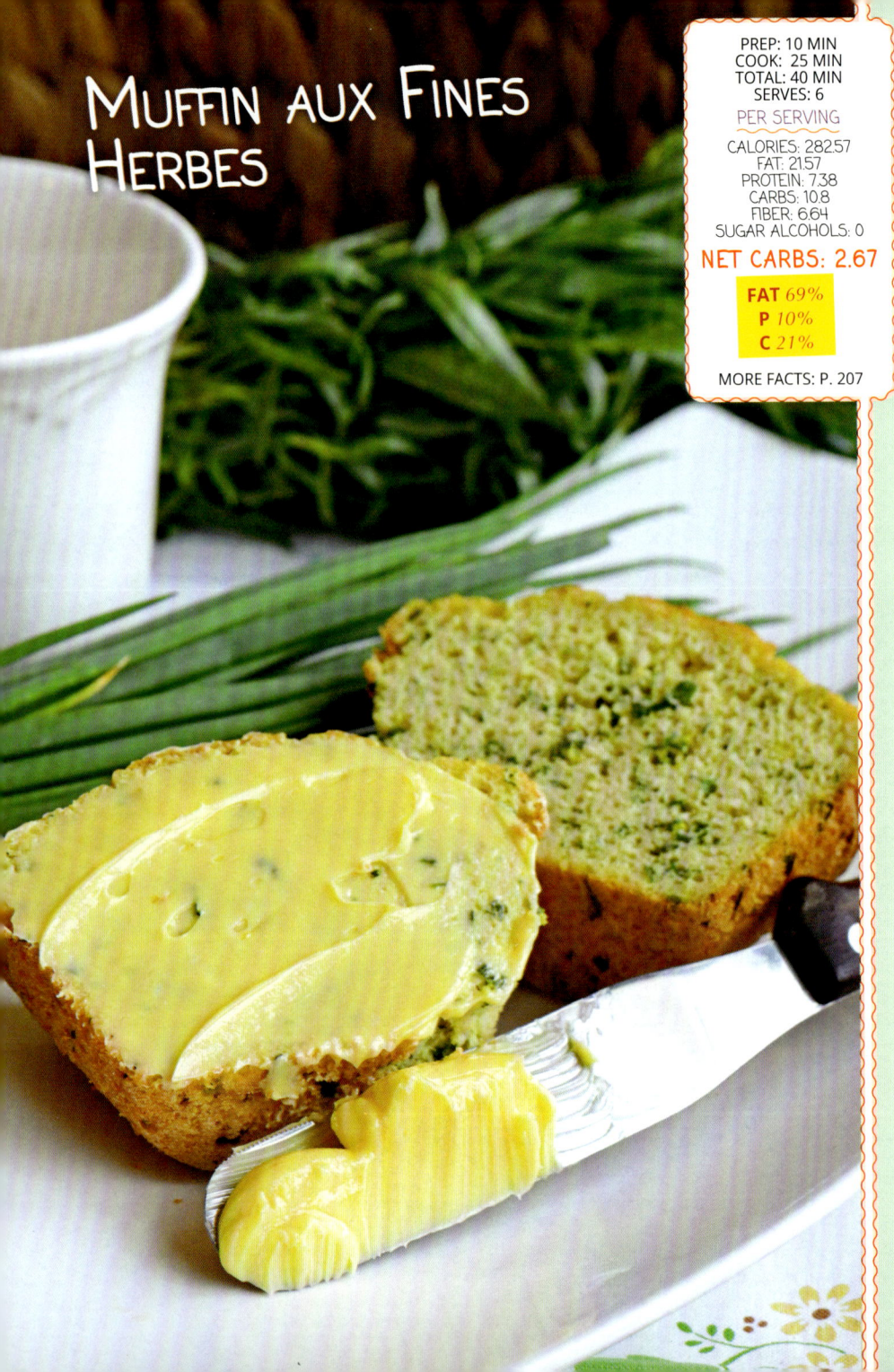

PREP: 10 MIN
COOK: 25 MIN
TOTAL: 40 MIN
SERVES: 6

PER SERVING

CALORIES: 282.57
FAT: 21.57
PROTEIN: 7.38
CARBS: 10.8
FIBER: 6.64
SUGAR ALCOHOLS: 0

NET CARBS: 2.67

FAT 69%
P 10%
C 21%

MORE FACTS: P. 207

A lot of the tastes in this book are big and bold. Being that the foundation of these faked goods tend to be calorie-dense nuts and seeds, they lend themselves well to heavier flavors. However, some of the time, all that heft can become a bit much. It's not uncommon for me to seek out lighter flavors.

Fines herbs (pronounced *feenz-AIRb*), is French for delicate greenery (fine herbs). It's classically a combination of aromatic fresh parsley, chervil, tarragon, and chives. It's not specifically a fixed blend, with some omitting the parsley and others adding the olfactory ticklers dill and basil.

I personally believe the addition of something sweet, salty, and acidic (tart or sour) can often enhance and elevate flavors. So I also added a squeeze of lemon and a smidgen of lemon zest. This allows me to use baking soda in place of the baking powder... and the tart lemon juice helps the sweeter notes of the herbs really shine! Nothing much to do with this other than smear some fancy French butter over all of it!

3/4 cup (180 mL)	almond flour
1/2 cup (120 mL)	ground white chia seed
1/4 cup (60 mL)	golden flaxseed meal
3/4 tsp (4 mL)	baking soda
3/4 tsp (4 mL)	salt
Dash	pepper
1	lemon
6 large	eggs
1/4 cup (60 mL)	unsweetened almond milk
3 tbsp (45 mL)	melted butter
*1 to 2 tbsp (15 to 30 mL)	fresh chopped parsley
1 tbsp (15 mL)	fresh chopped tarragon
1 tbsp (15 mL)	fresh chopped chives
1 tbsp (15 mL)	fresh chopped chervil (optional)

- Preheat oven to 350° F (177° C).

- Grease a standard 12-cup muffin pan (or two standard sized 6-cup muffin pans [We're looking for 12 smallish muffins.]). Set aside.

- In a large bowl, combine the almond, chia, flaxseed, baking soda, salt, and pepper. With a whisk or a fork, combine the dry ingredients so they are evenly mixed and distributed in and amongst one another.

- With a zester or a peeler, remove a small amount of the very outer yellow skin (the zest) of the lemon. Try not to get any of the bitter white pith. Chop the zest. You want about a teaspoon (5 mL) of chopped fresh lemon zest. Juice the lemon, as well. We are looking for about 2 tbsp (30 mL) of fresh lemon juice. Set the juice and chopped zest aside.

- In a separate smaller bowl, whisk together eggs with the almond milk. Pour into the dry ingredients. Whisk together, while pouring in the warm melted butter and fresh lemon juice. Set aside to allow your flax and chia to thicken and gel (about 2 to 3 minutes).

- Whisk in the chopped herbs and lemon zest. The batter should be like a thick pancake batter. These ingredients tend to be a bit inconsistent from brand to brand and grind to grind. You may need to add a little more almond milk to thin it out (just not too much!).

- Once the batter is well mixed, pour even amounts between the 12 muffin cups.

- Bake for about 18 to 21 minutes, or until the muffins have crowned and the surface is dry, beginning to crisp, and has turned golden.

- Remove from the oven and let rest for 5 minutes before removing from the pan. Enjoy warm!

- *Note: Because chervil can be so difficult to find, you may use 2 tbsp (30 mL) of fresh chopped parsley. However, if you ARE able to locate chervil, use 1 tbsp (15 mL) of each.

Pesto, Sausage and Parmesan Muffins

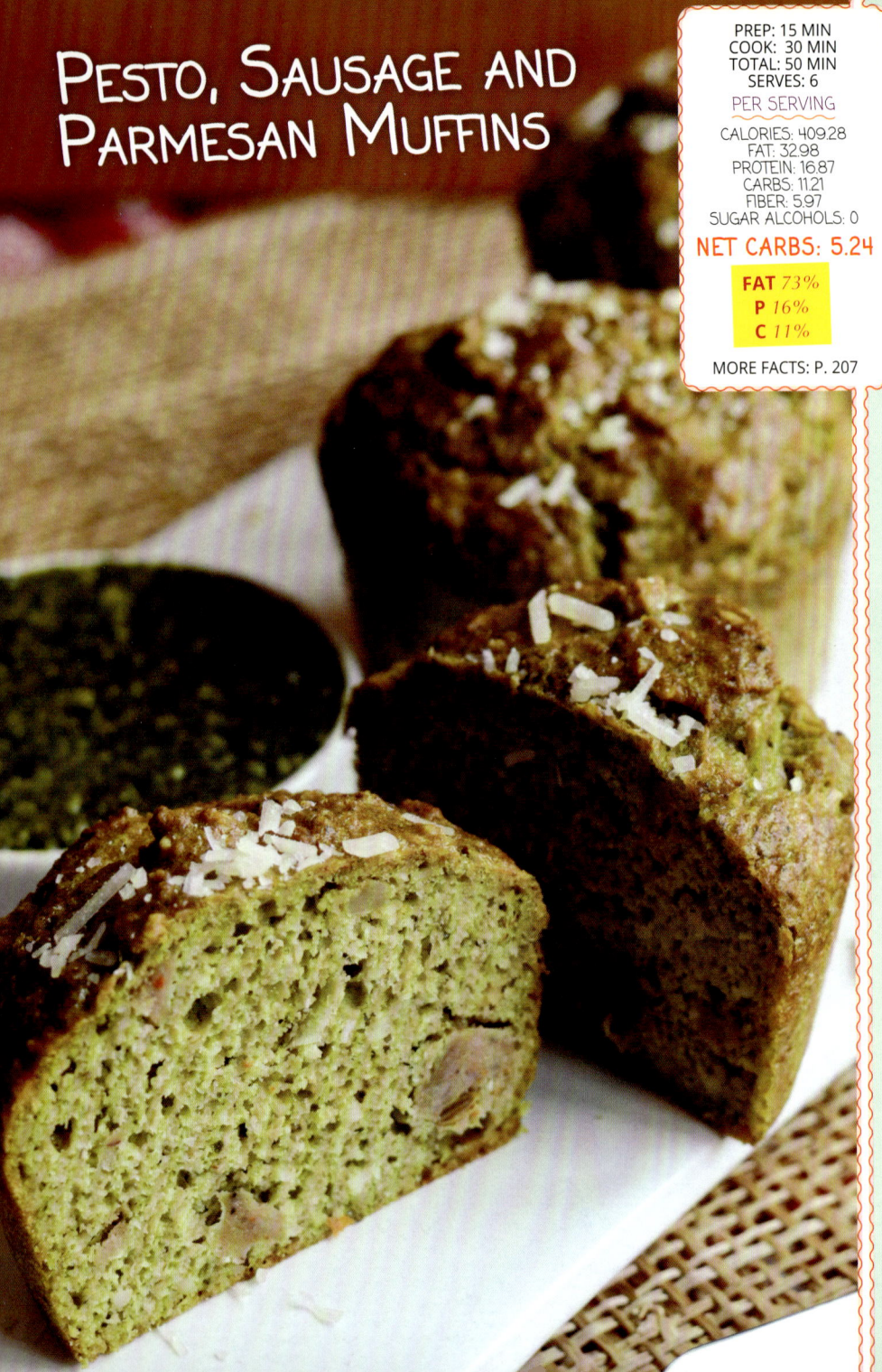

PREP: 15 MIN
COOK: 30 MIN
TOTAL: 50 MIN
SERVES: 6

PER SERVING

CALORIES: 409.28
FAT: 32.98
PROTEIN: 16.87
CARBS: 11.21
FIBER: 5.97
SUGAR ALCOHOLS: 0

NET CARBS: 5.24

FAT *73%*
P *16%*
C *11%*

MORE FACTS: P. 207

Much like the earlier Chorizo and Cotija Cheese muffins, this sassy delicacy is also infused with sausage. I'm a huge fan of sausage; it's prepared, is often already cooked and comes in a HUGE variety of flavors! Putting something like this together is easy, can be done in batches, and makes for a quick lunch!

Hey, if you really want to live life on the edge, slice it down the middle, toast it, and throw a fried egg and a lightly salted, thick-cut tomato slice into it for a sp-egg-tacular breakfast sandwich!

(Someone, somewhere is rolling their eyes and groaning, right now...)

Anywhoo... In this one, you'll notice I removed the addition of fat. Why? Because pesto has a huge amount of fat in it. Just add the pesto and this brings along with it some fat, cheese, and a keen basil flavor!

8 oz (227g)	Italian sausage links (sweet or spicy)
3/4 cup (180mL)	almond flour
1/2 cup (120mL)	ground white chia seed
1/4 cup (60mL)	golden flaxseed meal
1 tbsp (15mL)	baking powder
Dash	chili flakes (to taste)
Dash	salt and pepper
6 large	eggs
1/4 cup (60mL)	unsweetened almond milk
1/3 cup (80mL)	pesto (p. 194)
1/3 cup (80mL)	grated parmesan cheese

- Preheat oven to 350° F (177° C).
- Grease a standard 12-cup muffin pan (or two standard sized 6-cup muffin pans [We're looking for 12 smallish muffins.]). Set aside.
- Place a sauté pan on the stove over high heat.
- While the pan is heating, cut your sausage into little nibblets. Evenly spread the pieces along the bottom of the pan and cook until the edges begin to crisp and color. Remove and strain off any fat or liquid that accumulates. Discard the fat.
- In a large bowl, combine the almond, chia, flaxseed, baking powder, chili flakes, salt, and pepper. With a whisk or a fork, combine the dry ingredients so they are evenly mixed and distributed in and amongst one another.
- In a separate smaller bowl, whisk together eggs with the almond milk and pesto. Pour into the dry ingredients. Set aside to allow your flax and chia to thicken and gel (about 2 to 3 minutes).
- Add the sausage and grated cheese to the batter. Whisk. The batter should be like a thick pancake batter. These ingredients tend to be a bit inconsistent from brand to brand and grind to grind. You may need to add a little more almond milk to thin it out (just not too much!).
- Once the batter is well mixed, pour even amounts between the 12 muffin cups.
- Bake for about 18 to 21 minutes, or until the muffins have crowned and the surface is dry, beginning to crisp, and has turned golden.
- Remove from the oven and let rest for 5 minutes before removing from the pan. Enjoy warm!

Jalapeño Cheddar Muffins

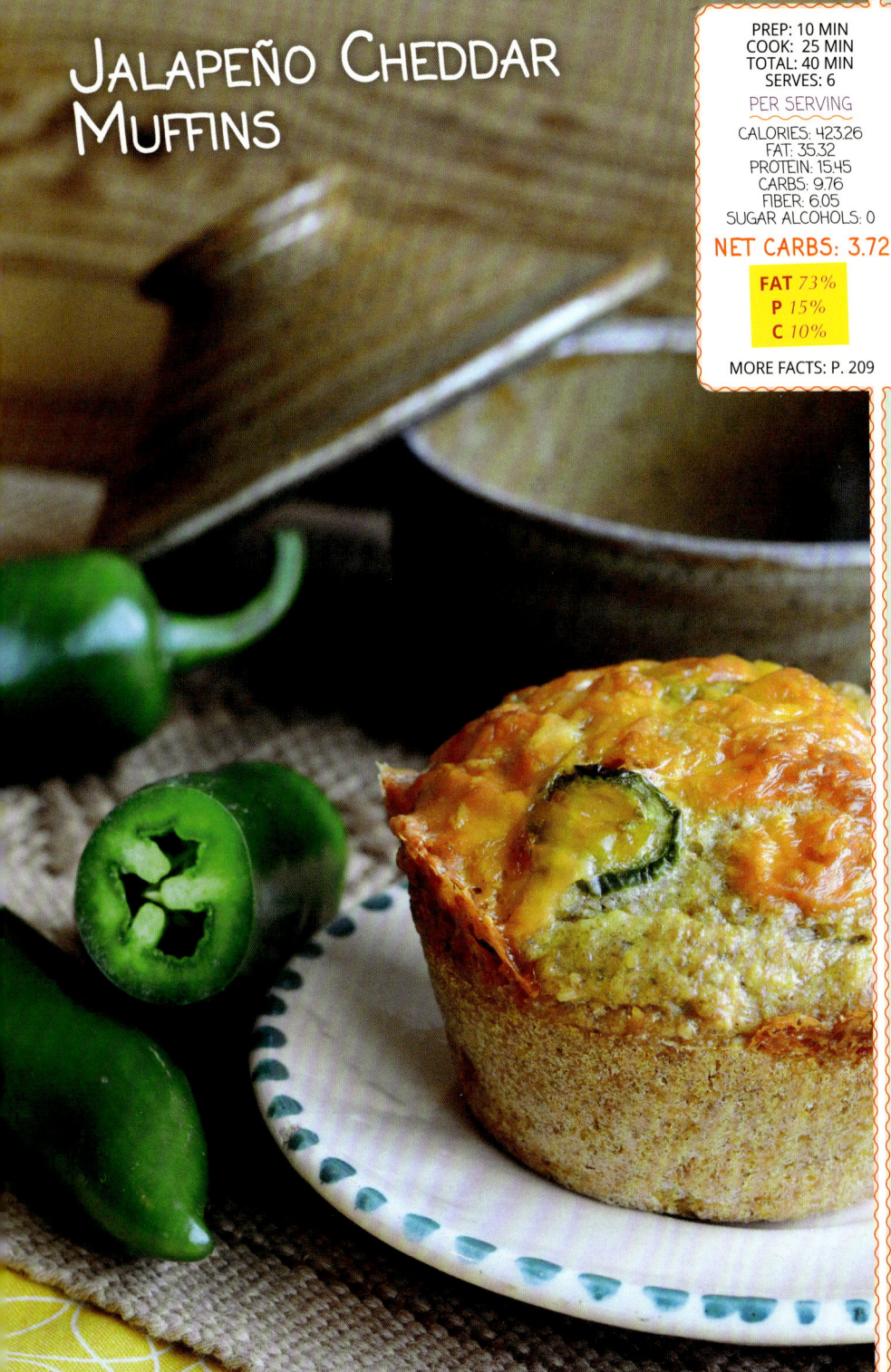

PREP: 10 MIN
COOK: 25 MIN
TOTAL: 40 MIN
SERVES: 6

PER SERVING

CALORIES: 423.26
FAT: 35.32
PROTEIN: 15.45
CARBS: 9.76
FIBER: 6.05
SUGAR ALCOHOLS: 0

NET CARBS: 3.72

FAT *73%*
P *15%*
C *10%*

MORE FACTS: P. 209

As stated earlier in the book, I was once a professional baker. Aside from the dazzling array of assorted breakfast treats, the true culmination of my skills erupted in the form of the most spectacular single bread basket you'd ever see in any restaurant. I hazard to romanticize the impressive list of steamy aromatic contents, as I don't want to trigger anyone, but I WILL say... "In your face, Olive Garden!"

I picture an oxymoronically fancy rustic restaurant dubbed Low Primal. One arrives and is greeted by a piping hot, grain-free bread basket and assorted compound butters and fatty spreads. One peek into the basket of hearty breadstuffs and the eyes cannot turn away from the crown of the spicy hot Jalapeño Cheddar Muffins as they blearily peek back, as if just woken from slumber.

I mixed this up and added a little bit of pecan flour. It's absolutely unnecessary, but I wanted to start playing with some grinding of nuts, and the pecan almond blend is perfect for this hot cheesy concoction.

1/2 cup (120mL)	pecan flour
1/2 cup (120mL)	ground white chia seed
1/4 cup (60mL)	golden flaxseed meal
1/4 cup (60mL)	almond flour
3/4 tsp (4mL)	baking soda
3/4 tsp (4mL)	salt
Dash	pepper
1 large	lime
6 large	eggs
1/4 cup (60mL)	unsweetened almond milk
3 tbsp (45mL)	melted butter or lard
8 oz (227g)	cheddar cheese
2	fresh jalapeño peppers

≥ Preheat oven to 350° F (177° C).

≥ Grease a standard 12-cup muffin pan (or two standard sized 6-cup muffin pans [We're looking for 12 smallish muffins.]). Set aside.

≥ In a large bowl, combine the pecan flour, chia, flaxseed, almond, baking soda, salt, and pepper. With a whisk or a fork, combine the dry ingredients so they are evenly mixed and distributed in and amongst one another.

≥ With a zester or a peeler, remove a small amount of the very outer green skin (the zest). Try not to get any of the bitter white pith. Chop the zest. You want about a scant teaspoon (4mL) of chopped fresh lime zest. Juice the lime, as well. We are looking for about 2 tbsp (30mL) of fresh lime juice.

≥ In a separate smaller bowl, whisk together lime juice, lime zest, eggs and the almond milk. Pour mixture into the dry ingredients. Whisk together while pouring in the warm melted butter or lard. Set aside to allow your flax and chia to thicken and gel (about 2 to 3 minutes).

≥ Cut your cheese into cubes. Grated cheese would be quite tasty, but I particularly enjoy the small pockets of melted cheese globs. Cut the cheese into rough 1/4 to 1/3-inch cubes (just shy of a centimeter).

≥ Slice the jalapeños into very thin rings.

≥ Add the cubed cheese and jalapeños to the batter. Whisk. The batter should be like a thick pancake batter. These ingredients tend to be a bit inconsistent from brand to brand and grind to grind. You may need to add a little more almond milk to thin it out (just not too much!).

≥ Once the batter is well mixed, pour even amounts between the 12 muffin cups.

≥ Bake for about 18 to 21 minutes, or until the muffins have crowned and the surface is dry, beginning to crisp, and has turned golden.

≥ Remove from the oven and let rest for 5 minutes before removing from the pan. Enjoy warm!

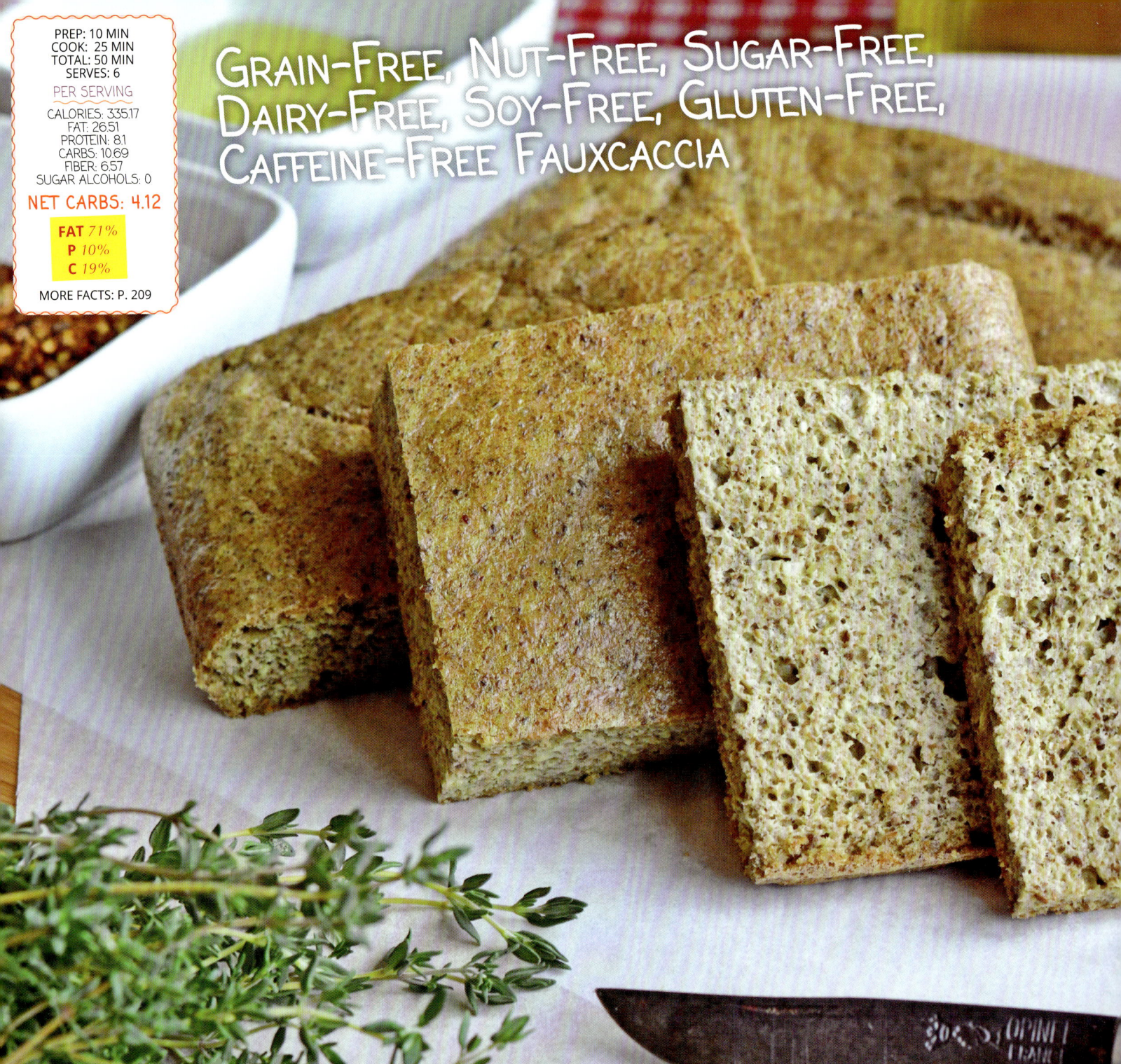

Grain-Free, Nut-Free, Sugar-Free, Dairy-Free, Soy-Free, Gluten-Free, Caffeine-Free Fauxcaccia

PREP: 10 MIN
COOK: 25 MIN
TOTAL: 50 MIN
SERVES: 6

PER SERVING
CALORIES: 335.17
FAT: 26.51
PROTEIN: 8.1
CARBS: 10.69
FIBER: 6.57
SUGAR ALCOHOLS: 0
NET CARBS: 4.12

FAT 71%
P 10%
C 19%

MORE FACTS: P. 209

Shortly after graduating college, I drove to San Francisco to begin my lofty career as the greatest chef the planet had ever seen (whoops!). On the way, I hung a right and took a pitstop in Seattle to visit my folks and see their new house. The first morning in Seattle, my mother talked me into joining her on a dog walk. She spun yarns about this *amazing* newfangled business venture called Starbucks, where they served a fancy hot Italian coffee drink called a latte. Having never heard of such a thing, I was intrigued and joined her.

We arrived at Starbucks, a small, clean-looking building on Mercer Island, WA. My mother ordered a "small decaf *caffè latte*, with soy milk and sugar-free vanilla syrup." This was a very foreign string of words to my early '90s self. Not knowing what was what, I sheepishly ordered a minty-sounding mocha-thing.

There are a few moments in my life that register as high in my list of happy moments. Very high on that list was my first sip of the minty-mocha thing, on a brisk cloudy morning with my mother in the Pacific Northwest. Nothing had ever complemented a nip in the air more than that toasty beverage. Sitting with my mother, now an adult, looking at the snow-capped mountains and enjoying the new culture, we got to talking about our drinks. She continued to explain Starbucks to me; explained her beverage and what it meant. Her latte was a sweet-tasting sugar-free and fat-free concoction, void of caffeine and dairy. She went on to explain that many people refer to her daily beverage as the "Why bother?"

It is with this that I frame my intention for this *wonderful* bread-like fakestuff.

This perfect and simple bread has no grains, no sugars, no gluten, no dairy, no caffeine... and doesn't even contain nuts. While I haven't tried it, I suspect it's possible to even take this a step further... using chia eggs to make this additionally egg-free.

Aw, heckfire! You could even remove the scant optional chili flakes to make it nightshade-free!

In all seriousness, this really is a banging recipe (I'm listening to an audiobook read by a British narrator). I use this variation of the recipe on *page 190* quite regularly, baking up a big batch, cutting into squares, and freezing them in a plastic zipper bag. It exists on the hearty side, tasting a bit like a whole-grain bread, heavy on the buckwheat, but in a good way! I use it to make a vast array of sandwiches (mostly griddled panini-like creatures).

I'm using this specific recipe to highlight how one can use seeds to make bread... no grains and no nuts. Why? Largely because of allergies. Loads of people struggle with nut allergies, but I ALSO think it's important to eat a wider variety of foodstuffs. Swapping out the ubiquitous almond flour for periodic alternatives is just the healthy thing to do. Too many almonds simply aren't good for anyone, anyway...

ANY of the preceding recipes could've been made in just the same manner; swapping out the nut flour for the gray and aromatic sunflower seed flour (sunflour). Nut-free fakery!

1 cup (240ᵐᴸ)	sunflower seed flour
1/2 cup (120ᵐᴸ)	flaxseed meal
1/2 cup (120ᵐᴸ)	ground chia
1 tbsp (15ᵐᴸ)	fresh chopped thyme
1 1/8 tsp (6ᵐᴸ)	baking soda
1 tsp (5ᵐᴸ)	salt
1/2 tsp (3ᵐᴸ)	crushed red chili flakes (or to taste)
8 large	eggs, beaten
1/4 cup + 2 tbsp (90ᵐᴸ)	water or unsweetened hempseed milk
1/4 cup (60ᵐᴸ)	extra-virgin olive oil
1 1/2 tbsp (23ᵐᴸ)	white vinegar or lemon juice
6 cloves (18ᵍ)	garlic, minced

- Preheat oven to 350° F (177° C).
- Grease a 9" x 9" (23ᶜᵐ x 23ᶜᵐ) square baking pan.
- In a large bowl, combine sunflour, flax, chia, thyme, baking soda, salt, and chili flakes. Mix well.
- Add the eggs, water (or hempseed milk), olive oil, vinegar (or lemon juice), and garlic to the mix. Mix well. Wait about 2 to 3 minutes, allowing the flax and chia to gel. The batter should resemble a thick pancake batter. If it does not, whisk in a bit of hempseed milk or water to thin it out.
- Pour the batter into the pan. With a spatula, smooth it out so that it is evenly distributed throughout the pan.
- Bake for about 23 to 28 minutes, or until lightly golden brown and nicely puffed.
- Place on a rack and cool for at least 10 minutes before slicing. Remove from pan, slice, and serve!

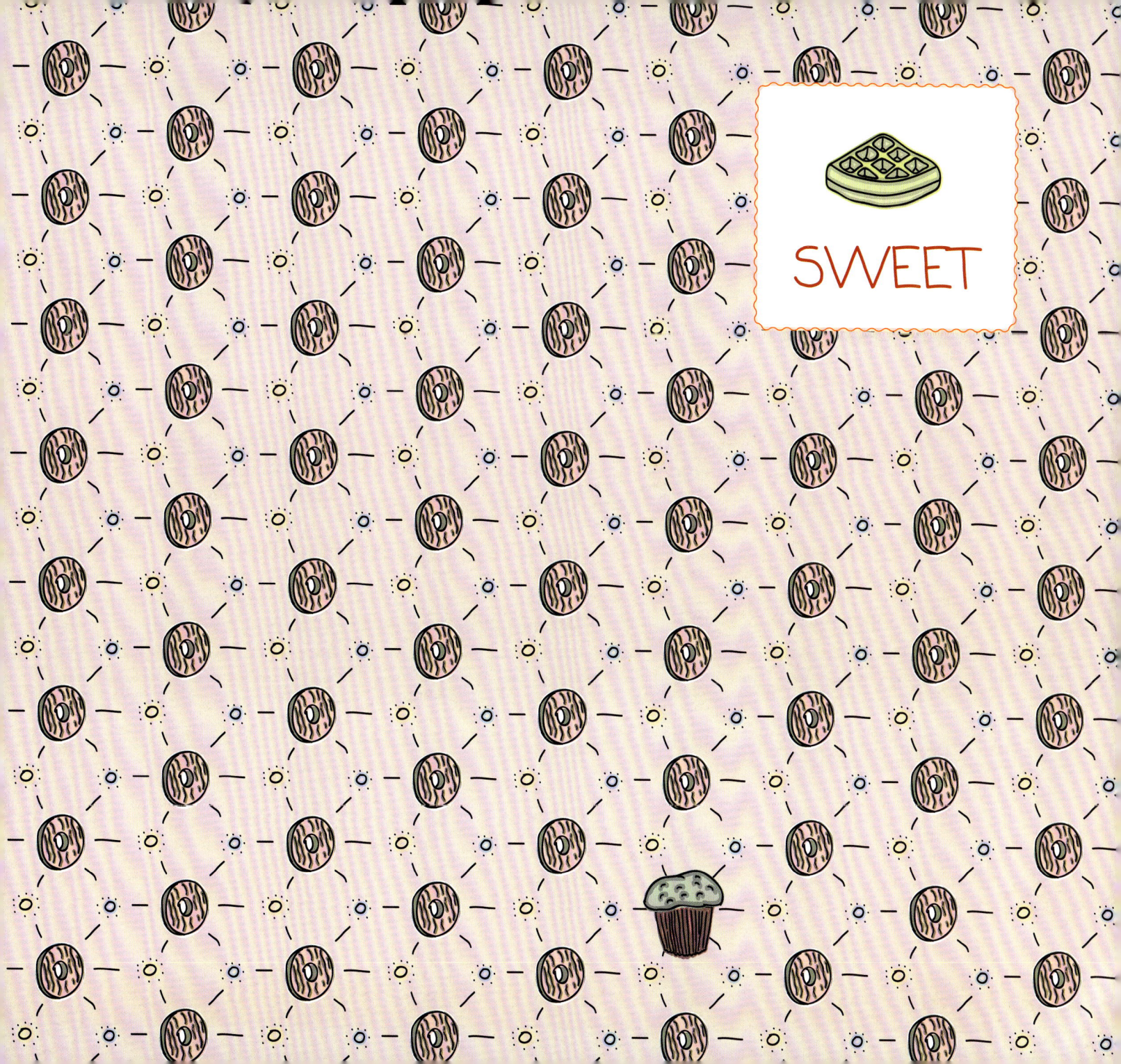

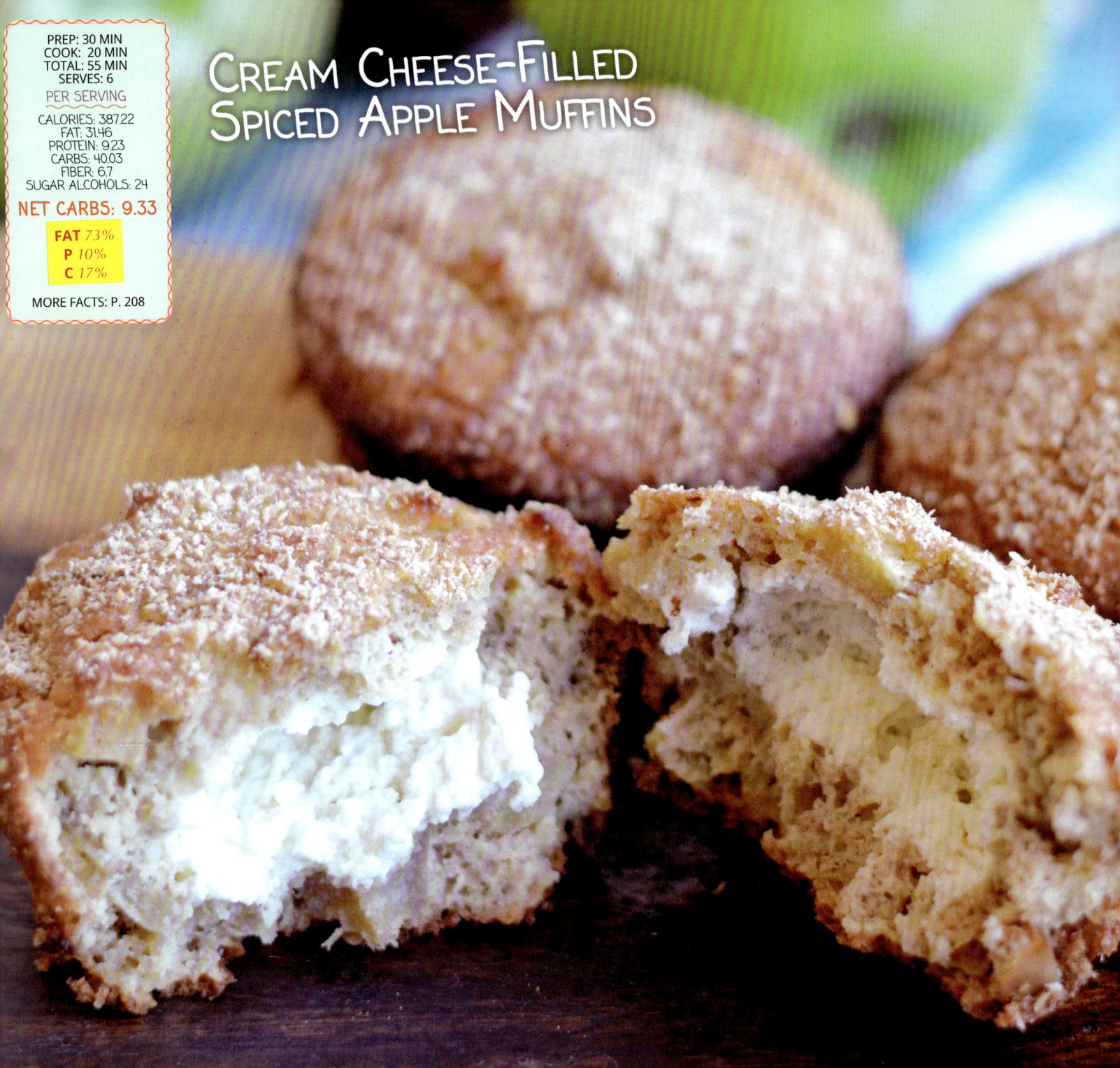

Cream Cheese-Filled Spiced Apple Muffins

PREP: 30 MIN
COOK: 20 MIN
TOTAL: 55 MIN
SERVES: 6

PER SERVING
CALORIES: 387.22
FAT: 31.46
PROTEIN: 9.23
CARBS: 40.03
FIBER: 6.7
SUGAR ALCOHOLS: 24

NET CARBS: 9.33

FAT 73%
P 10%
C 17%

MORE FACTS: P. 208

Before we get into the sweeter of the two main faking ratios, I thought it would make sense to bridge the two sections with a sweet-tasting muffin, but using the savory ratio. Why? Largely because I think of apples as a winter fruit, and winter is a season that tends toward heartier flavors.

See, the savory ratio has earthier notes than the more floral aromas of the sweet. I find it complements the flavors of this particular muffin quite well!

And, you know, to be *different*, I stuffed it!

1 large	apple (like a Fuji or Gala)
3 tbsp (45mL)	butter
1 tsp (5mL)	salt, divided
3/4 cup (180mL)	cream cheese, room-temperature
3/4 cup (180mL)	sugar replacement, divided
3/4 cup (180mL)	almond flour
1/2 cup (120mL)	ground white chia seed
1/4 cup (60mL)	golden flaxseed meal
1/2 tsp (3mL)	ground cinnamon
1/4 tsp (1mL)	ground nutmeg
3/4 tsp (4mL)	baking soda
6 large	eggs
1/4 cup (60mL)	unsweetened almond milk
1 tsp (5mL)	blackstrap molasses or yacón syrup
1 tbsp (15mL)	apple cider vinegar

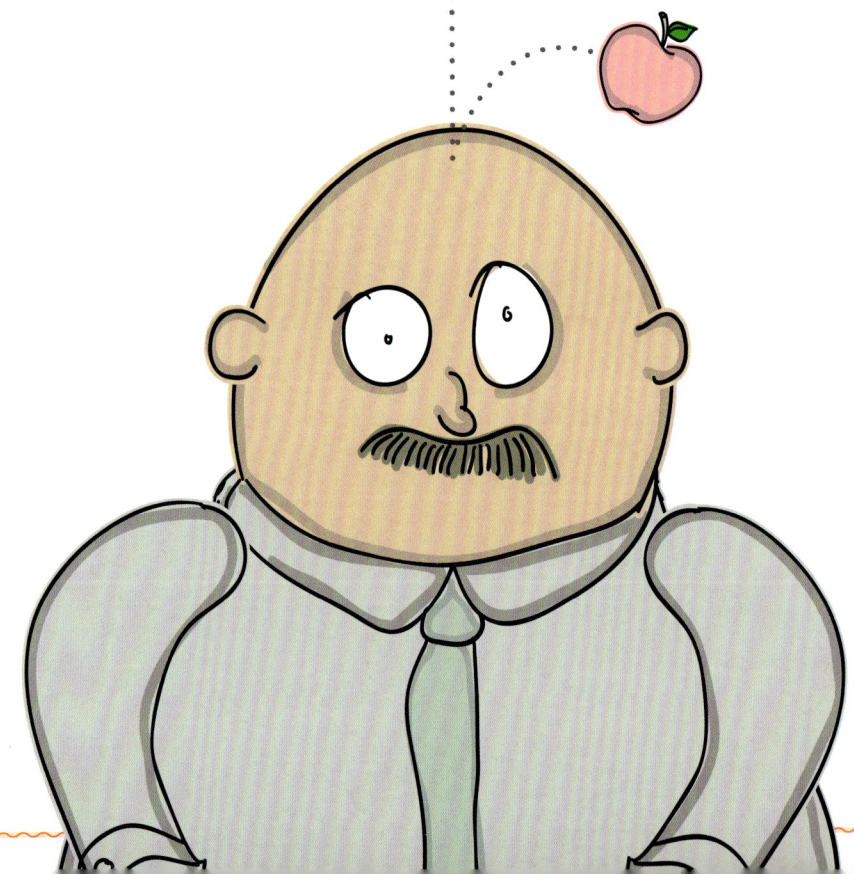

- Preheat oven to 350° F (177° C).
- Grease a standard 12-cup muffin pan (or two standard sized 6-cup muffin pans [We're looking for 12 smallish muffins.]). Set aside.
- Preheat a large sauté pan over medium-high heat.
- While the pan is heating, cut your apple into small cubes about 1/4 to 1/3-inch square (just short of 1 cm).
- Add your butter to the pan and swirl it around to coat the bottom. If it turns a little bit brown while you're doing this… super! Browned butter is a terrific flavor in this recipe (black butter, however, isn't). Once the butter coats the bottom of the pan, evenly sprinkle the apple cubes into the pan to form one clean layer. Sprinkle 1/4 tsp (1 mL) of salt over the apples. Let cook on one side, then toss the apples around. We are looking to brown (caramelize) the outside of the apples. After about 2 minutes over a medium-high heat, the apples should have a nice color. They will have begun to soften, but shouldn't be mushy. Remove the apples from the pan and spread evenly onto a plate to cool.
- In a small mixing bowl, combine the cream cheese with 1/4 cup (60 mL) of the sugar replacement. Set aside.
- In a large bowl, combine the almond flour, chia, flaxseed, cinnamon, nutmeg, the remaining 1/2 cup (120 mL) sugar replacement, and remaining 3/4 tsp (4 mL) salt. With a whisk or a fork, combine the dry ingredients so they are evenly mixed and distributed in and amongst one another. Remove about 1/4 cup (60 mL) of this mixture and set aside.
- Add the baking soda to the large bowl of dry ingredients. Incorporate with a whisk or fork.
- In a separate smaller bowl, whisk together eggs with the almond milk and molasses or yacón syrup. Pour into the large bowl of dry ingredients. Whisk together, while pouring in the vinegar. Set aside to allow your flax and chia to thicken and gel (about 2 to 3 minutes).
- Fold the cooked apples into the batter. The batter should be like a thick pancake batter. These ingredients tend to be a bit inconsistent from brand to brand and grind to grind. You may need to add a little more almond milk to thin it out (just not too much!).
- Once the batter is well mixed, evenly distribute half of the batter between the 12 muffin cups.
- With a spoon (I like to use a small ice cream scoop for this), spoon a hefty 1 tbsp (15+ mL) dollop of the warm cream cheese mixture into the direct center of each muffin, being sure to keep the cream cheese from touching the edge of the actual muffin pan. It should be perfectly suspended in the center of the batter in each muffin cup.
- Evenly cover the cream cheese dollops with the remaining batter.
- Evenly sprinkle the little bit of reserved dry ingredients on top, to give the muffins a fuzzy-rustic (fuzztic?) look.
- Bake for about 18 to 21 minutes, or until the muffins have crowned and the surface is dry, beginning to crisp, and has turned golden.
- Remove from the oven and let rest for 15 minutes before removing from the pan. Enjoy warm!

Blueberry, Lemon and Poppy Seed Muffins

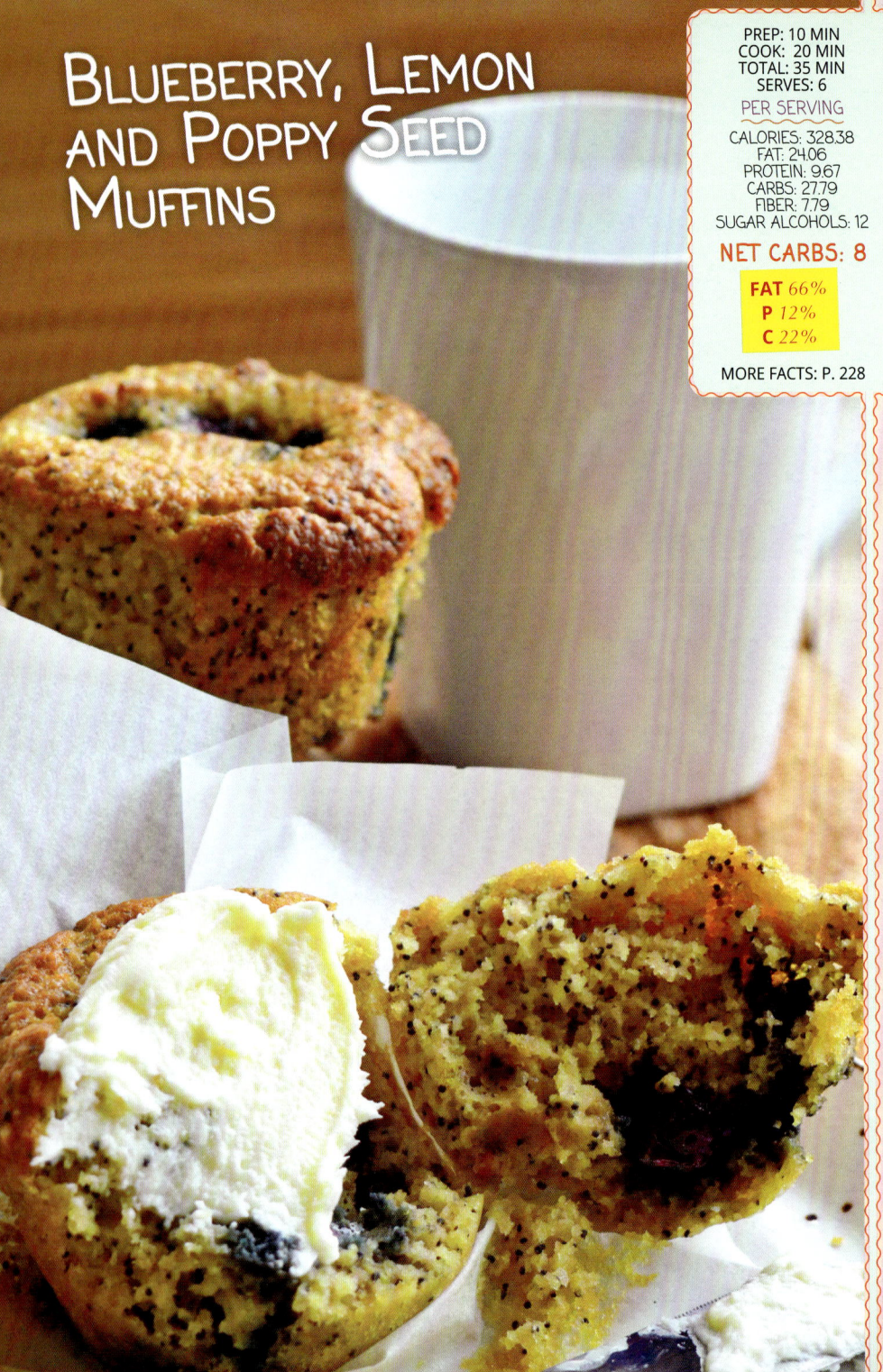

PREP: 10 MIN
COOK: 20 MIN
TOTAL: 35 MIN
SERVES: 6

PER SERVING
CALORIES: 328.38
FAT: 24.06
PROTEIN: 9.67
CARBS: 27.79
FIBER: 7.79
SUGAR ALCOHOLS: 12

NET CARBS: 8

FAT 66%
P 12%
C 22%

MORE FACTS: P. 228

Blueberry-lemon is a classic combination. Poppy seed muffins are also about as classic a muffin flavor as a muffin flavor can get. As long as we're going to work with classic flavors, why not just jump down a generation into the offspring of the two classics!

These flavors get some of their tart notes from the lemon (which also works as the acid to help the baking soda leaven the batter). The tart complements the sweeter bursts of berry. Poppy seeds? I mean... why not?!

Note: In the photo, I'm spreading mascarpone cheese all over those tasty sweet-tart critters.

1 cup + 2 tbsp (270ᵐᴸ)	almond flour
1/4 cup + 2 tbsp (90ᵐᴸ)	coconut flour
1/4 cup + 2 tbsp (90ᵐᴸ)	sugar replacement
3/4 tsp (4ᵐᴸ)	baking soda
3/4 tsp (4ᵐᴸ)	salt
1	lemon
6 large	eggs
1/4 cup (60ᵐᴸ)	unsweetened almond milk
3 tbsp (45ᵐᴸ)	melted butter
1 cup (240ᵐᴸ)	blueberries (I like mine frozen)
3 tbsp (45ᵐᴸ)	poppy seeds

≈ Preheat oven to 350° F (177° C).

≈ Grease a standard 12-cup muffin pan (or two standard sized 6-cup muffin pans [We're looking for 12 smallish muffins.]). Set aside.

≈ In a large bowl, combine the almond flour, coconut flour, sweetener, baking soda, and salt. With a whisk or a fork, combine the dry ingredients so they are evenly mixed and distributed in and amongst one another.

≈ With a zester or a peeler, peel or zest about a third of the very outer yellow skin (the zest). Try not to get any of the bitter white pith. Chop the zest. You want about a teaspoon (5ᵐᴸ) of finely chopped fresh lemon zest. Juice the lemon, as well. We are looking for about 2 tbsp (30ᵐᴸ) of fresh lemon juice. Set the juice and chopped zest aside.

≈ In a separate smaller bowl, whisk together eggs with the almond milk. Pour into the dry ingredients. Whisk together while pouring in the warm, melted fat and fresh lemon juice.

≈ Whisk in the blueberries (I like them frozen because I believe they bleed a bit less inside the muffins), poppy seeds, and reserved lemon zest. The batter should be like a thick pancake batter. These ingredients tend to be like a bit inconsistent from brand to brand and grind to grind. You may need to add a little more almond milk to thin it out (just not too much!).

≈ Once the batter is well mixed, pour even amounts between the 12 muffin cups.

≈ Bake for about 18 to 21 minutes, or until the muffins have crowned and the surface is dry, beginning to crisp, and has turned golden.

≈ Remove from the oven and let rest for 5 minutes before removing from the pan. Enjoy warm!

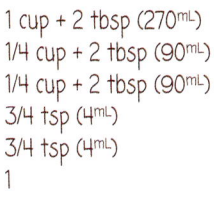

Mini Carrot Cakes with Cream Cheese Frosting

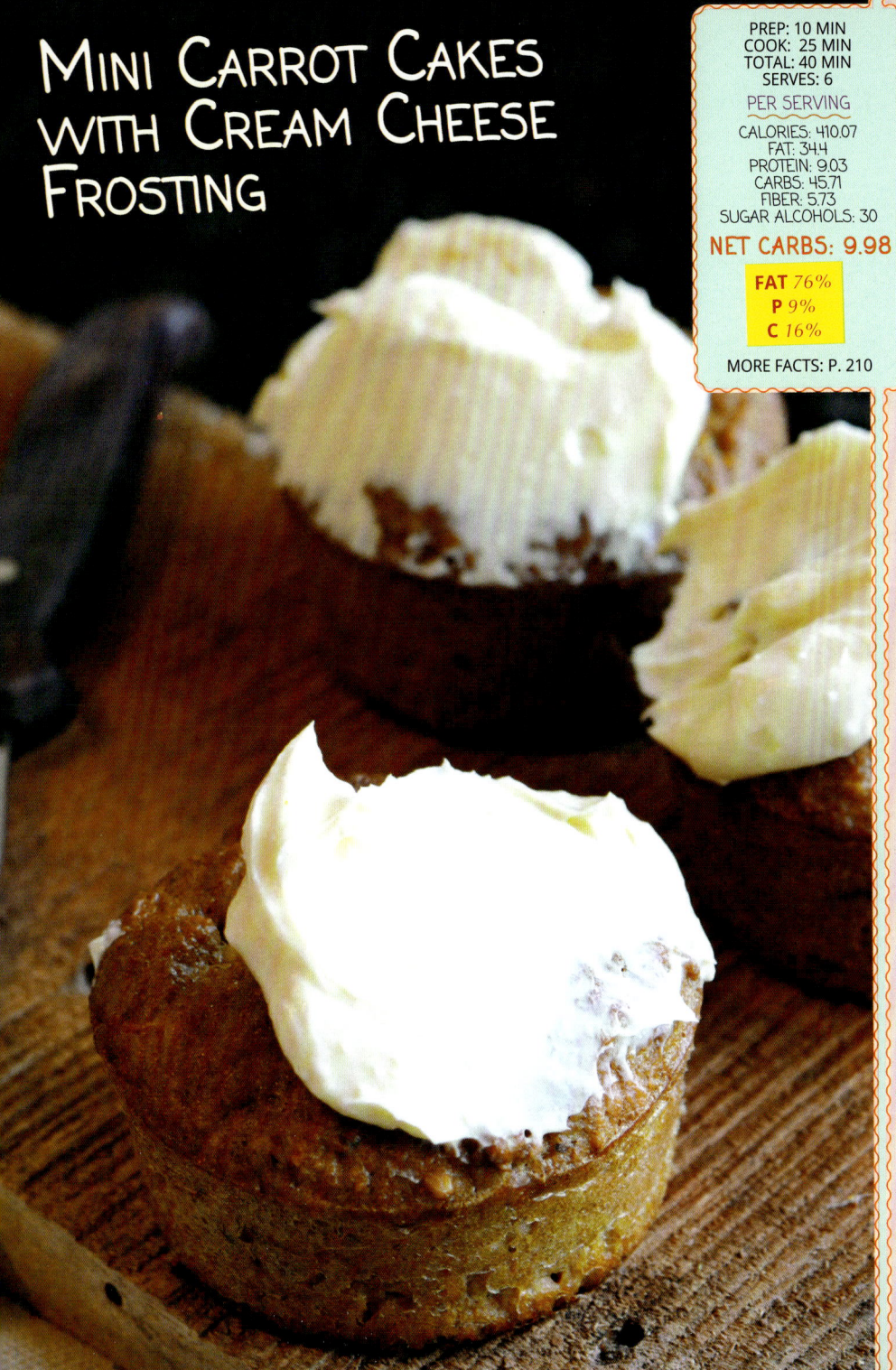

PREP: 10 MIN
COOK: 25 MIN
TOTAL: 40 MIN
SERVES: 6
PER SERVING
CALORIES: 410.07
FAT: 34.4
PROTEIN: 9.03
CARBS: 45.71
FIBER: 5.73
SUGAR ALCOHOLS: 30
NET CARBS: 9.98
FAT 76%
P 9%
C 16%
MORE FACTS: P. 210

Here's another classic muffin flavor: carrot.

Because one of the primary thrusts of this book is variety within a narrow range of ratios, this particular blob takes advantage of my mini muffin pan. The basic idea is to have lots of little tiny snow-capped muffins, easy to grab and eat, potentially for some form of social gathering. Bowling extravaganza? Waterski tournament? A holiday fiesta, perhaps?

In this one I use a mixture of walnuts and almonds. I just like the blend!

1 cup (240ᵐᴸ)	grated raw carrot
1 tsp (5ᵐᴸ)	salt, divided
1/2 cup + 2 tbsp (150ᵐᴸ)	walnut flour
1/2 cup (120ᵐᴸ)	almond flour
1/4 cup + 2 tbsp (90ᵐᴸ)	coconut flour
1/4 cup + 2 tbsp (90ᵐᴸ)	sugar replacement
1 tbsp (15ᵐᴸ)	baking powder
1/2 tsp (3ᵐᴸ)	ground cinnamon
1/4 tsp (1ᵐᴸ)	ground nutmeg
6 large	eggs
1/4 cup (60ᵐᴸ)	unsweetened almond milk
1 tsp (5ᵐᴸ)	blackstrap molasses or yacón syrup (optional)
2 tbsp (30ᵐᴸ)	coarsely chopped raisins
3 tbsp (45ᵐᴸ)	melted butter
1 recipe	cream cheese frosting (p. 196)

- Add your grated carrots to a medium sized mixing bowl. Add 1/4 tsp (1ᵐᴸ) salt. Mix and set the bowl aside. We're going to let the carrots sit for a few minutes while the salt macerates (softens) them and pulls some of the water out.

- Preheat oven to 350° F (177° C).

- Grease two miniature 12-cup muffin pans (for a total of 24 mini cakes). Alternatively, feel free to use two standard sized 6-cup muffin pans in order to arrive at the more common 12 regular-ish sized muffins. Set prepared pans aside.

- In a large bowl, combine the walnut flour, almond flour, coconut flour, sweetener, baking powder, cinnamon, nutmeg, and remaining 3/4 tsp (4ᵐᴸ) salt. With a whisk or a fork, combine the dry ingredients so they are evenly mixed and distributed in and amongst one another.

- To the macerated carrots in the smaller bowl, add eggs, almond milk, and optional molasses or yacón syrup. Whisk to combine.

- Pour carrot mixture into the dry ingredients. Add the raisins. Whisk together while pouring in the warm, melted butter. The batter should be like a thick pancake batter. These ingredients tend to be a bit inconsistent from brand to brand and grind to grind. You may need to add a little more almond milk to thin it out (just not too much!).

- Once the batter is well mixed, pour even amounts between the 12 muffin cups.

- Bake for about 18 to 21 minutes, or until the muffins have crowned and the surface is dry, beginning to crisp, and has turned golden.

- Remove from the oven and let rest for 5 minutes before removing from the pan. Enjoy warm or cool, topped with a heaping mound of frosting!

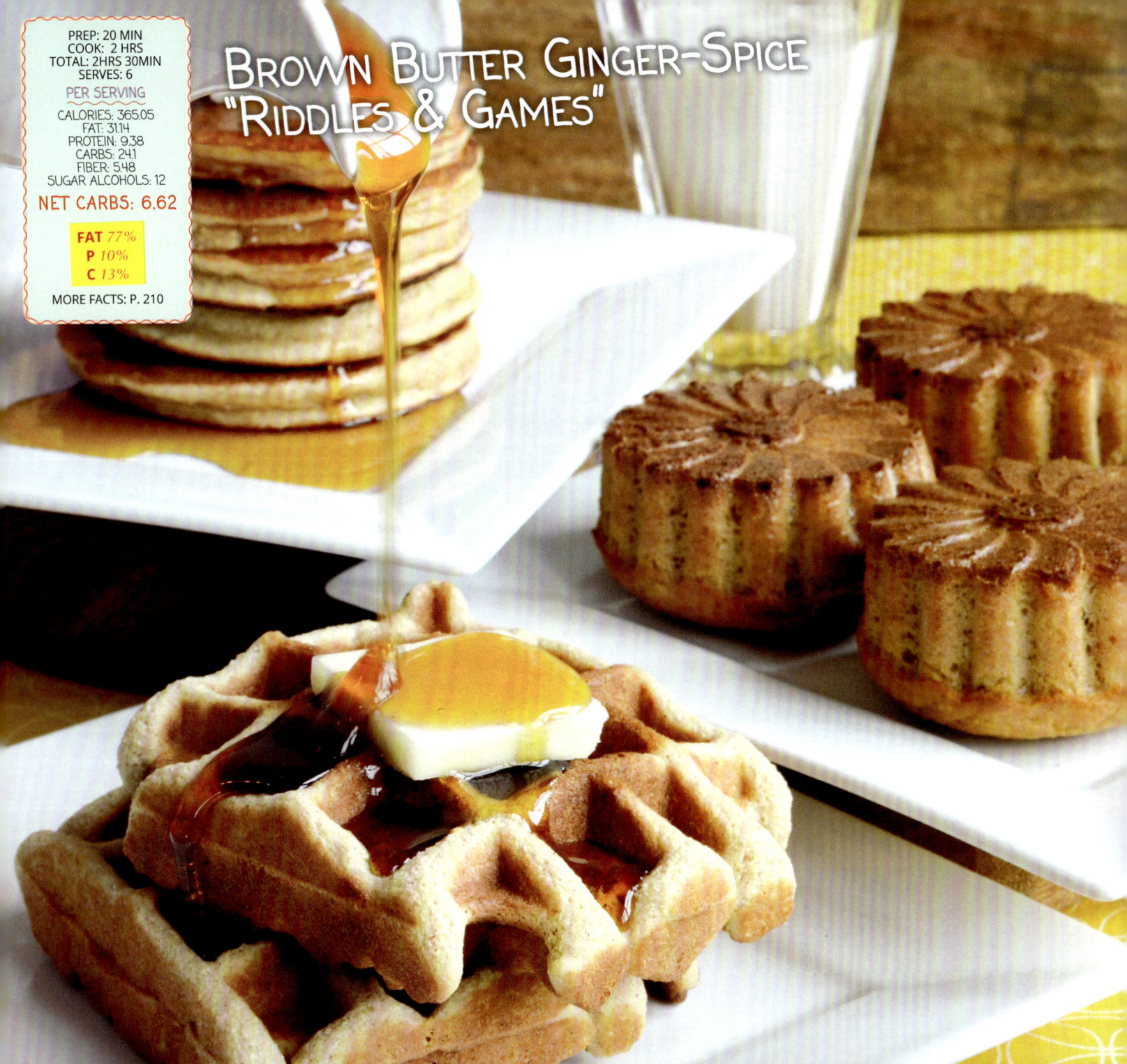

Brown Butter Ginger-Spice "Riddles & Games"

PREP: 20 MIN
COOK: 2 HRS
TOTAL: 2HRS 30MIN
SERVES: 6

PER SERVING
CALORIES: 365.05
FAT: 31.14
PROTEIN: 9.38
CARBS: 24.1
FIBER: 5.48
SUGAR ALCOHOLS: 12
NET CARBS: 6.62

FAT 77%
P 10%
C 13%

MORE FACTS: P. 210

As stated multiple times, this book is about taking a few core sets of rules (basic ratios) and pouring them into various shapes in order get different results. This tantalizing recipe perfectly showcases how one can take a flavorful blob and use it in a variety of ways.

With this one, I made a big batch of blob, poured a third into greased sunflower silicone pans, used a third to make pancakes, and then used the final third to make waffles. All literally thirds of the very same batter, just faked in a few different ways.

This recipe is written as if it's for standard muffins, but I encourage all y'all to pour your blobs into a variety of molds and shapes. Then cook or bake. If you have too much blob batter, just pour whatever remains into a separate faking vessel and make a snack!

Hence the name "Riddles and Games." Yes, I'm suggesting you play with your food. Don't tell anyone!

wink

In terms of flavor, just as molasses and yacón syrup lend a deeper, more charismatic flavor to foods... another approach can be found in caramelizing, or browning, some of the ingredients. What is the browned crust of a baked good, if not a caramelized and more robustly flavored part of the whole? No wonder people love the muffin tops. They're adorned with the more richly flavored crown!

In this case, we're going to brown "butter" in an effort to dial in a more complicated flavor to this particular blob. And when I say "butter," I actually mean "cream." What is cream, if not butter with the water all emulsified within it? Churn cream to make butter, right?

Store-bought cream typically has more milk solids than store-bought butter. It's the milk solids we want to caramelize for its darker flavor.

We're going start by slowly simmering the cream. Eventually the water will all evaporate, leaving about one third of its original volume. Near this point, the cream will "break" into a sandy yellow oil slick with soft, tasty milk solid nodules swimming, floating, and bobbing about. It's THIS concoction that will give us our fat, while also bringing a complex and magical caramel flavor.

Yes. It's *magical* and absolutely worth the trouble.

1 cup (240ᵐᴸ)	heavy cream
1 cup + 2 tbsp (270ᵐᴸ)	almond flour
1/4 cup + 2 tbsp (90ᵐᴸ)	coconut flour
1/4 cup + 2 tbsp (90ᵐᴸ)	sugar replacement
1 tbsp (15ᵐᴸ)	baking powder
3/4 tsp (4ᵐᴸ)	salt
1/2 tsp (3ᵐᴸ)	ground cinnamon
1/4 tsp (1ᵐᴸ)	ground nutmeg
1/8 tsp (5ᵐᴸ)	ground cloves
6 large	eggs
1/4 cup (60ᵐᴸ)	unsweetened almond milk
1 tbsp (15ᵐᴸ)	freshly grated ginger

- Place the heavy cream on the stove over low heat to start reducing. Do not try and go too fast or hurry the process, because the cream will boil up the sides of the pot, overflow, and make a big mess of your kitchen. You need to go with a very low simmer and simply allow it to gurgle away for a spell. It can take a good hour or two, but in my own personal opinion, it's absolutely worth it!

- Reduce (simmer while the water evaporates) the cream until it breaks and starts to color. ("Breaking" means that it will stop looking like cream. It will separate into clear liquid fat, with stuff floating in it... this is a good thing, in this case.) DO NOT burn it. Look for something that resembles a nice "sand at the beach." Much darker than a nice sandy color and it gets bitter. Too light in color and the flavors are not developed as well as they could be. It's a very fine line. Taste the richness!

- Once it's like little pebbles and the color of sand at the beach, set it aside. Keep it warm, but not hot.

- Preheat oven to 350° F (177° C).

- Assuming you're making muffins, grease a standard 12-cup muffin pan (or two standard sized 6-cup muffin pans [We're looking for 12 smallish muffins.]). Set aside.

- In a large bowl, combine the almond flour, coconut flour, sweetener, baking powder, salt, cinnamon, nutmeg, and cloves. With a whisk or a fork, combine the dry ingredients so they are evenly mixed and distributed in and amongst one another.

- In a separate smaller bowl, whisk together your brown butter (the broken cream), eggs, almond milk, and grated ginger.

- Add the gingered eggs to the larger bowl with the dry ingredients. Whisk and combine.

- The batter should be like a thick pancake batter. These ingredients tend to be a bit inconsistent from brand to brand and grind to grind. You may need to add a little more almond milk to thin it out (just not too much!).

≷ **Note:** It is at this point that you can pour your blob into virtually any manner of mold. Just remember that there is no gluten in this batter. It can very much collapse under its own weight. Try not to make anything over about 2 inches (5^cm) in height. If you do opt to go for something a little taller and grander, don't forget you can add things like xanthan gum, chia flour, and tapioca flour. A bit of each will give you a slightly lighter, cakier, and more structurally sound fakestuff.

≷ Assuming you're disregarding the previous paragraph, once the batter is well mixed, pour even amounts between the 12 muffin cups.

≷ Bake for about 18 to 21 minutes, or until the muffins have crowned and the surface is dry, beginning to crisp, and has turned golden.

≷ Remove from the oven and let rest for 5 minutes before removing from the pan. Enjoy warm, slathered with fresh salted butter, topped with a heaping mound of frosting *(p. 196)*, or just drizzled with pancake syrup all over it.

≷ Down the hatch!

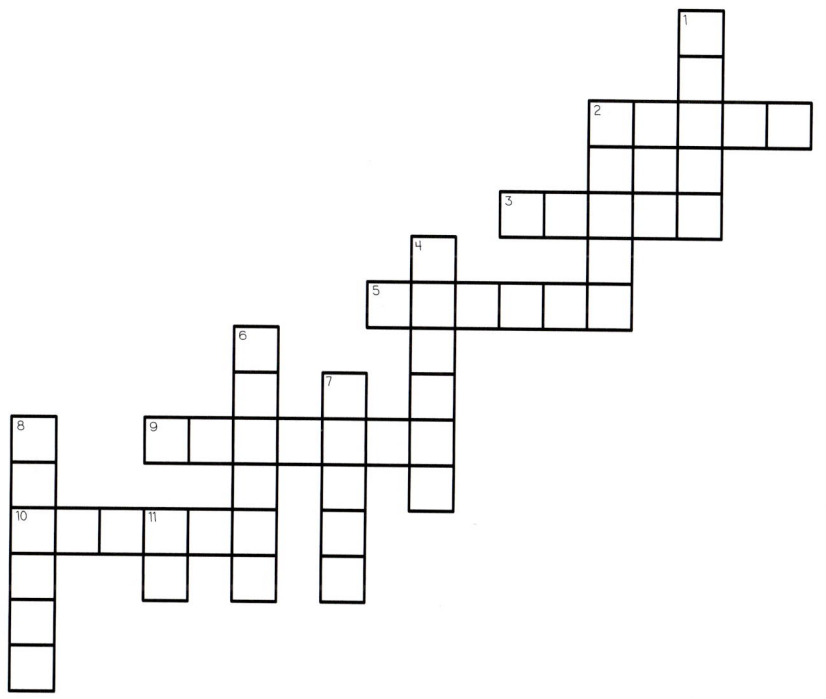

ACROSS

2 Streaky, Canadian, or Bits
3 Kevin _____
5 Do You Know the _____ Man?
9 Better than a waffle
10 Outdated term for culinary enthusiast

DOWN

1 Cured pork belly
2 Seriously, greatest food ever ever
4 It takes 21 pints of milk to make a pound of it
6 Aromatic rhizome
7 Greatest food ever
8 This is better than a pancake
11 A spinner of records

Carrot, Coconut and Macadamia Mega-Muffins

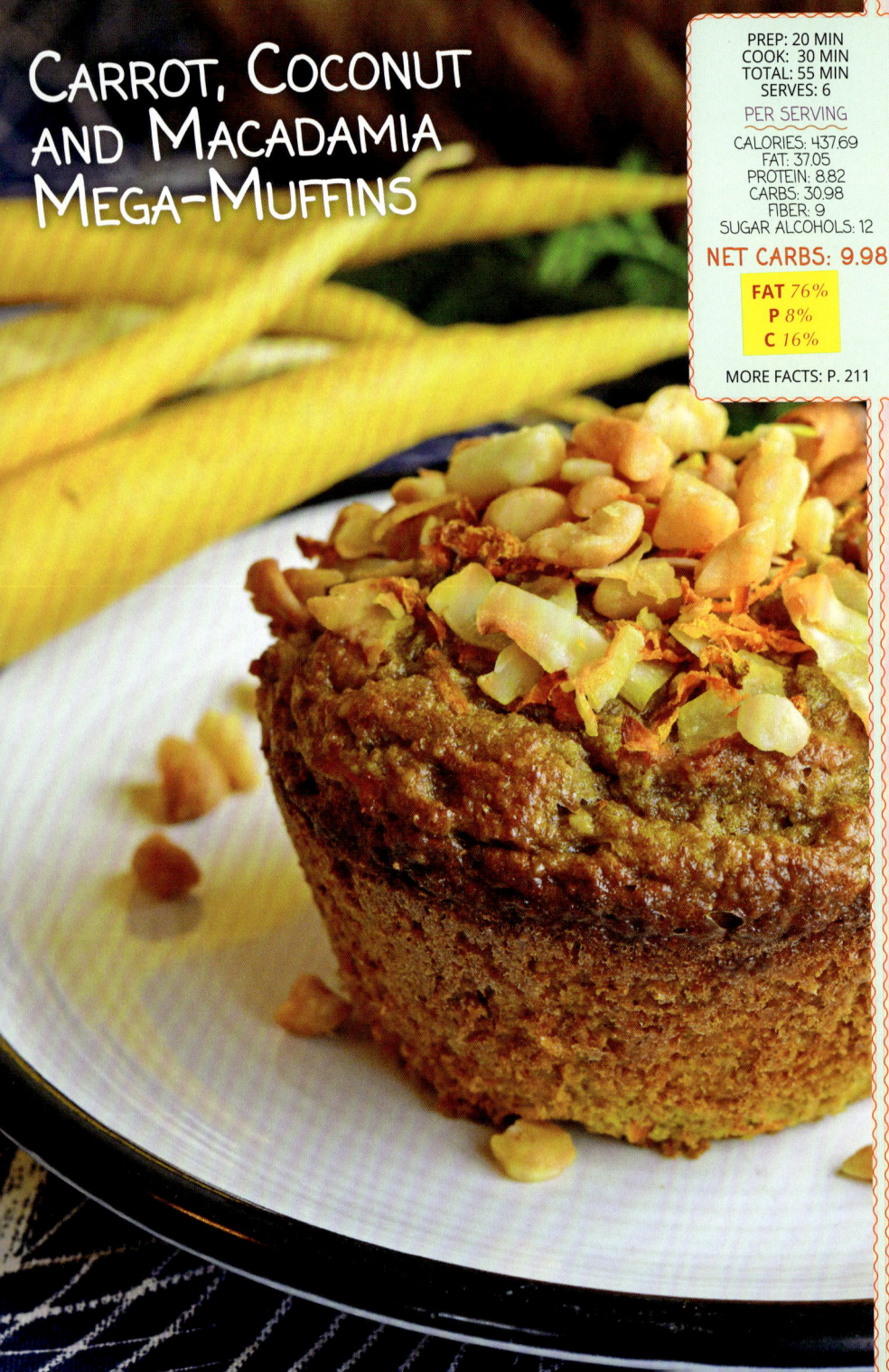

PREP: 20 MIN
COOK: 30 MIN
TOTAL: 55 MIN
SERVES: 6

PER SERVING
CALORIES: 437.69
FAT: 37.05
PROTEIN: 8.82
CARBS: 30.98
FIBER: 9
SUGAR ALCOHOLS: 12

NET CARBS: 9.98

FAT *76%*
P *8%*
C *16%*

MORE FACTS: P. 211

Here's one that should appeal greatly to those focusing on a ketogenic way of eating. The macadamia nut is the keto eater's best friend! While they're undoubtedly expensive, they're also incredibly calorie dense, from their unusually high fat content.

Add some coconut and a little bit of carrot for color contrast, a twinge of sweet, nice complementary flavors, and some added nutritional variety. What we have is a straight-up health food! I'm not the kind of guy who ever felt like I'd be writing about health food, but one of these a day is sure to keep the doctor away!

Note: This last bit was a joke. I'm *tooooooooootally* joking. Read the disclaimer at the front. I'm a fan of macadamia nuts and an absolute bacon enthusiast, but a doctor I am not. On that note, I'd bet some bacon bits tossed in this batter would be outstanding. 2 out of 10 doctors disagree!

1/2 cup (120ᵐᴸ)	grated raw carrot, divided
1 tsp (5ᵐᴸ)	salt
1/2 cup + 2 tbsp (150ᵐᴸ)	macadamia flour
1/2 cup (120ᵐᴸ)	almond flour
1/4 cup + 2 tbsp (90ᵐᴸ)	coconut flour
1/4 cup + 2 tbsp (90ᵐᴸ)	sugar replacement
3 tbsp (45ᵐᴸ)	tapioca flour (optional)
1 tsp (5ᵐᴸ)	xanthan gum (optional)
3/4 tsp (4ᵐᴸ)	baking soda
1 large	lime
6 large	eggs
1/4 cup (60ᵐᴸ)	unsweetened almond milk
1 tsp (5ᵐᴸ)	blackstrap molasses or yacón syrup (optional)
1/2 cup (120ᵐᴸ)	flaked unsweetened coconut, divided
1/2 cup (120ᵐᴸ)	chopped macadamia nuts, divided
2 tbsp (30ᵐᴸ)	coconut oil, melted

- Add your grated carrots to a medium sized mixing bowl with the salt. Mix and set the bowl aside.
- Preheat oven to 350° F (177° C).
- Grease a 6-cup large-cup muffin pan. Set prepared pan aside.
- In a large bowl, combine the macadamia flour, almond flour, coconut flour, sugar replacement, tapioca flour, xanthan gum and baking soda. With a whisk or a fork, combine the dry ingredients so they are evenly mixed and distributed in and amongst one another.
- With a zester or a peeler, remove about a third to half of the very outer green skin (the zest) of the lime. Try not to get any of the bitter white pith. Chop the zest. You want about a scant teaspoon (4ᵐᴸ) of chopped fresh lime zest. Juice the lime, as well. We are looking for about 2 tbsp (30ᵐᴸ) of fresh lime juice.
- Reach into the carrot bowl and pull out about one third of the total. Squeeze that third in your fist, removing and shaking any excess carrot water back into the bowl. Set this carrot wad aside.
- To the remaining wet, macerated carrots in the smaller bowl, add eggs and optional molasses or yacón syrup.
- Pour carrot mixture into the dry ingredients. Add about two thirds of both the flaked coconut and chopped macadamias. Whisk together, while pouring in the warm, melted coconut oil. The batter should be like a thick pancake batter. These ingredients tend to be a bit inconsistent from brand to brand and grind to grind. You may need to add a little more almond milk to thin it out (just not too much!).
- Once the batter is well mixed, pour even amounts between the 6 muffin cups.
- Break up the reserved carrot wad and mix it with the flaked coconut and chopped macadamias. Sprinkle evenly over the top of the muffins.
- Bake for about 23 to 28 minutes, or until the muffins have crowned and the surface is dry, beginning to crisp, and has turned golden. Careful not to let the coconut burn. It shouldn't, but if it starts to and the muffins aren't done, turn the heat down to 300° F (150° C) and bake until ready.
- Remove from the oven and let rest for 5 minutes before removing from the pan. Enjoy warm. I'd want to slather these with butter and a sweet, sugar-free orange marmalade!

Chocolate-Banana Muffcakes

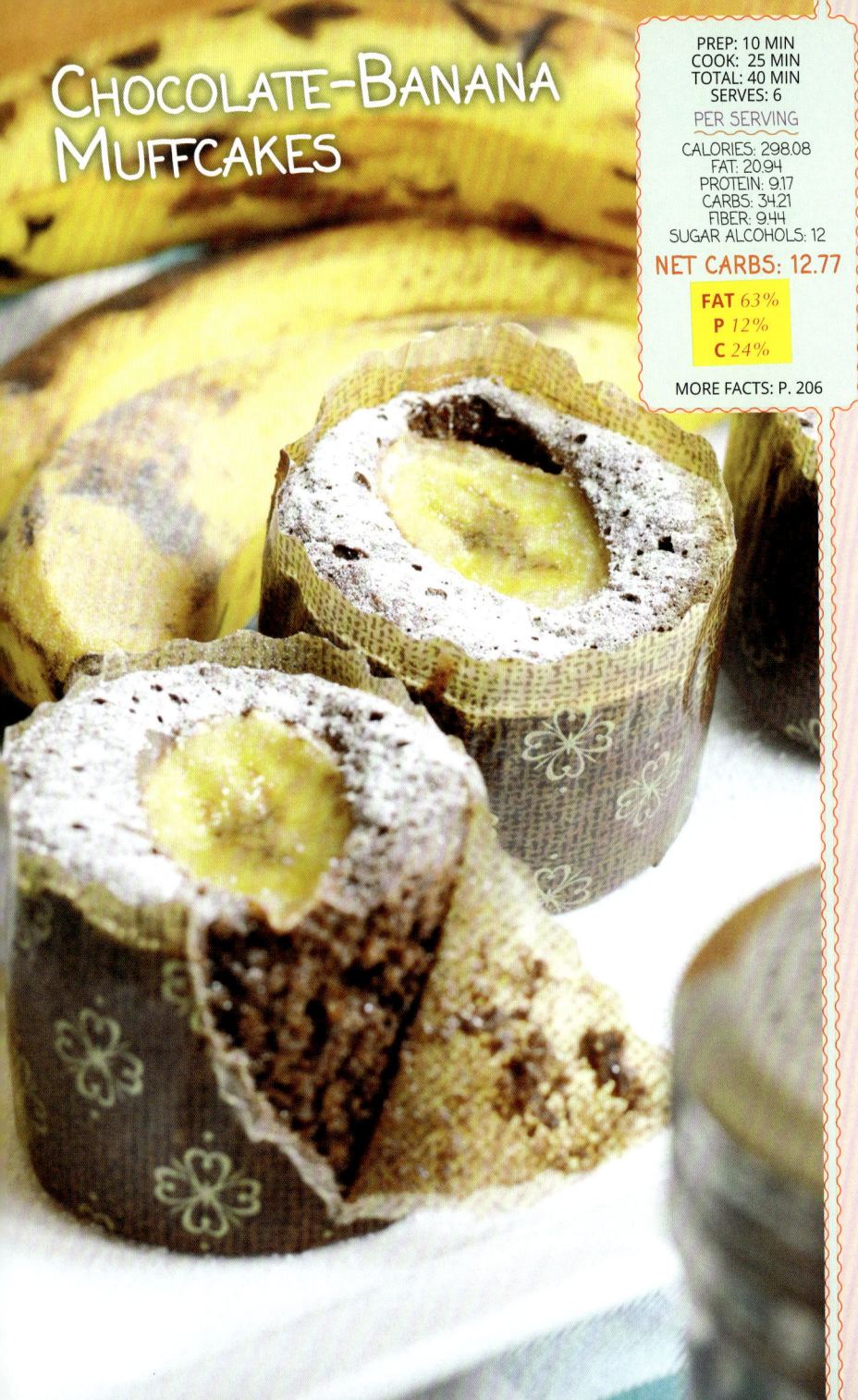

PREP: 10 MIN
COOK: 25 MIN
TOTAL: 40 MIN
SERVES: 6
PER SERVING
CALORIES: 298.08
FAT: 20.94
PROTEIN: 9.17
CARBS: 34.21
FIBER: 9.44
SUGAR ALCOHOLS: 12
NET CARBS: 12.77
FAT 63%
P 12%
C 24%

MORE FACTS: P. 206

When I eat out at fancy restaurants and am really trying to enjoy the experience unencumbered by limits, I will *still* try and skip dessert. I've never had a huge sweet tooth, but I confess to having a loose unwritten (until now) guideline: If the dessert menu has a chocolate and banana combination, I'm allowed to cave. I try not to and it doesn't happen often, but when it does, I relish it. I just need to accept the probability that the next day will be a haze of carb fog and cravings. I bite my leather strap and forge ahead.

Bananas are one of those taboo "forbidden fruits." So it's probably a bit shocking to see it here, but... firstly, I love chocolate and banana. Secondly, I find that finding stealthy ways to thoughtfully bake periodic taboos into my way of eating has dramatically decreased my feeling of limits, carrying me further into success and maintenance.

Now, in *reality*, when I make banana treats, I use half the amount of fresh banana, dropping the net carb count by about 3.5 per serving. Then I *stretch* that flavor with either sugar-free banana syrup (like for coffee drinks) and/or banana extract. I find it really quenches that particular thirst! For those who dabble in the dark arts (synthetic sweeteners and flavorings), I suggest cutting the sweetener in half, cutting the almond milk in half, and substituting with 1/4 cup (60^{mL}) of sugar-free banana syrup, as well as 1/2 tsp (3mL) of banana extract.

I also feel like pointing out that I tweaked the ratio on this one. I omitted some of the almond flour and replaced it with ground chia, as well as replacing 2 eggs with the spirit of chia eggs. Frankly, I love what ground chia does in sweet chocolate muffcakes, lending them a subtle pudding-like texture. The taste is exquisite with chocolate as well.

Finally... why "Muffcakes"? I made these with cupcake wrappers, but I'd never actually do this in real life. It's just to make the photo pretty. Also, I'm a fan of muffins, and I feel a bit like cupcakes have had their day. Muffcakes are where it's at. Move over Cronut®!

1 cup (240mL)	almond flour
1/4 cup + 2 tbsp (90mL)	coconut flour
1/4 cup + 2 tbsp (90mL)	sugar replacement
1/4 cup + 2 tbsp (90mL)	unsweetened cocoa powder
1/4 cup (60mL)	ground chia
1 tbsp (15mL)	baking powder
3/4 tsp (1mL)	salt
2 small	bananas
4 large	eggs
2 tbsp (30mL)	unsweetened almond milk
3 tbsp (45mL)	melted butter

- Preheat oven to 350° F (177° C).
- Grease a standard 12-cup muffin pan (or two standard sized 6-cup muffin pans [We're looking for 12 smallish muffins.]). Set aside.
- In a large bowl, combine the almond flour, coconut flour, sugar replacement, cocoa powder, ground chia, baking powder, and salt. With a whisk or a fork, combine the dry ingredients so they are evenly mixed and distributed in and amongst one another.
- Peel the two bananas and cut 12 very thin rounds from the middle section of one of them, leaving about 1 1/2 bananas. Set rounds aside.
- Place the remaining bananas into a medium sized bowl and smoosh them. Add eggs and almond milk to the bananas. Whisk until combined. A few small banana chunks are fine and potentially even fun!
- Pour egg mixture into the dry ingredients. Whisk together, while pouring in the warm melted butter. Let sit for about 2 minutes to allow time for the chia to gel.
- The batter should be like a thick pancake batter. These ingredients tend to be a bit inconsistent from brand to brand and grind to grind. You may need to add a little more liquid to thin it out (just not too much!).
- Once the batter is well mixed, pour even amounts between the 12 muffin cups.
- Place a banana round in the center of each muffcake.
- Bake for about 18 to 21 minutes, or until the muffcakes have risen and the surface is dry.
- Remove from the oven and let rest for 5 minutes before removing from the pan. Enjoy warm, potentially with a hefty dollop of whipped cream!

Chocolate-Chocolate Chunk with Chocolate Ganache

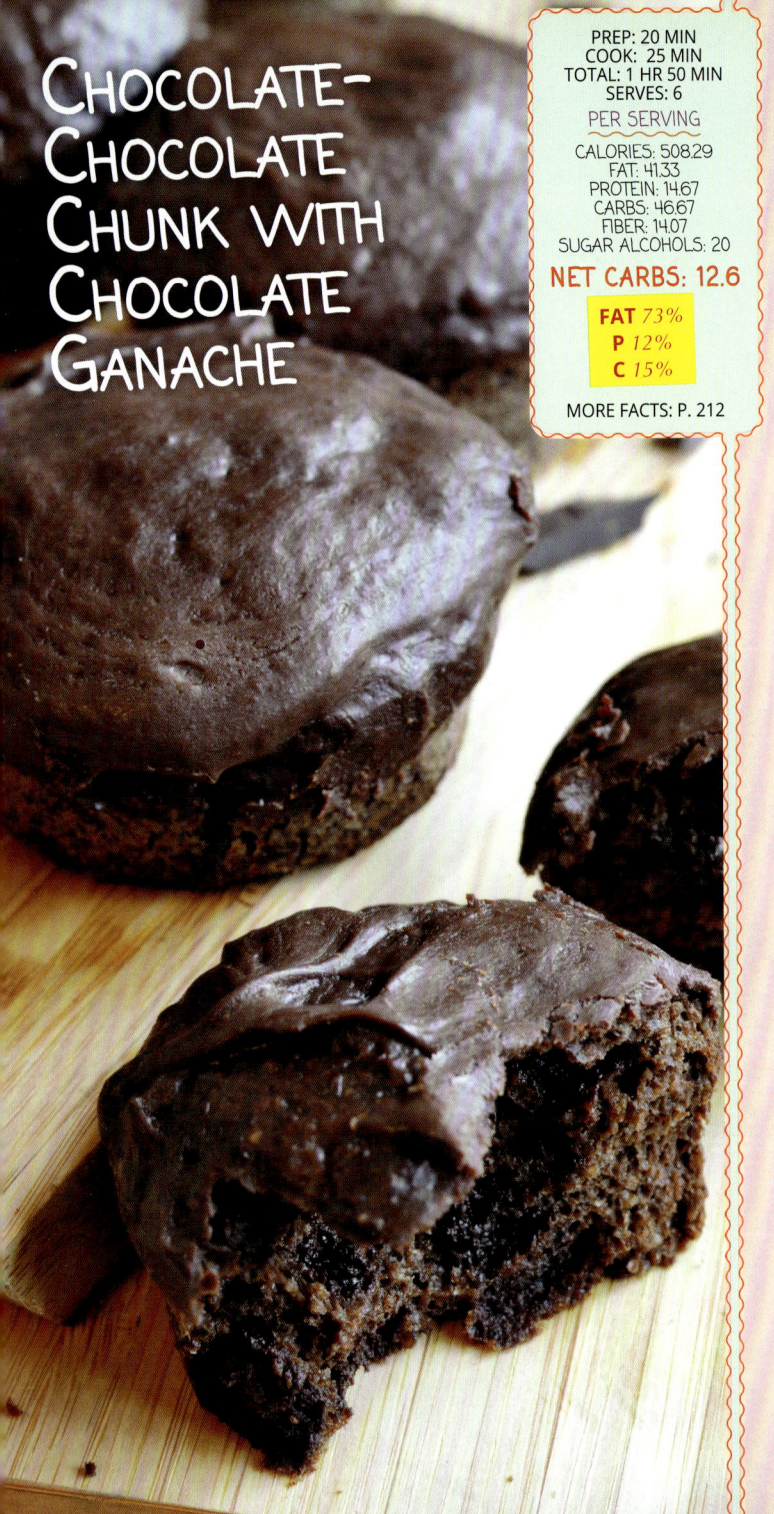

PREP: 20 MIN
COOK: 25 MIN
TOTAL: 1 HR 50 MIN
SERVES: 6

PER SERVING
CALORIES: 508.29
FAT: 41.33
PROTEIN: 14.67
CARBS: 46.67
FIBER: 14.07
SUGAR ALCOHOLS: 20

NET CARBS: 12.6

FAT 73%
P 12%
C 15%

MORE FACTS: P. 212

If you're a chocolate lover, you can stop reading the rest of this book. You have arrived! THIS is the recipe that will make your taste buds sing!

Now, this recipe is intensely chocolatey. I have a raspberry-cocoa sorbet in my first cookbook, which is equally intense. It's like being slapped in the tongue with a swift wave of cacao nibs. Granted, this holds a bit of sweet and a final vanilla note, but it's very bittersweet by design. To sweeten it up, double the sweetener in the muffin batter and the ganache.

Finally, the "chunk" can be a bit of a pickle to discuss. My personal favorite is to chop up *ChocoPerfection* bars, as I find they've got the best flavor, without using anything synthetic or sacrificing texture. The quick and obvious downside to these chocolate bars is the price. Many are dumbfounded when they see it, but like many things... you get what you pay for. They're very high quality and the taste is the *best* of the best!

To be fair, this recipe is based on a higher carb, still natural, easier to find and far more affordable, high-percentage chocolate. I try and stick to anything over 70% cacao when I eat a store-bought, sugar-sweetened chocolate bar. I've been known to dabble in 99%, but tend to hover around 80 to 85%. Lindt, Godiva and Ghirardelli are all fairly common and easy to find chocolate bars. There are MANY other options, but those are the biggies that come to mind.

Note: This recipe is written using a Lindt 3.5 oz (100 g) 85% Chocolate Bar. Two 50-gram ChocoPerfection bars, instead, would drop the net carb count of this recipe by over 3 net carbs per serving.

1 cup (240ᵐᴸ)	almond flour
1/4 cup + 2 tbsp (90ᵐᴸ)	coconut flour
1/4 cup + 2 tbsp (90ᵐᴸ)	sugar replacement
1/4 cup + 2 tbsp (90ᵐᴸ)	unsweetened cocoa powder
1/4 cup (60ᵐᴸ)	ground chia
1 tbsp (15ᵐᴸ)	baking powder
3/4 tsp (4ᵐᴸ)	salt
4 large	eggs
1/4 cup + 2 tbsp (90ᵐᴸ)	unsweetened almond milk
3 tbsp (45ᵐᴸ)	melted butter
1 3.5 oz (100ᵍ)	dark chocolate bar, chopped
1 recipe	warm chocolate ganache (p. 200)

- Preheat oven to 350° F (177° C).
- Grease a standard 12-cup muffin pan (or two standard sized 6-cup muffin pans [We're looking for 12 smallish muffins.]). Set aside.
- In a large bowl, combine the almond flour, coconut flour, sugar replacement, cocoa powder, ground chia, baking powder, and salt. With a whisk or a fork, combine the dry ingredients so they are evenly mixed and distributed in and amongst one another.
- Add eggs and almond milk to the dry ingredients. While whisking to combine, pour in warm melted butter. Allow to sit for about 2 minutes to allow time for the chia to gel.
- Making sure there are no chocolate chunks much bigger than a large chocolate chip, fold chopped chocolate bar into the blob.
- The batter should be like a thick pancake batter. These ingredients tend to be a bit inconsistent from brand to brand and grind to grind. You may need to add a little more liquid to thin it out (just not too much!).
- Once the batter is well mixed, pour even amounts between the 12 muffin cups.
- Bake for about 18 to 21 minutes, or until the muffins have risen and the surface is dry.
- Remove from the oven and let rest for 5 minutes before removing from the pan. Once removed, let them cool to room temperature (they're too soft to handle while still warm).
- Once the muffins are stable and at room temperature, make your ganache using the recipe on *page 200*. (Or, if you have leftover ganache, gently warm it).
- Dip the top of each muffin into the ganache. Set aside, with the ganache side up. Allow ganache to come to room temperature to dry and harden (or, just eat them all gloopy and warm!).
- Enjoy!

Crunchy Mocha-Zucchini Muffins

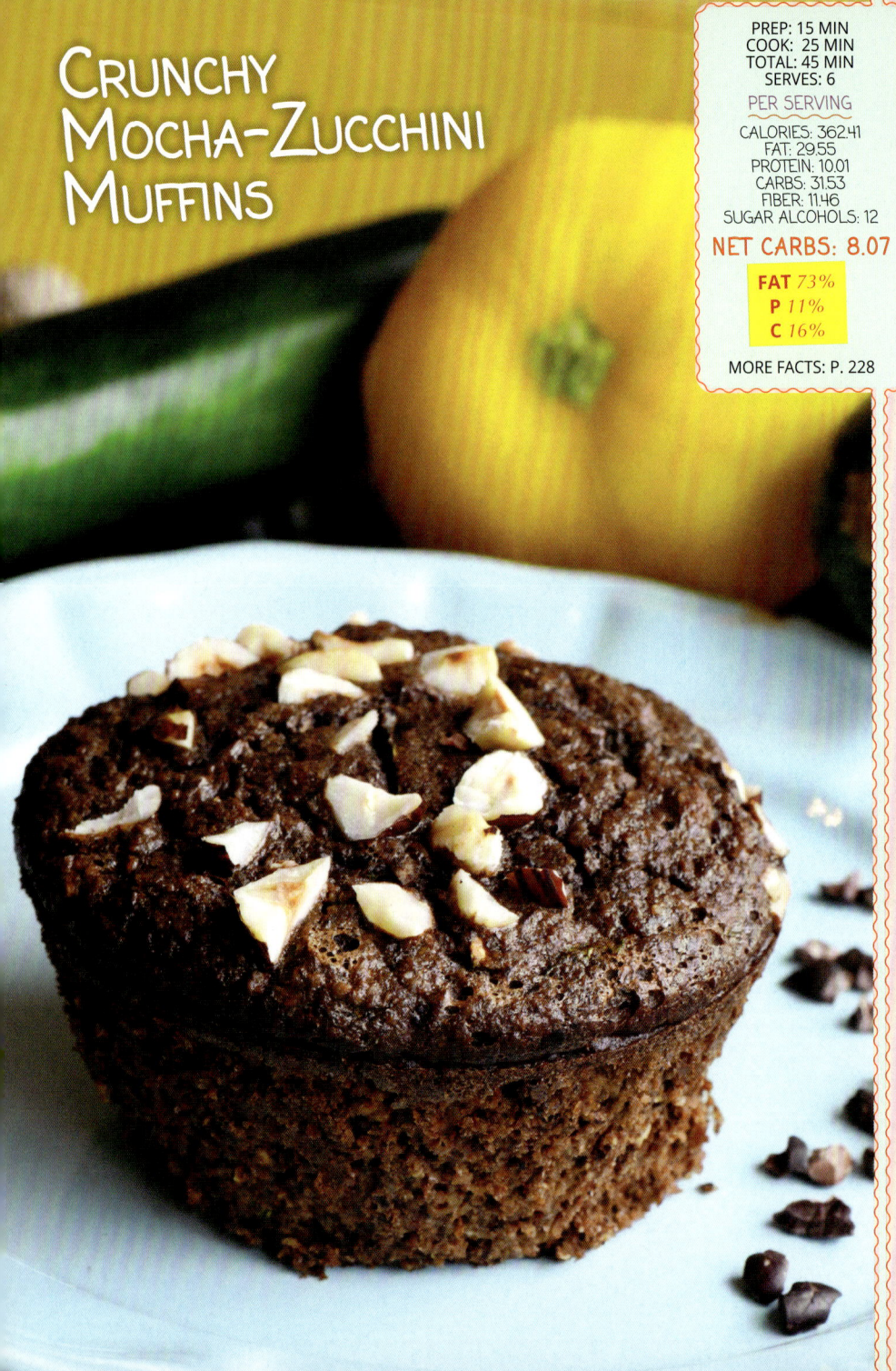

PREP: 15 MIN
COOK: 25 MIN
TOTAL: 45 MIN
SERVES: 6

PER SERVING
CALORIES: 362.41
FAT: 29.55
PROTEIN: 10.01
CARBS: 31.53
FIBER: 11.46
SUGAR ALCOHOLS: 12

NET CARBS: 8.07

FAT 73%
P 11%
C 16%

MORE FACTS: P. 228

I bake cookies. I've baked cookies for as long as I can remember. Even now, I have cookie batter balls frozen in my fridge. I like knowing that if I have visitors, I can pop some frozen doughballs in the oven and make totally fresh and homemade cookies, right then, *effortlessly*.

Much like the recipes in this book, my cookie dough recipe starts with a basic ratio (a slight twist of the Nestle-Toll House recipe). However, I'm known to toss different things into it, just to play or use up bits, pieces, this, that, odds and ends. Once, I whipped up a batch of "Kitchen Sink" Cookies containing cocoa powder, crushed nuts, chocolate chips, cacao nibs, and toasted crushed coffee beans. *That* idea came from my love of chocolate-coated coffee beans.

So, *here* I've decided to create a similarly tossed-together muffin... a Kitchen Sink/Zucchini hybrid, if you will. Will you?

I *thought* you would!

1 cup (240 mL)	hazelnut flour
1/4 cup + 2 tbsp (90 mL)	coconut flour
1/4 cup + 2 tbsp (90 mL)	sugar replacement
1/4 cup + 2 tbsp (90 mL)	unsweetened cocoa powder
1/4 cup (60 mL)	ground chia
1 tbsp (15 mL)	baking powder
3/4 tsp (4 mL)	salt
4 large	eggs
1 cup (240 mL)	grated zucchini
2 tbsp (30 mL)	unsweetened almond milk
3 tbsp (45 mL)	melted butter
3 tbsp (45 mL)	cacao nibs
3 tbsp (45 mL)	crushed toasted whole coffee beans
1/2 cup (120 mL)	coarsely chopped hazelnuts, divided

- Preheat oven to 350° F (177° C).
- Grease a standard 12-cup muffin pan (or two standard sized 6-cup muffin pans [We're looking for 12 smallish muffins.]). Set aside.
- In a large bowl, combine the hazelnut flour, coconut flour, sugar replacement, cocoa powder, ground chia, baking powder and salt. With a whisk or a fork, combine the dry ingredients so they are evenly mixed and distributed in and amongst one another.
- Add eggs, zucchini, and almond milk to the dry ingredients. While whisking to combine, pour in warm melted butter. Allow to sit for about 2 minutes to allow time for the chia to gel.
- Fold the cacao nibs, coffee beans and *half* of the chopped hazelnuts into the batter.
- The batter should be like a thick pancake batter. These ingredients tend to be a bit inconsistent from brand to brand and grind to grind. You may need to add a little more almond milk to thin it out (just not too much!).
- Once the batter is well mixed, pour even amounts between the 12 muffin cups.
- Evenly distribute the remaining hazelnuts over the top of the raw muffins.
- Bake for about 18 to 21 minutes, or until the muffins have risen and the surface is dry.
- Remove from the oven and let rest for 5 minutes before removing from the pan.
- Enjoy!

Mini Coconut Muffaroons

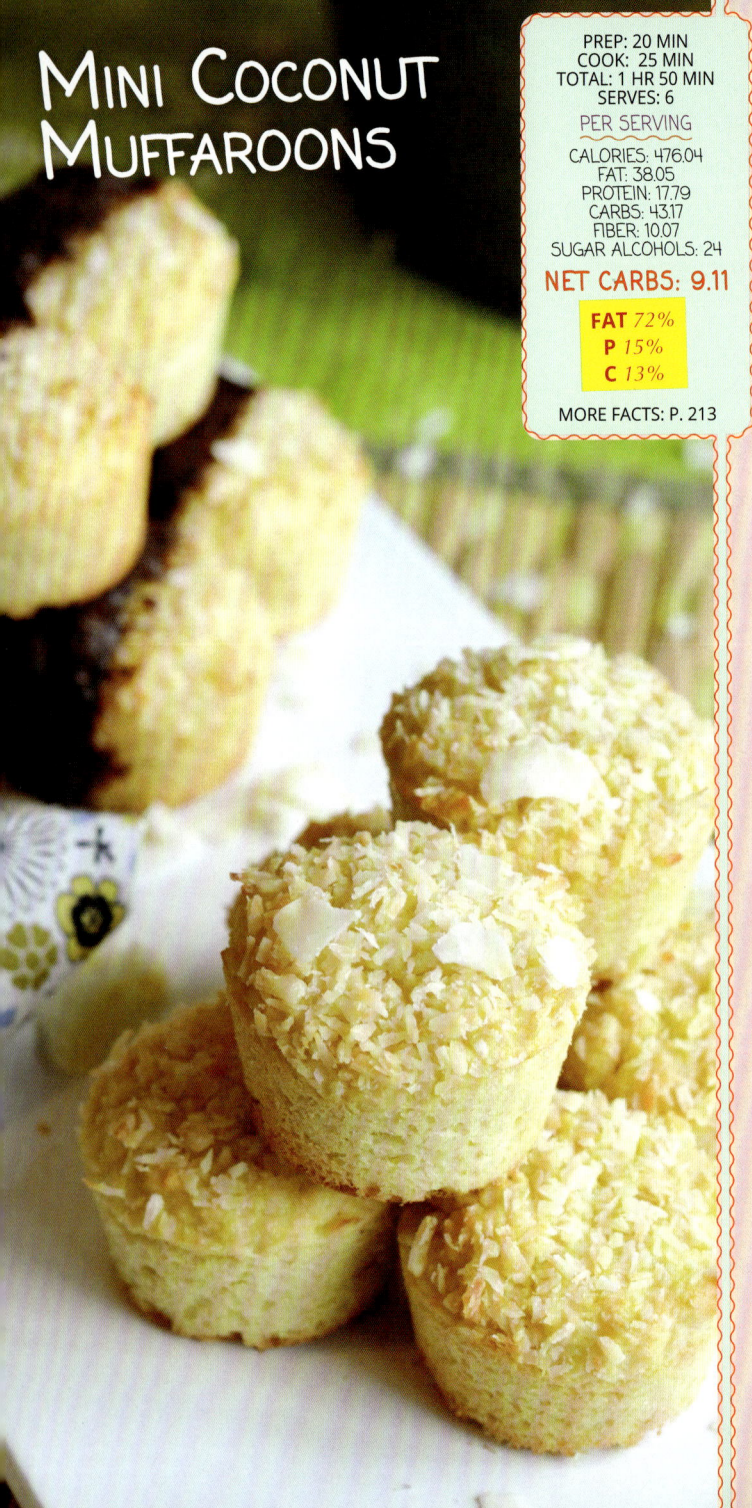

PREP: 20 MIN
COOK: 25 MIN
TOTAL: 1 HR 50 MIN
SERVES: 6

PER SERVING
CALORIES: 476.04
FAT: 38.05
PROTEIN: 17.79
CARBS: 43.17
FIBER: 10.07
SUGAR ALCOHOLS: 24

NET CARBS: 9.11

FAT 72%
P 15%
C 13%

MORE FACTS: P. 213

I'm a big fan of macaroons. They're *chewy*. Much like my distant memories of Mounds bars, I love sweetened coconut treats. I love to gnaw and chew the coco-cud for a good 10 minutes while sucking the sugary coconut nectar from the fiber in my cheek. Ok, I agree it doesn't read very well, but it's absolutely heaven in my mouth!

I've tried to make multiple low-primal macaroons, but have yet to come up with one that holds anywhere near the same allure. They're always dry, slightly bitter, barely holding it together and a skosh depressing. I thought that maybe if I made them into little muffaroons, instead, that perhaps I'd find something lovely and sweet to suck and gnaw on.

See, sugar has a very specific mouthfeel. It's its own magical form of viscous lubrication. The feeling is thick, smooth, and seems to cure everything! Sugar-free treats are also sweet, but the pleasant syrupy thickness is simply not there, often feeling a bit hollow or empty. This is quickly covered up by other ingredients in most goodies, but sugar-free *coconut* treats really need that true sugary lube job. The only other way to achieve a similar mouthfeel is to begin layering in all kinds of madness like vegetable glycerin, poly-dextrose, and gastrically distressing sugar-alcohols like maltitol and isomalt. No one really wants that.

I give up on true macaroons, for now. Some are better than others, but none I've tried are worth writing home about. Let's make it a series of little muffins, instead!

The end result? Sweet little coconut cakes. The fat and texture from the nuts, combined with the cakier elements brought in by the coconut flour, really help restore much of what is lost without the sugar. Not *quite* a macaroon, but with just enough sweet fatty chewing to make me happy. For those planning to go the extra mile, dipping them into some melted chocolate or ganache really brings them that much closer to a macaroon. Or fold in some chocolate chunks (see notes on *p. 126* about chocolate chunks).

Note: I included the protein powder because I love the flavor, but also believe its heartiness stands up well to the coconut. If you don't have any, you can substitute an equivalent amount of almond flour. The optional molasses or yacón is to give it some chewiness at the atomic level, while also lending some of the charisma lost from the more common use of sweetened condensed milk.

1/2 cup + 2 tbsp (150ᵐᴸ)	almond flour
1/2 cup (120ᵐᴸ)	sugar replacement
1/4 cup + 2 tbsp (90ᵐᴸ)	sugar-free vanilla whey protein isolate
1/4 cup + 2 tbsp (90ᵐᴸ)	coconut flour
1 tbsp (15ᵐᴸ)	baking powder
3/4 tsp (4ᵐᴸ)	salt
1 cup (240ᵐᴸ)	unsweetened shredded coconut
6 large	eggs
1/4 cup + 2 tbsp (90ᵐᴸ)	unsweetened almond milk
1 tsp (5ᵐᴸ)	blackstrap molasses or yacón syrup (optional)
3 tbsp (45ᵐᴸ)	melted butter
1 recipe	chocolate ganache (optional - p. 200)

- Preheat oven to 350° F (177° C).
- Grease two miniature 12-cup muffin pans (for a total of 24 mini muffins). Alternatively, feel free to use two standard sized 6-cup muffin pans in order to arrive at the more common 12 regular-ish sized muffins. Set prepared pans aside.
- In a large bowl, combine the almond flour, sweetener, protein powder, coconut flour, baking powder, and salt. With a whisk or a fork, combine the dry ingredients so they are evenly mixed and distributed in and amongst one another.
- Mix the shredded coconut into the dried ingredients.
- In a separate smaller bowl, whisk together eggs with the almond milk and molasses or yacón syrup.
- Pour egg mixture into the large bowl of dry ingredients. Whisk together, while pouring in the melted butter.
- The batter should be thicker than most recipes in this book. A *little* too thick to make pancakes with, but not by much. You *may* need to add a little more liquid to thin it out, but I doubt it (unless the coconut is SUPER hungry, which can happen).
- Once the batter is well mixed, evenly distribute the batter between the 24 mini muffin cups.
- Bake for about 13 to 18 minutes, or until the muffins have crowned and the surface is dry, beginning to crisp, and has turned golden.
- Remove from the oven and let rest for 5 minutes before removing from the pan. Enjoy warm, or dip into a warm batch of chocolate ganache!

Sour Cream Coffee Cake with Hazelnut Streusel

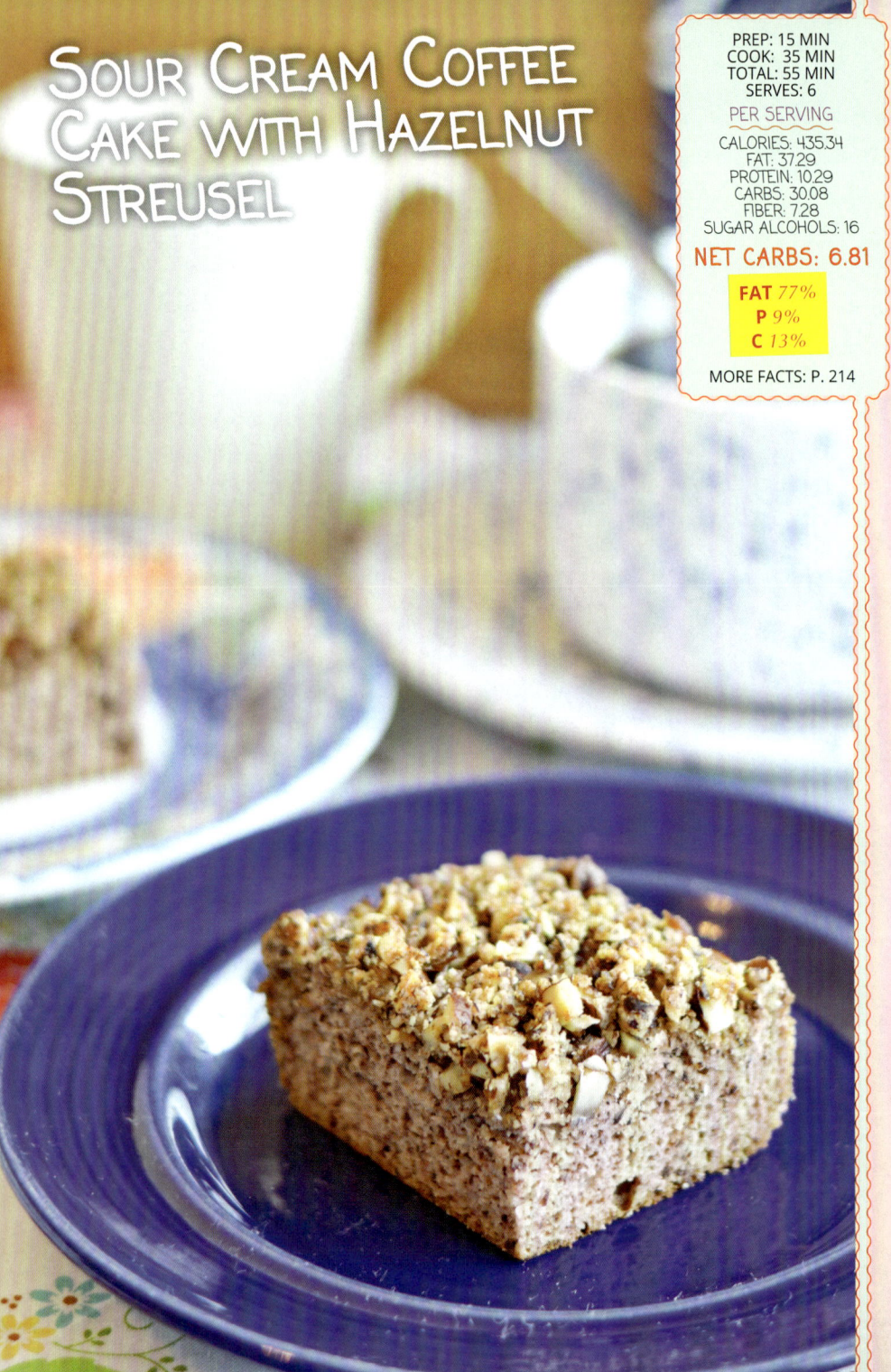

PREP: 15 MIN
COOK: 35 MIN
TOTAL: 55 MIN
SERVES: 6

PER SERVING
CALORIES: 435.34
FAT: 37.29
PROTEIN: 10.29
CARBS: 30.08
FIBER: 7.28
SUGAR ALCOHOLS: 16

NET CARBS: 6.81

FAT 77%
P 9%
C 13%

MORE FACTS: P. 214

This recipe also reminds me of my times as a professional baker. One of my more popular items was this massive overflowing sour cream coffee cake, erupting with boulders of the most divine crispy and craggly streusel ever baked.

Unfortunately, because we're limited to ingredients that don't quite erupt or craggle in the same ways, we're going to tone all that down to make a more simplistic version. I do truly love this one, though. It's quick and easy to throw together, it keeps and freezes very well, and is just lovely for breakfast with a sugar-free cinnamon Bulletproof® Coffee!

COFFEE CAKE

1 cup + 2 tbsp (270mL)	hazelnut flour
1/4 cup + 2 tbsp (90mL)	coconut flour
1/4 cup + 2 tbsp (90mL)	sugar replacement
3/4 tsp (4mL)	baking soda
3/4 tsp (4mL)	salt
6 large	eggs
1 tsp (5mL)	vanilla extract
3/4 cup (180mL)	sour cream

HAZELNUT STREUSEL

1/2 cup (120mL)	hazelnut flour
1/2 cup (120mL)	chopped hazelnuts
2 tbsp (30mL)	sugar replacement
1 tbsp (15mL)	melted butter
1 tsp (5mL)	blackstrap molasses, honey or yacón syrup
1/2 tsp (3mL)	ground cinnamon
Dash	salt

- Preheat oven to 350° F (177° C).

- Grease a 9" x 9" (23cm x 23cm) square baking pan.

- In a large bowl, combine the hazelnut flour, coconut flour, sugar replacement, baking soda, and salt. With a whisk or a fork, combine the dry ingredients so they are evenly mixed and distributed in and amongst one another.

- In a separate bowl, whisk together the eggs and vanilla until eggs are lemony in color. Whisk in sour cream.

- Whisk egg mixture into dry ingredients in the larger bowl. The batter should be like a thick pancake batter. These ingredients tend to be a bit inconsistent from brand to brand and grind to grind. You may need to add a little water (or almond milk, if you have any lying around) to thin it out.

- Once the batter is well mixed, pour into the prepared pan and spread evenly.

- In a separate bowl, combine the hazelnut flour, chopped hazelnuts, sugar replacement, melted butter, molasses (or honey or yacón), cinnamon, and salt. Mix until the mixture is evenly coated with butter and molasses.

- **Note:** In this case we need the molasses, honey or yacón because they function like glue, holding the streusel together in clumps. You CAN omit this, but the result will be a bit flatter in appearance (potentially more refined, if that's your goal).

- Squeeze small handfuls of the streusel inside your fist, compressing little boulders of it. *Gently* break these up and scatter evenly over the top of the batter. Continue forming fist-boulders, then breaking them into craggly crogs all over the top of the batter, until there is no more streusel in the bowl.

- Bake for about 30 to 35 minutes, or until the surface is dry and the streusel is clearly beginning to crisp and turn golden.

- Remove from the oven and let rest for 5 minutes before removing from the pan. Enjoy warm with a hot "Why Bother."

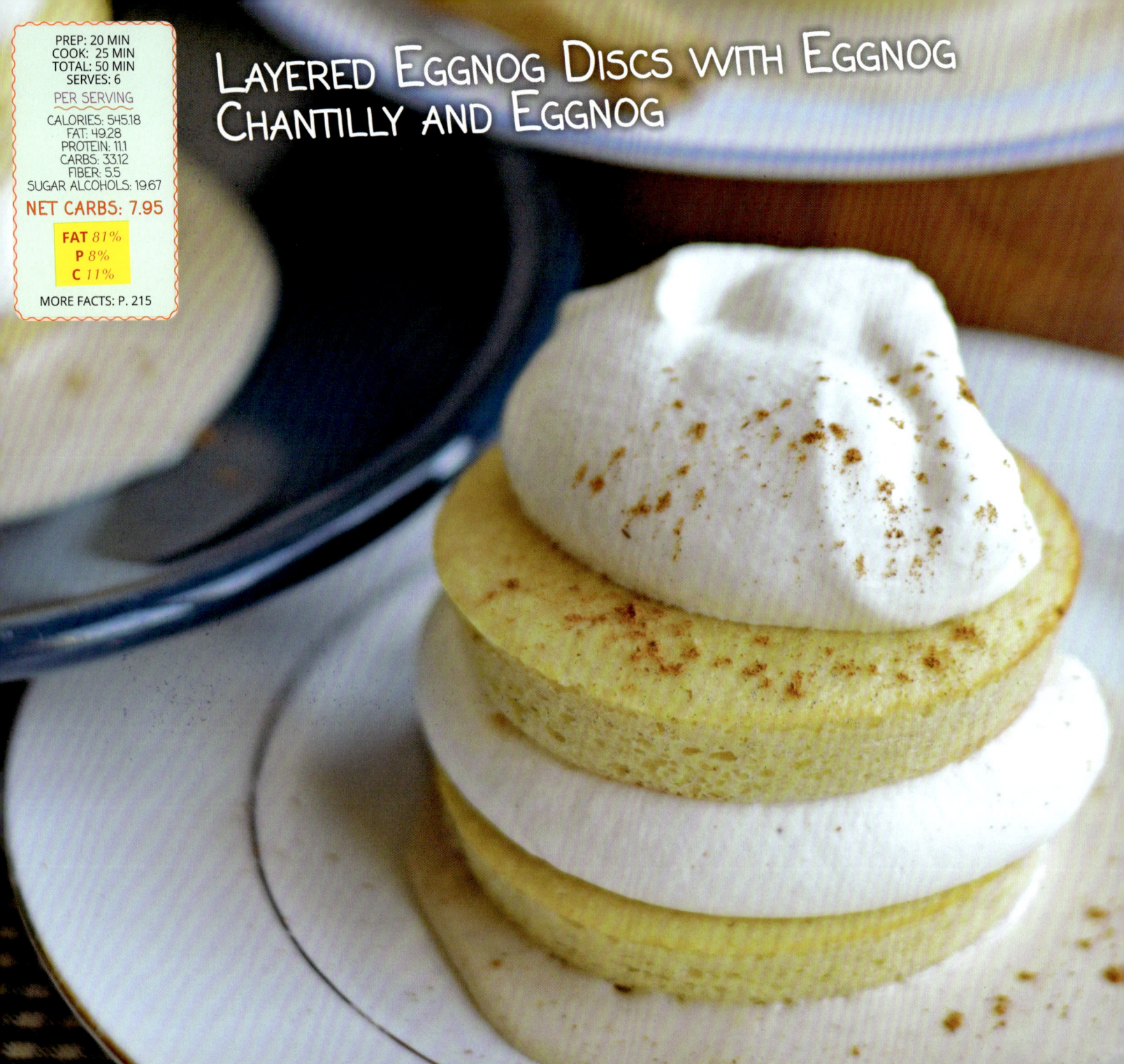

Layered Eggnog Discs with Eggnog Chantilly and Eggnog

PREP: 20 MIN
COOK: 25 MIN
TOTAL: 50 MIN
SERVES: 6

PER SERVING
CALORIES: 545.18
FAT: 49.28
PROTEIN: 11.1
CARBS: 33.12
FIBER: 5.5
SUGAR ALCOHOLS: 19.67
NET CARBS: 7.95

FAT *81%*
P *8%*
C *11%*

MORE FACTS: P. 215

I sometimes buy random stuff I want to play with. I like toys. One impulse purchase was for two strange silicone baking pans. The mold for each cup is about 3 inches (7.5cm) in diameter and maybe 1/2-inch (1.3cm) deep. Each pan has 6 cups. The pans are red and super wobbly.

I've had them for years and wanted to use them for something. Being that this is a book about pouring random blobs into variously shaped molds, it seemed only logical to use them for my upcoming blob-based fakery book. But, what to do?

In Mexico, there's a rich, sweet, and ubiquitous dessert known as Pastel de Tres Leches. It's a cake soaked in three kinds of milk: evaporated, condensed, and heavy cream. Mexico hasn't cornered the market on these, mind you. Trifles, rum cakes, and even tiramisu are all wet, cakey desserts that are soaked in some kind of liquidy goodness, but it was the Tres Leches that got my noggin eggnoggin'.

Maybe I could combine the idea of cake soaking with eggnog? Stranger things have happened. Let's do it!

To be clear, this book is intentionally flimsy in its descriptions. I envision it a bit like a "choose your own adventure" type of book, such as those I read as a child. The idea being, I'm presenting guidelines and suggestions to build confidence in the kitchen.

My hope is that you, dear reader, create something special, wonderful, and uniquely your own, while also keeping you (mostly) out of trouble. I aim more to instruct and teach actual cooking and baking rather than write a clear, bland list of ingredients and steps—resulting in a single, perfectly formed *hootenanny*.

The hope is that you can read this book, then start envisioning pouring this batter into wide-mouthed ramekins, ceramic soup bowls, or in the rings of a muffin-top pan. Perhaps it'll work in a casserole pan, then chilled, cut, and soaked? What about making pancakes, then stacking them? What about *blueberry* pancakes? What about blueberry pancakes, strawberry Chantilly (fold jelly into whipped cream) and a strained blackberry crème anglaise (basically eggnog without the spices [whisk pureed and strained blackberries into the crème anglaise])?

I don't actually want y'all to go out and purchase a special red wobbly pan just for this. All too often I see the comments that people can't find the right ingredients or don't have the right equipment. My hope is that I'm laying the groundwork for you to take these ideas, a small subset of ingredients and equipment, and go hog-wild with them.

Time and experience permitting, start really stretching what you can do!

1 cup + 2 tbsp (270mL)	almond flour
1/2 cup (120mL)	sugar replacement, divided
1/4 cup + 2 tbsp (90mL)	coconut flour
1 tbsp (15mL)	baking powder
3/4 tsp (4mL)	salt
1/2 tsp (3mL)	ground cinnamon
1/4 tsp (1mL)	ground nutmeg
6 large	eggs
1 1/4 cup (300mL)	heavy whipping cream, divided
1 tsp (5mL)	vanilla extract
2 cups (480mL)	eggnog (p. 202), divided

≥ Preheat oven to 350° F (177° C).

≥ Assuming you're making muffins, grease a standard 12-cup muffin pan (or two standard sized 6-cup muffin pans). We're looking for 12 smallish muffins. I used two 6-cup thin *disc*-shaped silicone pans. Set aside.

≥ In a large bowl, combine the almond flour, 1/4 cup + 2 tbsp (90mL) sugar replacement, coconut flour, baking powder, cinnamon, nutmeg, and salt. With a whisk or a fork, combine the dry ingredients so they are evenly mixed and distributed in and amongst one another.

≥ In a separate smaller bowl, whisk together eggs and 1/2 cup (120mL) of the cream, until consistent and lemony in color. (**Note:** from a ratio perspective, the cream is serving as both the fat AND liquid in this recipe.)

≥ Pour the egg mixture into the dry and whisk together.

≥ The batter should be like pancake batter, thinner than most in this book, but still thick enough to make a nice pancake. These ingredients tend to be a bit inconsistent from brand to brand and grind to grind. You may need to add a little more cream to thin it out (just not too much!).

≥ **Note:** It is at this point that you can pour your blob into virtually any manner of mold. Just remember that there is no gluten in this blob, so it can very much collapse under its own weight. Try not to make anything over about 2 inches (5cm) in height. If you do opt to go for something a little taller and grander, don't forget you can add things like xanthan gum, chia flour, and tapioca flour. A bit of each will give you a slightly lighter, cakier, and slightly more structurally sound fakestuff.

≥ Disregarding the previous paragraph, once the batter is well mixed, pour even amounts between the 12 muffin cups.

≥ Bake for about 18 to 21 minutes, or until the muffins have crowned and the surface is dry, beginning to crisp, and has turned golden.

- Remove from the oven and let rest for 5 minutes before removing from the pan. Let cool completely.
- A Chantilly is a fancy word for sweetened and flavored whipped cream. To make the Eggnog Chantilly, begin by lacing the remaining 3/4 cup (180^{mL}) cream, 2 tbsp (30^{mL}) of sugar replacement, and vanilla into a bowl or electric mixer. Whip the cream until stiff peaks form.
- Gently fold 1/2 cup (120^{mL}) of the eggnog into the sweetened whipped cream.
- Place the remaining 1 1/2 cups (360^{mL}) eggnog into a bowl.
- Set out upwards of 12 plates (probably 6, though).
- (My discs were wide and thin. I soaked 6, then put a heavy dollop of eggnog Chantilly on each one, then placed a second soaked disc on the dollop, followed by another dollop… you could split your muffins in half to accomplish a similar result).
- Submerge each muffin in the eggnog to fully coat. Allow to sit in the liquid for a few seconds to absorb some of the liquid (too long and the cake becomes difficult to hold, as it falls apart).
- Place each muffin on a plate.
- Garnish with the eggnog Chantilly and spoon the remaining eggnog around the base of the cakes. Feel free to sprinkle a small amount of cinnamon on there as well. Call some friends!

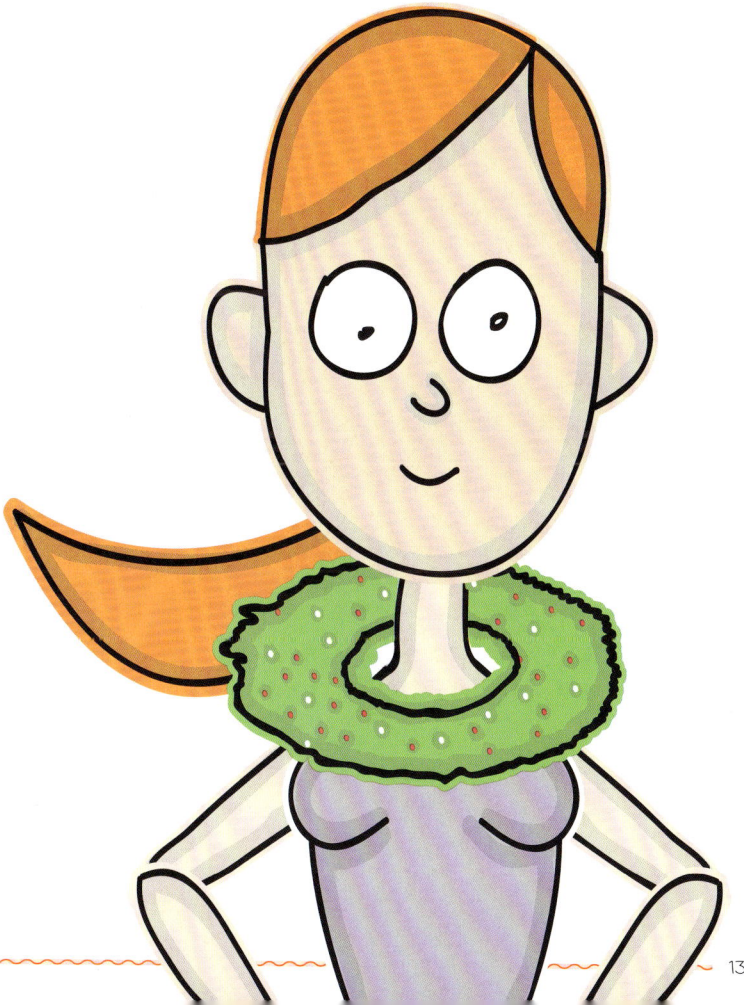

Mini Gingerbread Loaves

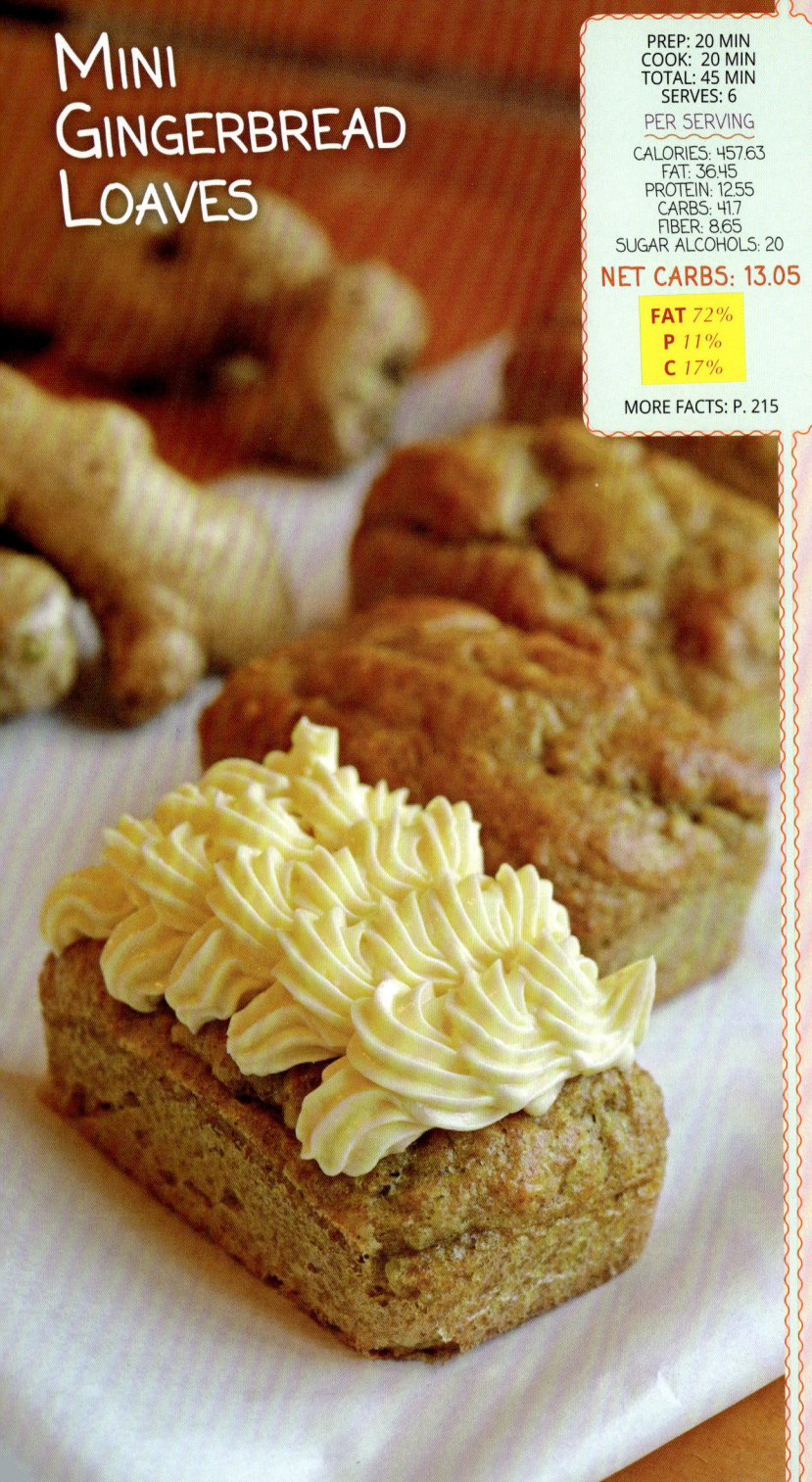

PREP: 20 MIN
COOK: 20 MIN
TOTAL: 45 MIN
SERVES: 6

PER SERVING

CALORIES: 457.63
FAT: 36.45
PROTEIN: 12.55
CARBS: 41.7
FIBER: 8.65
SUGAR ALCOHOLS: 20

NET CARBS: 13.05

FAT 72%
P 11%
C 17%

MORE FACTS: P. 215

As we get deeper into the book, we'll start seeing more shapes and sizes. In this case, I had purchased 2 wobbly red silicone baking pans, each containing 12 little rectangles, maybe 1- by 2-inches (2.5^{cm} x 5^{cm}), and maybe an inch (2.5^{cm}) deep. They'd be a bit like cornpone pans, if corn cobs were rectangular and had only 4 large substantial kernels.

I thought tossing some gingerbread blobs in there would be just the ticket. I LOVED the idea of little mini gingerbreads!

This recipe uses a lot of molasses. If I had my druthers, I'd add even more, but this is already really pushing it. See, what I'm aiming for is a dankly strong loaf. A lot of this deep-tasting backbone comes from the molasses. Molasses, unfortunately, is basically just sugar (which can be fine in small, reasonable amounts). However, in *this* case, it's REALLY pushing the limits. I COULD make the argument that this recipe is little more than an advertisement for yacón syrup, which has a very similar flavor, texture, and behavior as molasses, but is purported to have a glycemic index of zero. You could pour a good 1/4 cup (60^{mL}) of yacón syrup into this blob (cutting back a teensy bit on the cream and sweetener). This would boost the flavor, complexity and hot-diggity-dankness of it, without raising the net carb count. Yacón syrup would drop each serving of this recipe by a full 5 net carbs.

I used molasses in this recipe because it's easier to find, more affordable, and there's a chance it's already sitting in your kitchen. However, I might extend the suggestion that yacón syrup is tasty stuff you may actually use. It has a great shelf life and is wonderful in baked goods, sauces, BBQ sauce, etc. Mix some with coconut aminos and marinate a steak. You'll love it! I don't use my yacón daily, but I am often glad I have a bottle lying around.

Note: If I weren't playing with my toys, I'd probably just simplify and pour this blob into a greased 9-inch (23^{cm} x 23^{cm}) square pan, then just cut squares out of it, like coffee cake.

 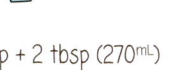

1 cup + 2 tbsp (270^{mL})	almond flour
1/4 cup + 2 tbsp (90^{mL})	coconut flour
1/4 cup + 2 tbsp (90^{mL})	sugar replacement
1 tsp (5^{mL})	ground cinnamon
3/4 tsp (4 ^{mL})	baking soda
3/4 tsp (4^{mL})	salt
1/2 tsp (3^{mL})	ground nutmeg
1/8 tsp (5^{mL})	ground cloves
6 large	eggs
1/2 cup (120^{mL})	heavy whipping cream
2 tbsp (30^{mL})	blackstrap molasses or yacón syrup
2 tbsp (30^{mL})	apple cider vinegar
1 tbsp (15^{mL})	fresh grated ginger
1 recipe	cream cheese frosting (optional - p. 196)

> Preheat oven to 350° F (177° C).

> Grease two miniature 12-cup muffin pans (for a total of 24 mini muffins). Alternatively, feel free to use two *standard* sized 6-cup muffin pans, in order to arrive at the more common 12 regular-ish sized muffins. Set prepared pans aside.

> In a large bowl, combine the almond flour, coconut flour, sugar replacement, cinnamon, baking soda, salt, nutmeg, and cloves. With a whisk or a fork, combine the dry ingredients so they are evenly mixed and distributed in and amongst one another.

> In a separate smaller bowl, whisk together eggs, cream, molasses or yacón, vinegar, and grated ginger.

> Add the gingered eggs to the larger bowl with the dry ingredients. Whisk and combine.

> The batter should be like a thick pancake batter. These ingredients tend to be a bit inconsistent from brand to brand and grind to grind. You may need to add a little more cream to thin it out (just not too much!).

> Bake for about 13 to 18 minutes, or until the muffins have crowned and the surface is dry, beginning to crisp, and has turned golden.

> Remove from the oven and let rest for 5 minutes before removing from the pan. Enjoy warm, slathered with fresh salted butter, topped with a heaping mound of frosting *(p. 196)*, a giant dollop of whipped cream— or just drizzle pancake syrup all over 'em.

Fried Blob

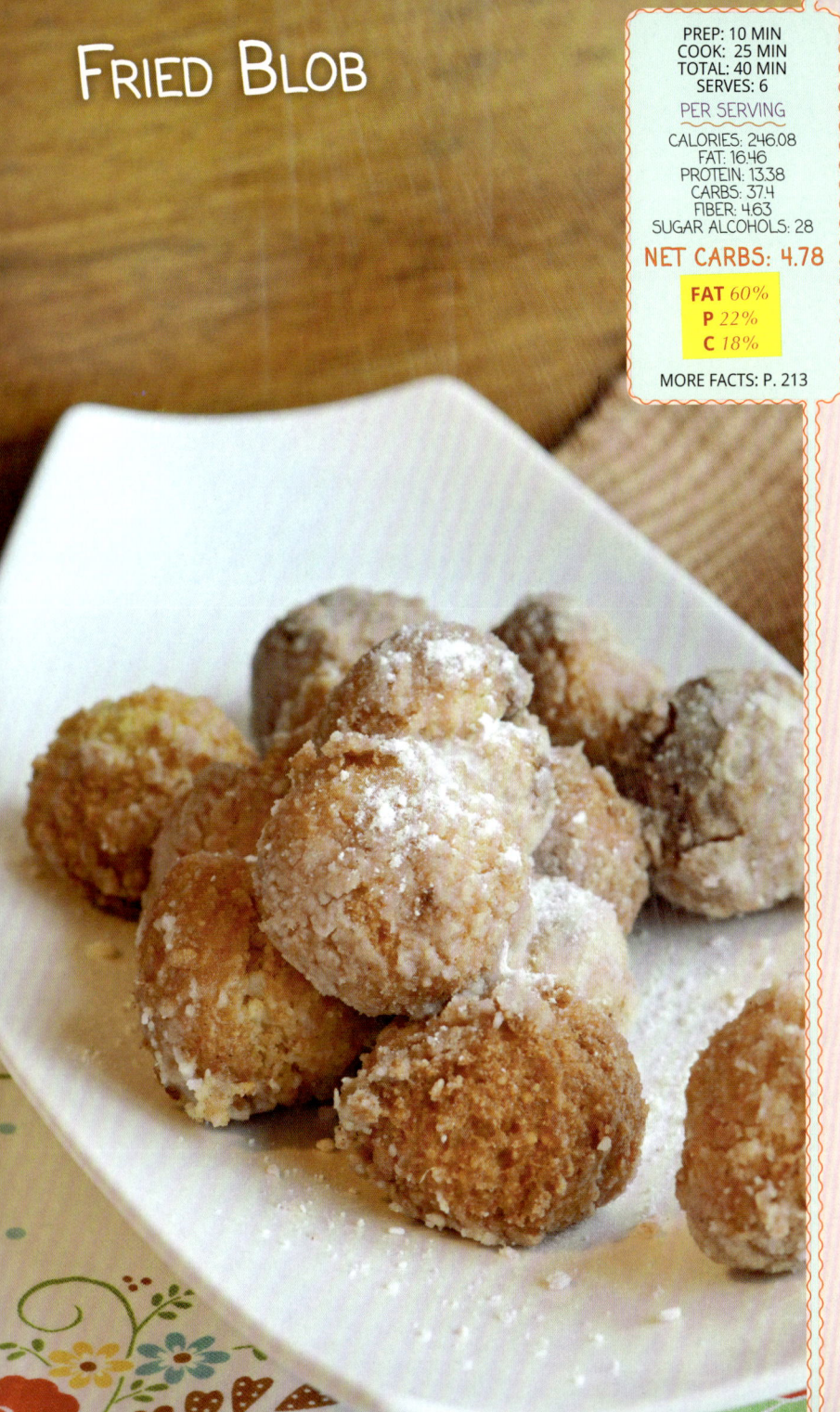

PREP: 10 MIN
COOK: 25 MIN
TOTAL: 40 MIN
SERVES: 6

PER SERVING

CALORIES: 246.08
FAT: 16.46
PROTEIN: 13.38
CARBS: 37.4
FIBER: 4.63
SUGAR ALCOHOLS: 28

NET CARBS: 4.78

FAT 60%
P 22%
C 18%

MORE FACTS: P. 213

So, now we're REALLY going to mix it up. Rather than baking formed blobs into the shape of our will, we're going to FRY, instead!

As a kid, I remember my mother doing most of the cooking. However, I do remember that my father would occasionally fry stuff. Taco night? He was on the fried taco shell duty. Another one, which was a rarity, but one that stuck with me: tasty dough, fried piping hot, then tossed in a paper sack filled with powdered sugar and cinnamon and tossed to coat.

Now to be clear... he didn't *make* the dough. No, it was biscuit dough, already prepared in the refrigerated cardboard tubes next to the cinnamon rolls. He'd heat oil, open the tube, poke holes in the dough pucks, drop them in the hot oil, fry 'em, powder 'em and we'd gobble 'em down!

The only part of this story that's really relevant is the frying and the powdering. Ignore the part about the can of dough, because it was *awful*... terrible (and if you believe that, I've got some magic beans I'll sell you!).

The reality is, these batters fry up quite well! They're not quite as "self-contained" as normal, in that they bleed oil faster than the standard doughnut hole might, and the outer texture isn't quite as springy. But they're no less delicious. Try it!

4 cups (960mL)	refined coconut oil or ghee
3/4 cup (180mL)	almond flour
1/4 cup + 2 tbsp (90mL)	sugar-free vanilla whey protein isolate
1/4 cup + 2 tbsp (90mL)	coconut flour
1/4 cup + 2 tbsp (90mL)	sugar replacement
1 tbsp (15mL)	baking powder
3/4 tsp (4mL)	salt
6 large	eggs
1/4 cup (60mL)	heavy whipping cream
1/2 cup (120mL)	powdered sugar replacement
1/2 tsp (3mL)	ground cinnamon
1/4 tsp (1mL)	ground nutmeg

- In a fryer or large wide-mouthed pot, slowly bring your oil up to 350° F (177° C).

- While the oil is heating, in a large bowl, combine the almond flour, protein powder, coconut flour, sugar replacement, baking powder, and salt. With a whisk or a fork, combine the dry ingredients so they are evenly mixed and distributed in and amongst one another.

- In a separate smaller bowl, whisk together eggs and cream until consistent and lemony in color.

- Pour the egg mixture into the dry and whisk together.

- The batter should be thick enough to form balls with a scooper or spoon (a similar consistency as the Muffaroons, *p. 130*). It's almost a dough.

- Before frying the batter, add powdered sugar replacement, cinnamon, and nutmeg to the bottom of a paper sack. Also, set up a plate with 3 or 4 layers of paper towels and have a slotted metal spoon close by.

- I like to use a very small ice cream scoop for this, but you could use a small metal spoon, as well. Scoop small balls or football shapes from the batter and gently place them into the oil. It helps to quickly dunk the spoon or scoop into the hot oil first, to get a thin coat of oil on it. When dropping the dough into the hot oil, make sure your spoon is close to the surface of the oil, or else you may get a big splash. I also wouldn't recommend frying more than about 10 blob balls at a time, or else the oil cools too much, as well as having inconsistent cooking times between them. Try and quickly get 10 balls into the hot oil, then let them sit and fry, making sure the oil stays at a steady 350° F (177° C). Use tongs or the slotted spoon to turn them occasionally, making sure they fry evenly on all sides.

- When the balls are golden, quickly remove them from the oil and place them on the prepared paper towels. Only drop them there long enough to get most of the glaring surface oil off of them.

- After a few seconds, transport them into the paper sack and shake them around, so they are evenly coated with spiced powdered sugar. Wake one of the kids (not the bad one) and share!

- Continue frying, blotting, tossing, and enjoying in rough batches of 8 to 10, until all the batter is gone.

- Try slathered with jam!

Mexican Chocolate Muffins

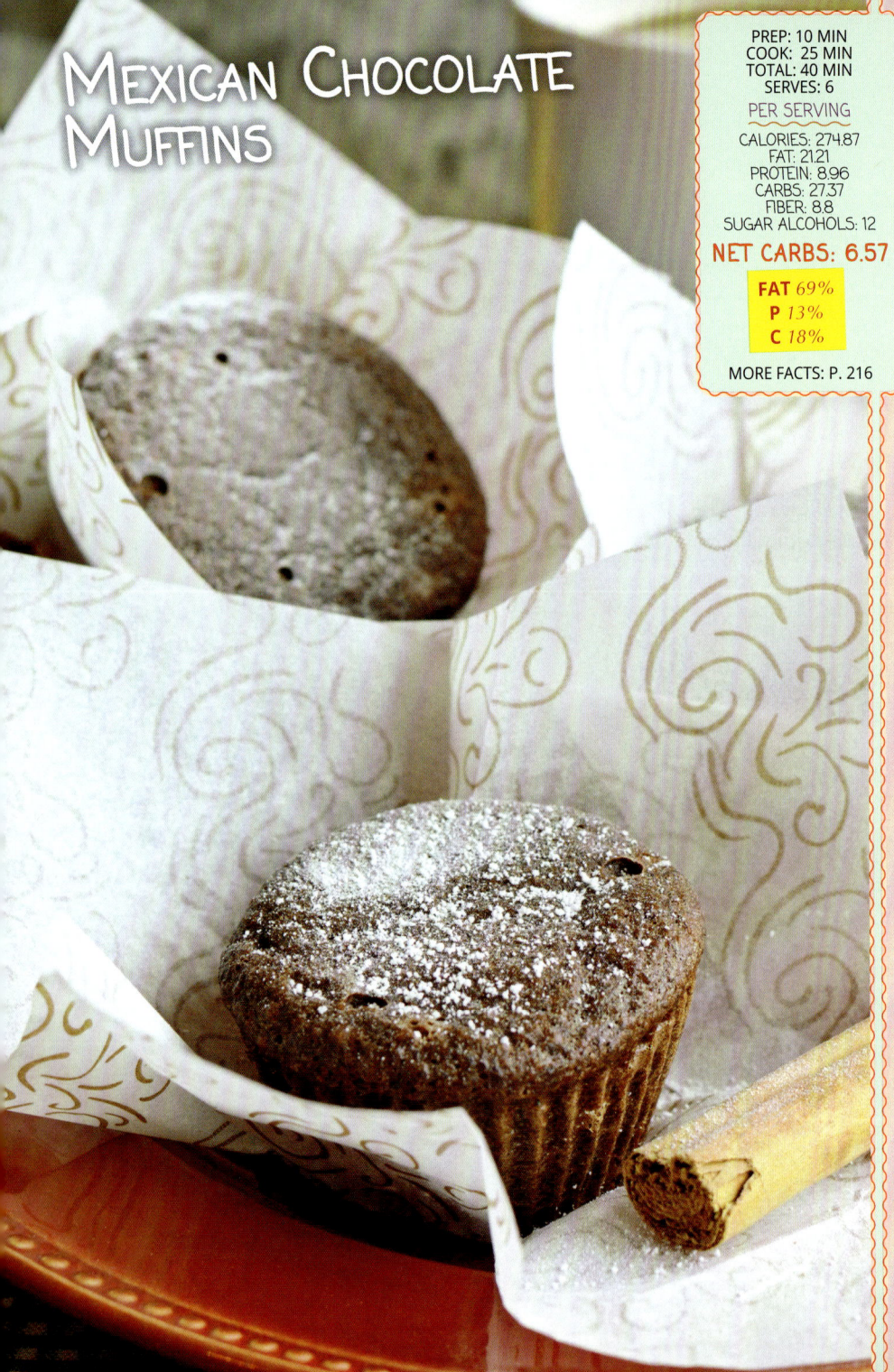

PREP: 10 MIN
COOK: 25 MIN
TOTAL: 40 MIN
SERVES: 6

PER SERVING
CALORIES: 274.87
FAT: 21.21
PROTEIN: 8.96
CARBS: 27.37
FIBER: 8.8
SUGAR ALCOHOLS: 12

NET CARBS: 6.57

FAT 69%
P 13%
C 18%

MORE FACTS: P. 216

Chocolate is a MASSIVE subject and could easily fill the contents of multiple books. In fact, I own two books focused solely on chocolate: one on the history of chocolate and another on chocolate confections—and neither put a dent in the scope of the topic.

It would be impossible to get into any depth on the subject in this relatively small book, but I'd be remiss to have a Mexican Chocolate Muffin recipe without first acknowledging that chocolate originated in Mexico (and Central America). The Pre-Olmec people were making beverages with it around 4,000 years ago. About 3,400 years ago, the Aztecs were making frothy fermented drinks. Both intense and bitter, they were mixed with spices, chilies, wine, and/or corn, and were considered to have aphrodisiacal powers and give the drinker strength (I still believe this). Even the word *chocolate* comes from the Nahuatl word *xocolātl*.

Interestingly, though, it was the Europeans who added sugar to chocolate just a few hundred years ago.

Most Mexican chocolate today is sold as a sweet, gritty chocolate puck with cinnamon flavoring. However, its use is often enhanced to more reflect its colorful history, with the addition of various nuts, chilies, and spices. It's in this spirit that I'm tying these flavors together!

1 cup (240ᵐᴸ)	almond flour
1/4 cup + 2 tbsp (90ᵐᴸ)	coconut flour
1/4 cup + 2 tbsp (90ᵐᴸ)	sugar replacement
1/4 cup + 2 tbsp (90ᵐᴸ)	unsweetened cocoa powder
1/4 cup (60ᵐᴸ)	ground chia
1 tbsp (15ᵐᴸ)	baking powder
1 tsp (5ᵐᴸ)	ground cinnamon
3/4 tsp (4ᵐᴸ)	salt
1/2 tsp (3ᵐᴸ)	grated nutmeg
1/2 tsp (3ᵐᴸ)	ground allspice
1/2 tsp (3ᵐᴸ)	powdered cayenne or ancho chili pepper
4 large	eggs
1/4 cup + 2 tbsp (90ᵐᴸ)	unsweetened almond milk
1 tsp (5ᵐᴸ)	vanilla extract
3 tbsp (45ᵐᴸ)	melted butter

- Preheat oven to 350° F (177° C).
- Grease a standard 12-cup muffin pan (or two standard sized 6-cup muffin pans [We're looking for 12 smallish muffins.]). Set aside.
- In a large bowl, combine the almond flour, coconut flour, sugar replacement, cocoa powder, ground chia, baking powder, cinnamon, salt, nutmeg, allspice, and chili powder. With a whisk or a fork, combine the dry ingredients so they are evenly mixed and distributed in and amongst one another.
- Add eggs, almond milk, and vanilla to the dry ingredients. While whisking to combine, pour in the warm melted butter. Allow to sit for about 2 minutes to allow time for the chia to gel.
- The batter should be like a thick pancake batter. These ingredients tend to be a bit inconsistent from brand to brand and grind to grind. You may need to add a little more liquid to thin it out (just not too much!).
- Once the batter is well mixed, pour even amounts between the 12 muffin cups.
- Bake for about 18 to 21 minutes, or until the muffins have risen and the surface is dry.
- Remove from the oven and let rest for 5 minutes before removing from the pan. Once removed, let them cool to room temperature (they're too soft to handle while still warm).
- Enjoy!

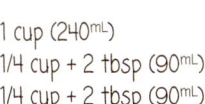

Mocha Mint Muffins

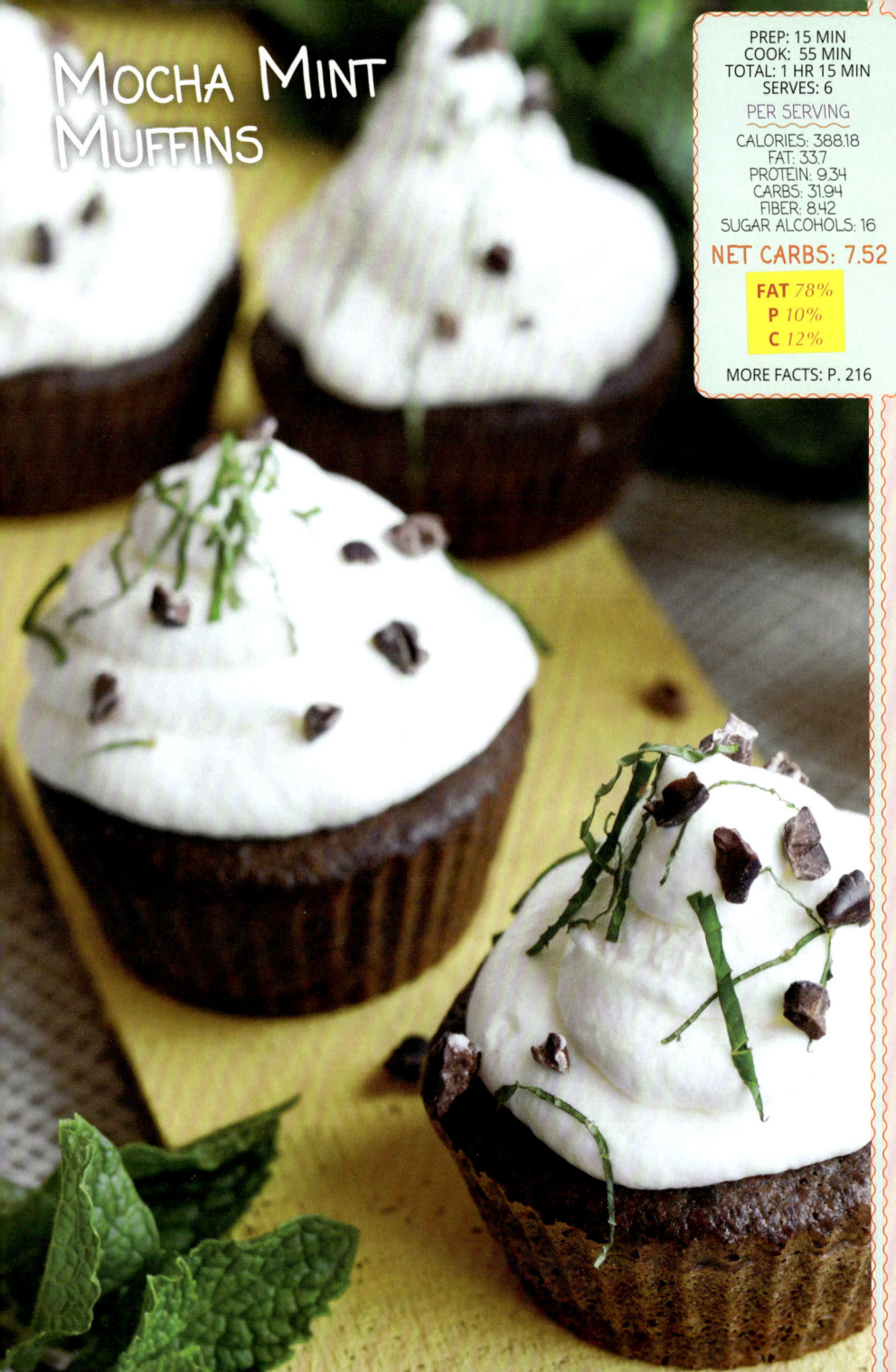

PREP: 15 MIN
COOK: 55 MIN
TOTAL: 1 HR 15 MIN
SERVES: 6

PER SERVING
CALORIES: 388.18
FAT: 33.7
PROTEIN: 9.34
CARBS: 31.94
FIBER: 8.42
SUGAR ALCOHOLS: 16

NET CARBS: 7.52

FAT 78%
P 10%
C 12%

MORE FACTS: P. 216

One of my absolute favorite flavor combinations is that of chocolate and mint. It's not uncommon for me to whip up a batch of mint-chocolate ice cream, sometimes using cream steeped with fresh organic peppermint and topped with crunchy cacao nibs, other times using mint flavoring and chopped high-percentage chocolate bars.

I once made a jaw-dropping batch of mocha mint chip using those Starbucks VIA instant coffee packets. As much as I loved it, it kept me up tossing and turning all night (as I fantasized about another couple of scoops).

So, while chocolate does contain some caffeine, the one-two punch of the two was just too much. However, combining those two for a BREAKFAST muffin, alongside my massive mug of coffee... sets me up for a beautiful day!

Note: While most grocery stores carry fresh mint (typically spearmint), I have farmer friends who grow peppermint (along with other radical herbs, like lemon thyme and pineapple sage). Finding these kinds of herbs at some high-end stores and farmers' markets will bring these kinds of recipes to new heights. HIGHLY recommended if you can find them.

1 1/4 cup (300 mL)	heavy cream
1 bunch (about 3.5 oz [100g])	fresh mint (peppermint, if you can find it), divided
1 cup (240 mL)	almond flour
1/2 cup (120 mL)	powdered sugar replacement, divided
1/4 cup + 2 tbsp (90 mL)	coconut flour
1/4 cup + 2 tbsp (90 mL)	unsweetened cocoa powder
1/4 cup (60 mL)	ground chia
1 tbsp (15 mL)	baking powder
3/4 tsp (4 mL)	salt
4 large	eggs

- Place the cream on the stove in a medium sized pot, over low heat. You want to bring it up to a point where it's *juuuuuuuust* about to simmer (don't let it boil). Watch for little bubbles around the edge of the pot.

- While waiting for the cream to simmer, prepare the mint by removing the mint leaves from the stems. Wash and dry the leaves. Set about 12 nice mint leaves aside for garnish. Wrap in a moist paper towel and place in the fridge. Tear or very coarsely chop the rest (essentially cutting/tearing each leaf into halves or thirds).

- Once the cream is hot but hasn't really simmered, turn off the heat and add the chopped mint. Stir the mint in the cream to allow it to wilt. Cover and allow to sit for about 15 minutes. Stir, cover, and allow to sit for 15 more minutes. The mint is steeping and will impart an AMAZING flavor into the cream. It's basically like making tea, but with cream!

- Strain the mint from the cream, discarding the mint and setting the mint-infused cream aside.

- Preheat oven to 350° F (177° C).

- Grease a standard 12-cup muffin pan (or two standard sized 6-cup muffin pans [We're looking for 12 smallish muffins.]). Set aside.

- In a large bowl, combine the almond flour, 1/4 cup + 2 tbsp (90 mL) powdered sugar replacement, coconut flour, cocoa powder, ground chia, baking powder, and salt. With a whisk or a fork, combine the dry ingredients so they are evenly mixed and distributed in and amongst one another.

- Add eggs and 1/2 cup (120 mL) of the minted cream to the dry ingredients. Whisk to combine well. Allow to sit for about 2 minutes to allow time for the chia to gel. Place the remainder of the cream in the refrigerator to cool.

- The batter should be like a thick pancake batter. These ingredients tend to be a bit inconsistent from brand to brand and grind to grind. You may need to add a little more minted cream to thin it out (just not too much!).

- Once the batter is well mixed, pour even amounts between the 12 muffin cups.

- Bake for about 18 to 21 minutes, or until the muffins have risen and the surface is dry.

- Remove from the oven and let rest for 5 minutes before removing from the pan. Let them cool to room temperature.

- Once the muffins are cool, whip the chilled minted cream with the remaining 2 tbsp (30 mL) powdered sugar replacement.

- Garnish each muffin with the cream and a mint leaf! (I cut mine into noodles and tossed a few cacao nibs on there … I LOVE the texture!)

- Enjoy!

Mini Notella Muffnuts

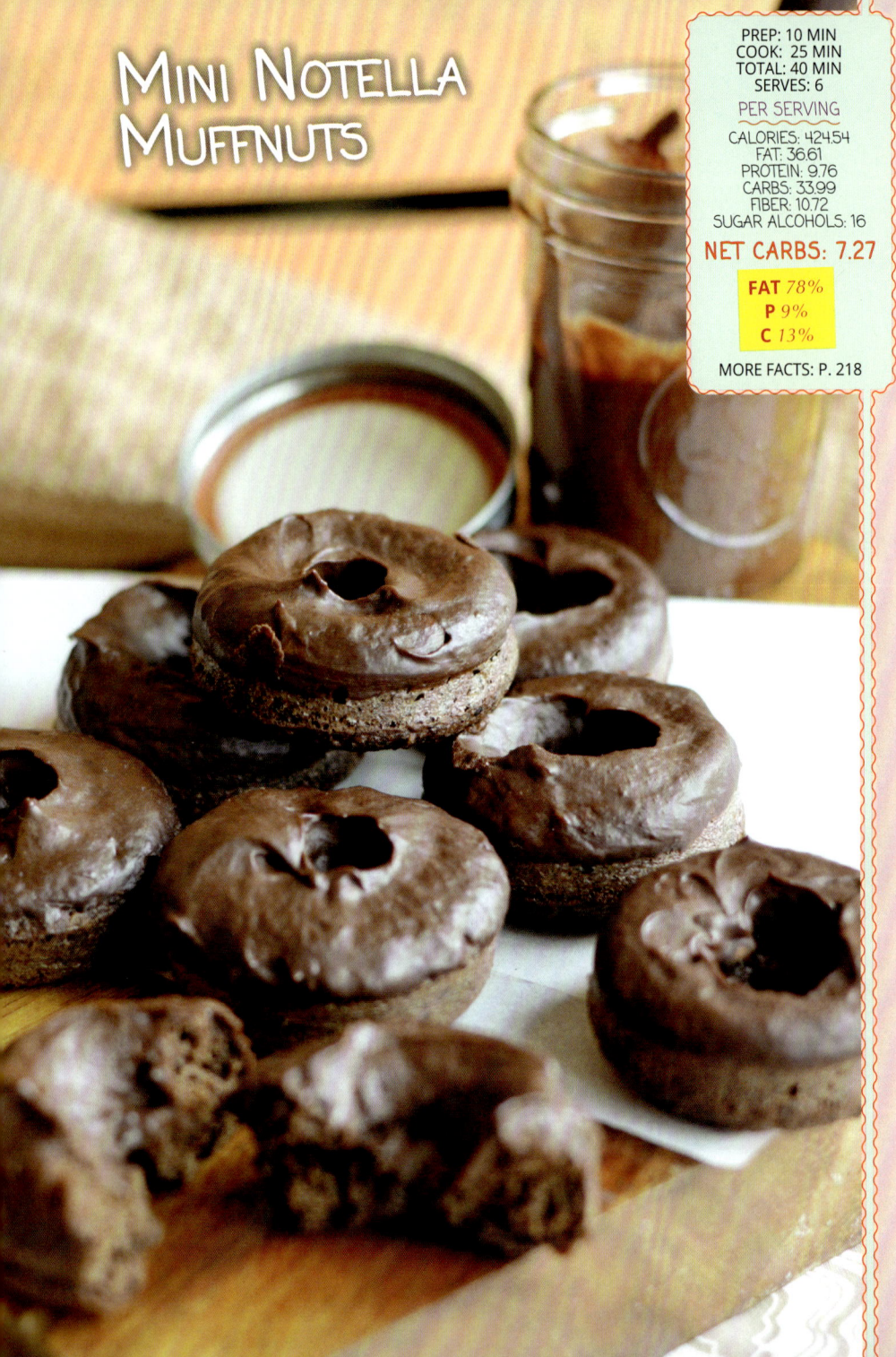

PREP: 10 MIN
COOK: 25 MIN
TOTAL: 40 MIN
SERVES: 6

PER SERVING
CALORIES: 424.54
FAT: 36.61
PROTEIN: 9.76
CARBS: 33.99
FIBER: 10.72
SUGAR ALCOHOLS: 16

NET CARBS: 7.27

FAT *78%*
P *9%*
C *13%*

MORE FACTS: P. 218

I really don't have a sweet tooth. I swear!

I remember driving with a buddy in upstate New York about 5 years ago. It was my first real trip after dropping all my weight. I wanted to be good, but was QUICKLY undone by all the options that exist outside my little Mexican town in Baja Sur. My friend had a family reunion in the very same town I'd attended college. A trip down memory lane? Sure, why not!

What I didn't know, expect, or anticipate was the sheer overwhelming ubiquitousness of Dunkin' Doughnuts in the Northeast of the United States. It was so overwhelming that it was my sole undoing, to the point that my buddy still cracks doughnut jokes whenever he sees me.

See, I'm either good or bad. I've never been very good at the middle ground. If I'm going to walk into a Dunkin' Doughnuts, I'm not going to eat a single doughnut hole. No, I'm going to eat ALL the holes. I'm going to look at the menu, scan the cases, take a big whiff and a deep breath, then casually and nonchalantly tell the Dunkin' staff member, "Yes."

Dunkin' Doughnuts also has a terrible

habit of always being open! Late at night, tweaking with doughnut fever, I'd sneak out for a bag of goodies.

Doughnuts have been scientifically proven to be the absolute perfect blend of fat and sugar. No. I don't have a problem! ***denial***

Really, if I were to be deeply, painfully, and brutally honest, this recipe was developed less because I wanted a doughnut, and more because I wanted Nutella, anyway. MMMmmmmm ....

I once had a writing instructor suggest that the best stuff *hurts* to write. Sometimes, I feel I'm a little too forthright. ***shame***

1 cup (240ᵐᴸ)	hazelnut flour
1/4 cup + 2 tbsp (90ᵐᴸ)	coconut flour
1/4 cup + 2 tbsp (90ᵐᴸ)	sugar replacement
1/4 cup + 2 tbsp (90ᵐᴸ)	unsweetened cocoa powder
1/4 cup (60ᵐᴸ)	ground chia
1 tbsp (15ᵐᴸ)	baking powder
1 tsp (5ᵐᴸ)	xanthan gum (optional)
3/4 tsp (4ᵐᴸ)	salt
4 large	eggs
1/2 cup + 2 tbsp (150ᵐᴸ)	heavy cream
1 recipe	Notella (p. 198)

⋛ Preheat oven to 350° F (177° C).

⋛ Grease a standard 12-cup doughnut baking pan (or two standard sized 6-cup muffin pans [We're looking for 12 smallish doughnut-muffins.]). Set aside.

⋛ In a large bowl, combine the hazelnut flour, coconut flour, sugar replacement, cocoa powder, ground chia, baking powder, optional xanthan gum, and salt. With a whisk or a fork, combine the dry ingredients so they are evenly mixed and distributed in and amongst one another.

⋛ Add eggs and cream to the dry ingredients. Whisk to combine well. Allow to sit for about 2 minutes to allow time for the chia to gel.

⋛ The batter should be like a thick pancake batter. These ingredients tend to be a bit inconsistent from brand to brand and grind to grind. You may need to add a little more cream to thin it out (just not too much!).

⋛ Once the batter is well mixed, pour even amounts between the 12 doughnut/muffin cups.

⋛ Bake for about 18 to 21 minutes, or until the muffins have risen and the surface is dry.

⋛ Remove from the oven and let rest for 5 minutes before removing from the pan. Once removed, let them cool to room temperature.

⋛ Once cool, slather them with Notella. Call no one and turn on the TV to something with loads of empty calories (*Modern Family?*). Enjoy!

Bacon and Orange Muffins with Pecan Streusel & Sour Cream Glaze

PREP: 20 MIN
COOK: 25 MIN
TOTAL: 50 MIN
SERVES: 6

PER SERVING
CALORIES: 498.45
FAT: 40.95
PROTEIN: 17.38
CARBS: 39.65
FIBER: 7.48
SUGAR ALCOHOLS: 24

NET CARBS: 8.17

FAT 74%
P 14%
C 12%

MORE FACTS: P. 217

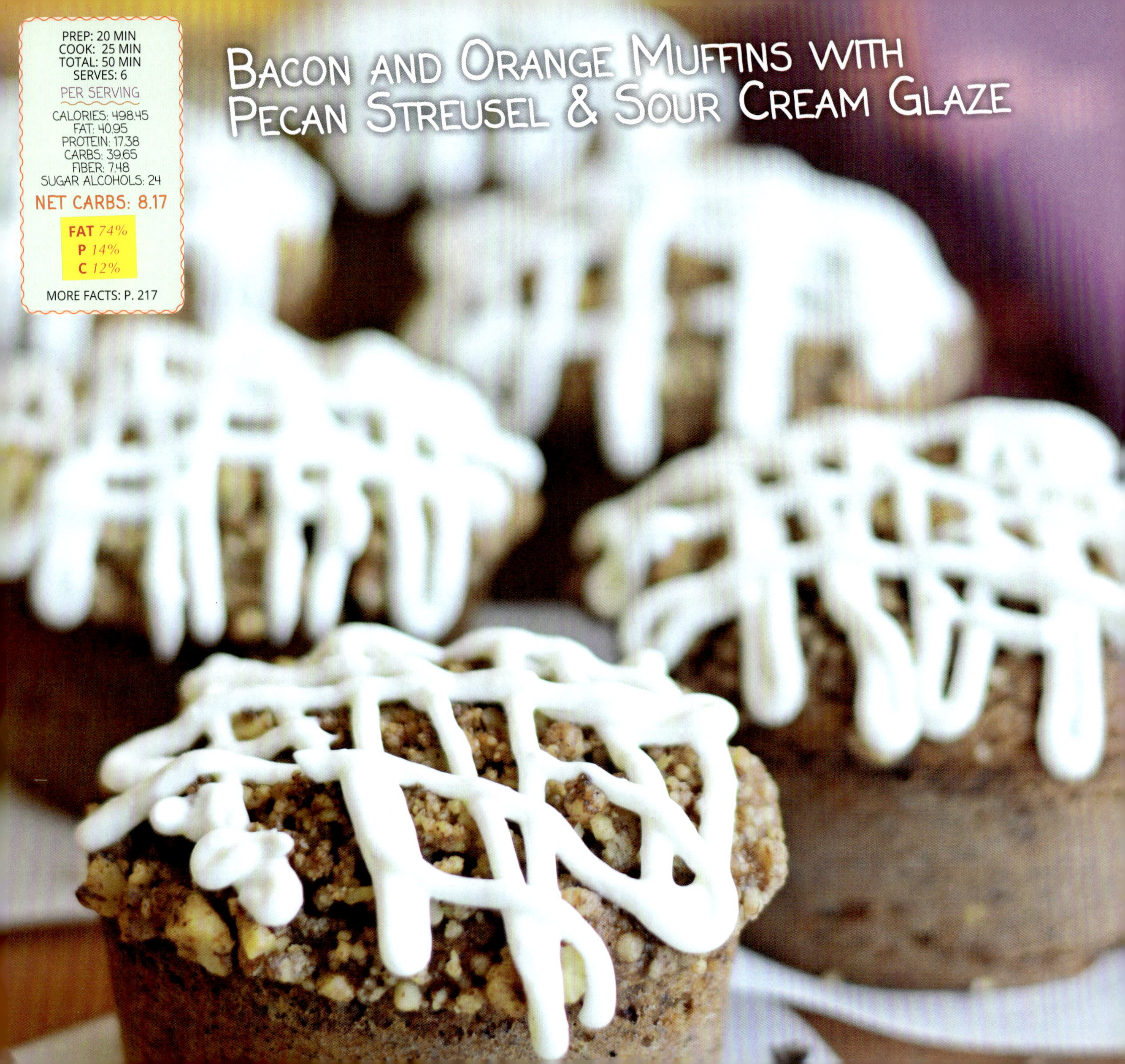

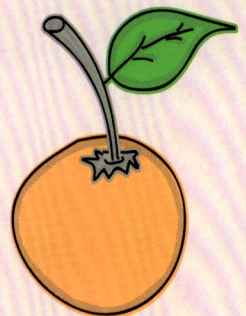

I repeatedly state (lie to myself) that I don't have much of a sweet tooth. What I DO have, though, is a sweet/savory tooth. I am a massive fan of the combination of sweet and salty. Think peanut butter cups or chocolate coated pretzels. Okay, now STOP thinking about those things, else you may make an unscheduled trip to a convenience store. Seriously, put your head in the freezer for a second. Cool off!

One of my favorite ice cream flavors is orange marmalade with bacon and rosemary. Think orange Creamsicle® dipped in bacon and served on a wreath. The only way to make this flavor combination just that much tastier would be to add a flavor enhancing acid, like... oh... say... sour cream!

Note: If you REALLY want to live on the edge, make your own bacon bits from a thick-cut *pepper* bacon!

Bacon & Orange Muffin

1/2 cup + 2 tbsp (150 mL)	pecan flour
1/4 cup + 2 tbsp (90 mL)	sugar-free vanilla protein isolate
1/4 cup + 2 tbsp (90 mL)	coconut flour
1/4 cup + 2 tbsp (90 mL)	sugar replacement
3/4 tsp (4 mL)	baking soda
3/4 tsp (4 mL)	salt
1	orange, divided
6 large	eggs
1/2 cup + 2 tbsp (150 mL)	sour cream
1/4 cup + 2 tbsp (90 mL)	bacon bits
1 tbsp (15 mL)	fresh chopped rosemary

Pecan Streusel

1/2 cup (120 mL)	pecan flour
1/2 cup (120 mL)	chopped pecans
2 tbsp (30 mL)	sugar replacement
1 tbsp (15 mL)	melted butter
1/4 tsp (1 mL)	ground cloves
Dash	salt

Sour Cream Glaze

1/2 cup (120 mL)	sour cream
1/4 cup (60 mL)	powdered sugar replacement
1 tsp (5 mL)	orange zest (from the orange in the muffin batter section)
1 tsp (5 mL)	vanilla extract
Dribble	orange juice (from the orange in the muffin batter section)
Dash	salt

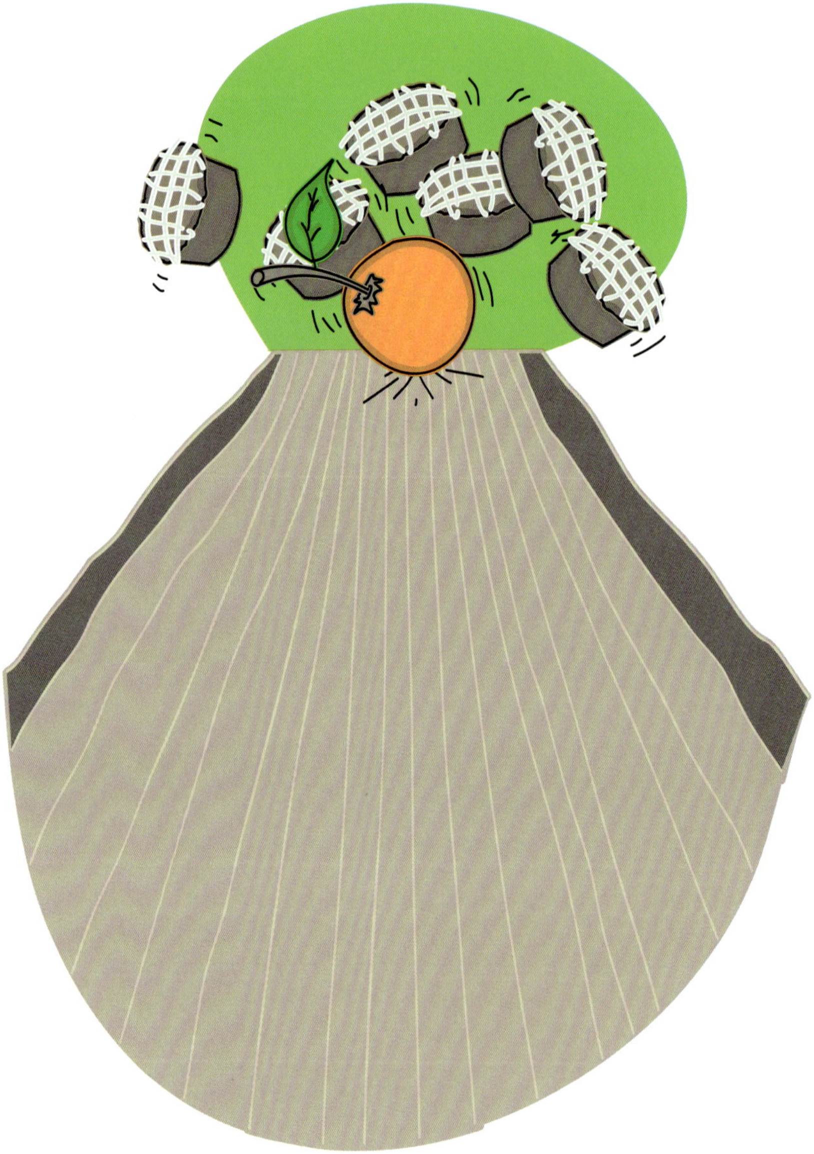

- Preheat oven to 350° F (177° C).
- **Note:** It's somewhat difficult to tell from the angle of the photo, but I used another random red silicone muffin pan. This particular shape was essentially oval, but as before, really any similarly sized muffin pan will do the trick!
- Grease a standard 12-cup muffin pan (or two standard sized 6-cup muffin pans [We're looking for 12 smallish muffins.]). Set aside.
- In a large bowl, combine the pecan flour, protein powder, coconut flour, sugar replacement, baking soda, and salt. With a whisk or a fork, combine the dry ingredients so they are evenly mixed and distributed in and amongst one another.
- With a zester or a peeler, remove about a third of the very outer orange skin (the zest) of the orange. Try not to get any of the bitter white pith. Chop the zest. You want about 1 tbsp (15 mL) of chopped fresh orange zest. Juice the orange, as well. Strain out the seeds. We are looking for about 1/4 cup (60 mL) of fresh orange juice.
- In a separate smaller bowl, whisk together eggs with sour cream, about half of the orange juice, about 2 tsp (10 mL) of the orange zest, the bacon bits, and chopped rosemary.
- Pour egg mixture into the large bowl of dry ingredients. Whisk together and combine well.
- The batter should be like a thick pancake batter. These ingredients tend to be a bit inconsistent from brand to brand and grind to grind. You may need to add a little water to thin it out (just not too much!).
- Once the batter is well mixed, pour even amounts between the 12 muffin cups.
- **For the streusel**, in a separate bowl, combine the pecan flour, chopped pecans, sugar replacement, melted butter, cloves and salt. Mix until the mixture is evenly coated. Scatter streusel evenly over the top of the batter.
- Bake for about 18 to 21 minutes, or until the muffins have crowned, the surface is dry, beginning to crisp, and has turned golden.
- Remove from the oven and let rest for 5 minutes before removing from the pan. Allow to cool to room temperature.
- While the muffins cool, **make the glaze** by combining and whisking together the sour cream, the powdered sugar replacement, the remaining orange zest, the vanilla, and salt.
- At this point, the glaze is pretty thick, which can make for a nice spread or a lovely sour cream dollop. I personally used a fine-tipped piping bag and squeezed little lattice lines across the top of the muffins in this photo. To do this, I used a little bit of the remaining orange juice to *gently* thin the sour cream mixture down to the right consistency. Be careful adding the orange juice. Once you've added it, you can't take it out if it's too thin. However, if it's too thick, you can still fix it by adding a touch more orange juice.
- Carefully adjust the consistency of your glaze with orange juice. When happy, glaze your muffins and enjoy!

Orange-Cranberry Muffins

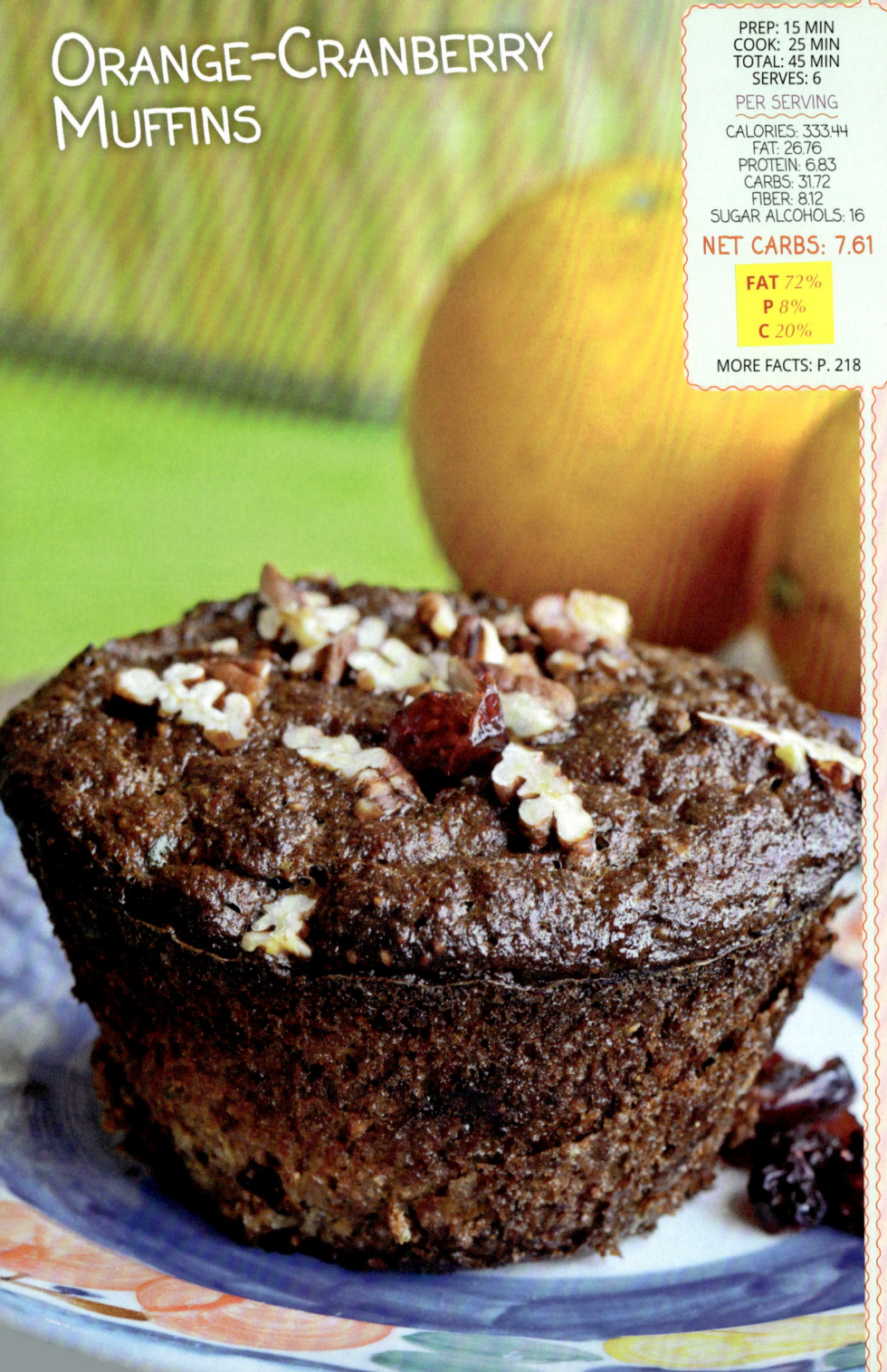

PREP: 15 MIN
COOK: 25 MIN
TOTAL: 45 MIN
SERVES: 6

PER SERVING

CALORIES: 333.44
FAT: 26.76
PROTEIN: 6.83
CARBS: 31.72
FIBER: 8.12
SUGAR ALCOHOLS: 16

NET CARBS: 7.61

FAT 72%
P 8%
C 20%

MORE FACTS: P. 218

Here's one I'd serve at a holiday feast! I envision it at the Thanksgiving dinner table, but really it's just something I see appearing somewhere in the fall and winter seasons.

I've taken this one back to a chia and flax blend, closer to those found in the front of the book. I just find those heartier earthy flavors match a colder climate. I also get a bit squingy when I think of coconuts and cranberries. It's tough for me to picture the two ever coexisting in the same muffin.

1/2 cup (120 mL)	ground chia seed
1/2 cup (120 mL)	pecan flour
1/2 cup (120 mL)	sugar replacement
1/4 cup (60 mL)	flaxseed meal
1/4 cup (60 mL)	almond flour
3/4 tsp (4 mL)	baking soda
3/4 tsp (4 mL)	salt
1	orange
6 large	eggs
3 tbsp (45 mL)	melted butter
1 tsp (5 mL)	blackstrap molasses or yacón syrup
1 cup (240 mL)	coarsely chopped cranberries
2 tbsp (30 mL)	chopped fresh sage
1/4 cup (60 mL)	chopped pecans

- Preheat oven to 350° F (177° C).
- Grease a standard 12-cup muffin pan (or two standard sized 6-cup muffin pans [We're looking for 12 smallish muffins.]). Set aside.
- In a large bowl, combine the chia flour, pecan flour, sugar replacement, flaxseed meal, almond flour, baking soda, and salt. With a whisk or a fork, combine the dry ingredients so they are evenly mixed and distributed in and amongst one another.
- With a zester or a peeler, remove about a third of the very outer orange skin (the zest) of the orange. Try not to get any of the bitter white pith. Chop the zest. You want about 1 tbsp (15 mL) of chopped fresh orange zest. Juice the orange, as well. Strain out the seeds. We are looking for about 1/4 cup (60 mL) of fresh orange juice.
- In a separate smaller bowl, whisk together eggs with the orange juice, orange zest, melted butter, and yacón or molasses.
- Pour egg mixture into the large bowl of dry ingredients. Whisk together and combine well.
- Fold in cranberries and sage. Allow to sit for about 5 minutes, allowing the chia and flax to gel and thicken.
- The batter should be like a thick pancake batter. These ingredients tend to be a bit inconsistent from brand to brand and grind to grind. You may need to add a little water (and/or orange juice, if you have any left) to thin it out (just not too much!).
- Once the batter is well mixed, pour even amounts between the 12 muffin cups.
- Top each muffin with a little bit of the chopped pecan.
- Bake for about 18 to 21 minutes, or until the muffins have crowned and the surface is dry, beginning to crisp, and has turned golden.
- Remove from the oven and let rest for 5 minutes before removing from the pan. Allow to cool to room temperature.
- Add to a bread basket and serve with roast turkey or a brined, chestnut-stuffed pork loin!

Pear, Walnut and Blue Cheese Tart Fauxtan

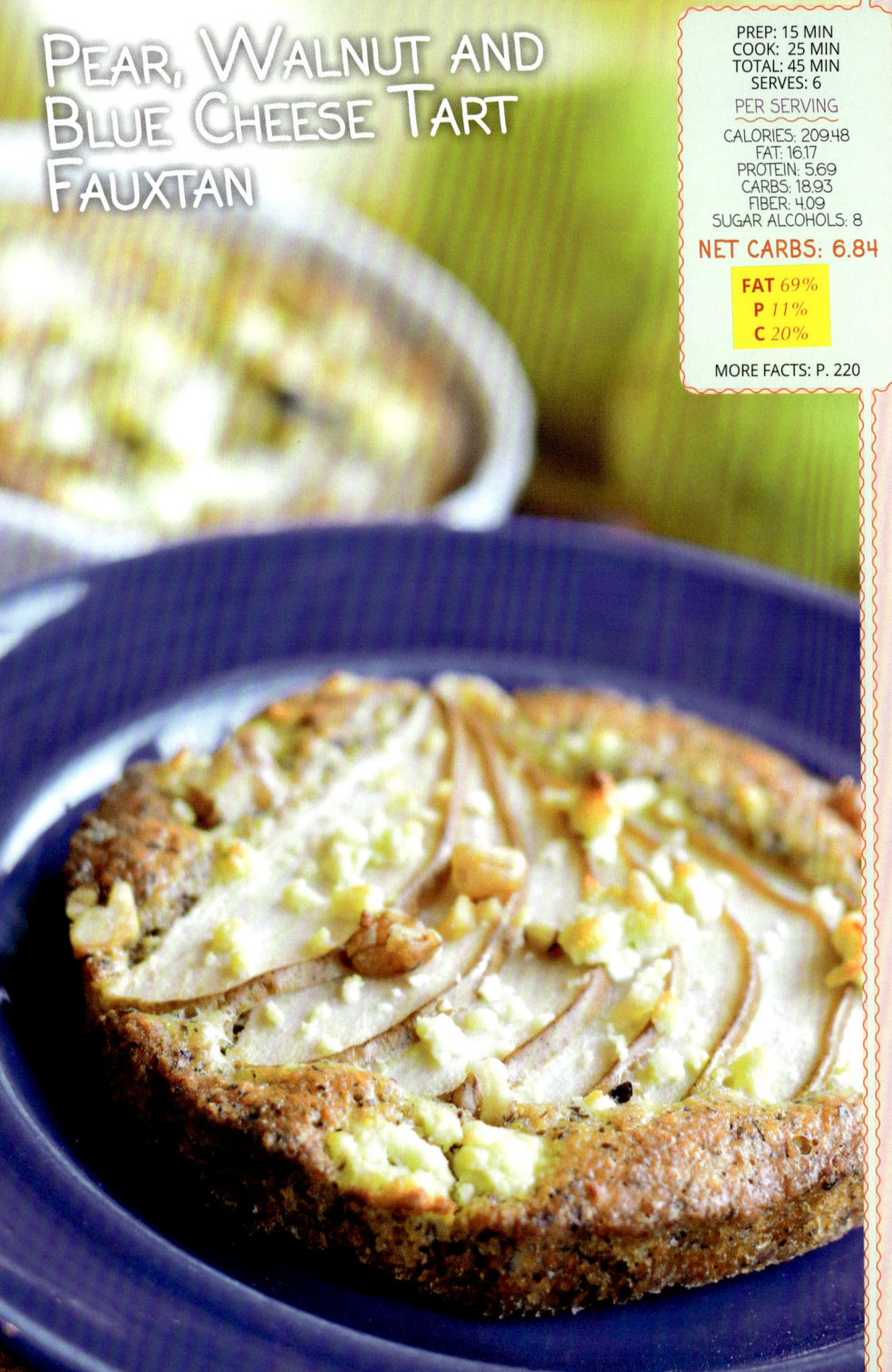

PREP: 15 MIN
COOK: 25 MIN
TOTAL: 45 MIN
SERVES: 6

PER SERVING
CALORIES: 209.48
FAT: 16.17
PROTEIN: 5.69
CARBS: 18.93
FIBER: 4.09
SUGAR ALCOHOLS: 8

NET CARBS: 6.84

FAT 69%
P 11%
C 20%

MORE FACTS: P. 220

The inspiration for this dish came from a port-braised endive tart tatin, from a restaurant in my youth. That recipe has been stripped down and simplified. It's no longer an upside-down tarte tatin... so I've dubbed it a Faux-Tan. Fitting for a book on faking! *wink*

Note: This recipe is roughly half the size of most of the other recipes in this book. It's intended as more of a small snack, pretty little appeteezer, or a small dessert. If you de-squint and un-focus on the back of the photo, you'll see the thin, wide and fluted ceramic tart pan for this dish. Another fun way to go would be to use something like two 9" (23cm) pie or cake pans. Pour a thin layer of batter into each greased pan, then top with fanned, sliced pears or apples, then crumbled or grated cheese (blue, cheddar, goat, Swiss, parmesan, etc. all would be wonderful!), then some chopped nuts. Bake. Remove from pan, slice wedges and... fruity cheese pizza with nuts. Serve with a nice salad on a rolling hill in the French Alps!

1/4 cup (60ᵐᴸ)	ground chia seed
1/4 cup (60ᵐᴸ)	walnut flour
1/4 cup (60ᵐᴸ)	sugar replacement
2 tbsp (30ᵐᴸ)	flaxseed meal
2 tbsp (30ᵐᴸ)	almond flour
1 tsp (5ᵐᴸ)	baking powder
Dash	salt
3 large	eggs
1/4 cup (60ᵐᴸ)	heavy cream
1 large	pear
1/4 cup (60ᵐᴸ)	crumbled blue cheese
2 tbsp (30ᵐᴸ)	chopped walnuts

≽ Preheat oven to 350° F (177° C).

≽ Grease 6 small shallow tart pans (3-inch by 1/2-inch [7.5ᶜᵐ x 1.25ᶜᵐ]) Set aside.

≽ In a large bowl, combine the chia flour, walnut flour, sugar replacement, flaxseed meal, almond flour, baking powder, and salt. With a whisk or a fork, combine the dry ingredients so they are evenly mixed and distributed in and amongst one another.

≽ In a separate smaller bowl, whisk together eggs with the cream.

≽ Pour egg mixture into the large bowl of dry ingredients. Whisk together and combine well. Allow the batter to sit for about 5 minutes, while it thickens as the chia and flax gel.

≽ The batter should be like a thick pancake batter. These ingredients tend to be a bit inconsistent from brand to brand and grind to grind. You may need to add a little cream to thin it out (just not too much!).

≽ Once the batter is well mixed, pour even amounts between your greased baking pans.

≽ Wash and dry the pear, then cut into halves from the top to the bottom. Cut out the core. Cut each half into 3 equal wedges. Then slice each wedge into about 5 equally thin wedges.

≽ Put your 5 thin slices on top of each blob.

≽ Sprinkle crumbled cheese and chopped nuts on the top of each peared blob.

≽ Bake for about 18 to 21 minutes, or until the top is golden and dry.

≽ Remove from the oven and let rest for 5 minutes before removing from the pan. Eat hot. Would be great with a salad!

Pumpkin Cheesecake Swirl Muffin

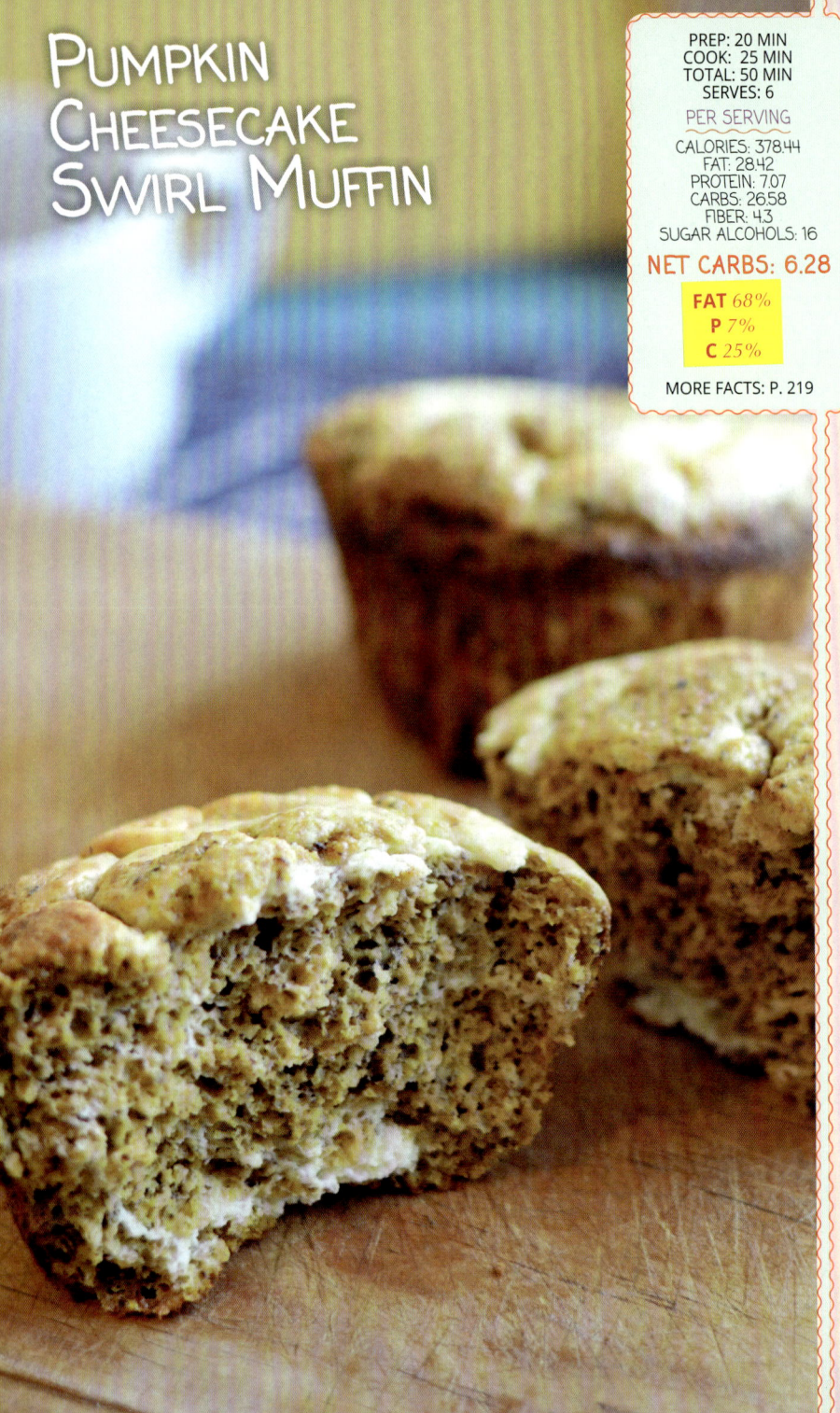

PREP: 20 MIN
COOK: 25 MIN
TOTAL: 50 MIN
SERVES: 6

PER SERVING

CALORIES: 378.44
FAT: 28.42
PROTEIN: 7.07
CARBS: 26.58
FIBER: 4.3
SUGAR ALCOHOLS: 16

NET CARBS: 6.28

FAT 68%
P 7%
C 25%

MORE FACTS: P. 219

This one is a bit different than the rest. Most are either straightforward quick breads or they're quick breads stuffed or filled, topped or riddled with nuts or berries.

This one reaches a little bit outside that scope. Sure, a pumpkin muffin is all fine and dandy, but hopefully at this point in the book, it should be obvious how to make a pumpkin muffin, pumpkin pancake, pumpkin doughnut, or pumpkin waffle... all without needing my help. However, what if you wanted to infuse said treat with a cheesecake? Could it be done?!

Yes! Of course!

See, here's the thing... You can fold similarly textured things together and bake them. Now, a cheesecake's texture isn't the same as a muffin, but they both start as batters and then end up firm enough to hold their shape. Why not let them do it, intertwined?!

Really, you could take any two or three batters from this book and fold them together. Let's say we're talking about the Mexican Chocolate Muffins *(p. 142)*. You could make the batter without the chocolate and spices, split it in half, add the chocolate to one half and the spices to the other. Swirl them together and you'd have a Mexican Chocolate Chimera! My point? Swirls are fun. Mix it up!

Pumpkin Muffin

3/4 cup (180 mL)	hazelnut flour
1/4 cup (60 mL)	coconut flour
1/4 cup (60 mL)	sugar replacement
2 tsp (10 mL)	baking powder
1/2 tsp (3 mL)	salt
1/2 tsp (3 mL)	ground cinnamon
1/4 tsp (1 mL)	ground nutmeg
1/8 tsp (.5 mL)	ground cloves
4 large	eggs
1/2 cup (120 mL)	canned or mashed pumpkin
2 tbsp (30 mL)	melted butter
1 tsp (5 mL)	blackstrap molasses or yacón syrup

Cheesecake

6 oz (168 g)	full fat cream cheese, room temperature
1 large	egg, room temperature
1/2 tsp (3 mL)	vanilla extract
Dash	salt
1/4 cup (60 mL)	powdered sugar replacement
1/2 tsp (3 mL)	lemon juice
1/4 cup (60 mL)	sour cream

⋛ Grease a standard 12-cup muffin pan (or two standard sized 6-cup muffin pans [We're looking for 12 smallish muffins.]). Set aside.

⋛ In a large bowl, combine the hazelnut flour, coconut flour, sugar replacement, baking powder, salt, cinnamon, nutmeg, and cloves. With a whisk or a fork, combine the dry ingredients so they are evenly mixed and distributed in and amongst one another.

⋛ In a separate smaller bowl, whisk together eggs with the pumpkin mash, melted butter, and molasses or yacón syrup.

⋛ Pour egg mixture into the large bowl of dry ingredients. Whisk together and combine well.

⋛ The batter should be like a thick pancake batter. These ingredients tend to be a bit inconsistent from brand to brand and grind to grind. You may need to add a little water to thin it out (just not too much!).

⋛ With an electric mixer in a fresh large bowl, beat the cream cheese until light and airy.

⋛ Add the egg and beat until well combined.

⋛ Add the vanilla and a dash of salt. Beat until well combined.

⋛ Slowly add the powdered sugar replacement to the cream cheese mixture while it beats.

⋛ Add the lemon juice and sour cream. Mix for another moment or two. Make sure everything is very well mixed and that there are no lumps. *If* there are lumps you can strain the mixture through a fine mesh (optional, but it does increase the silky-smooth quality).

⋛ Pour the cheesecake batter into the pumpkin muffin batter bowl.

⋛ With a spatula, *gently* fold the two batters together with 2 or 3 good passes through the two batters. We don't want to mix them, so much as create a general marble or swirl effect. The two batters should still be separate from one another, while being inextricably intertwined.

⋛ Once the batter is marbled, scoop even amounts between the 12 muffin cups.

⋛ Bake for about 18 to 21 minutes, or until the muffins have crowned and the tops are golden and dry.

⋛ Remove from the oven and let rest for 5 minutes before removing from the pan.

⋛ Enjoy!

Spiced Pumpkin-Sour Cream Muffin Pies

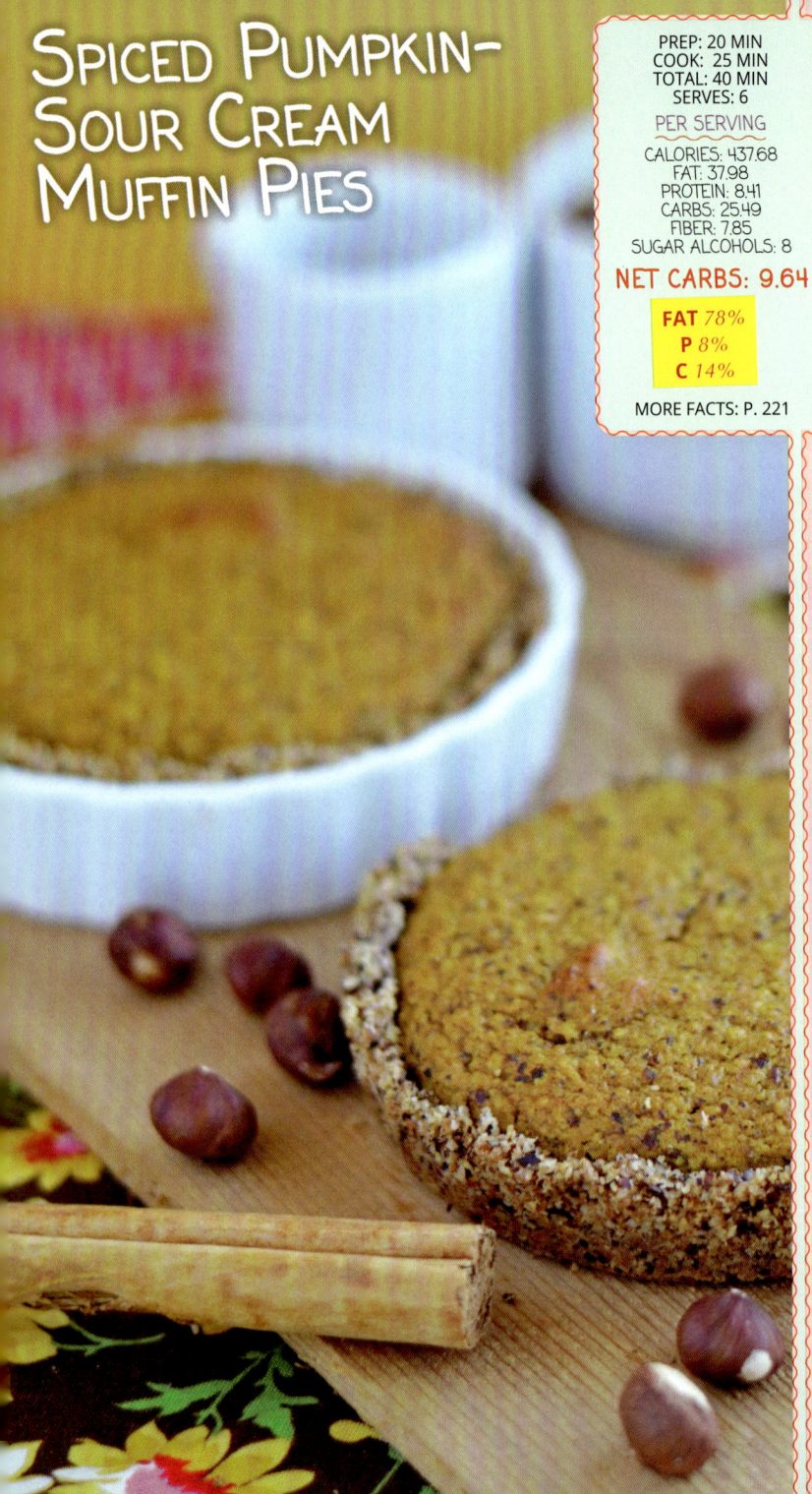

PREP: 20 MIN
COOK: 25 MIN
TOTAL: 40 MIN
SERVES: 6

PER SERVING
CALORIES: 437.68
FAT: 37.98
PROTEIN: 8.41
CARBS: 25.49
FIBER: 7.85
SUGAR ALCOHOLS: 8

NET CARBS: 9.64

FAT 78%
P 8%
C 14%

MORE FACTS: P. 221

Like the preceding recipe, I'm using a pumpkin muffin batter to showcase another unique way in which these blobs can be baked. In this case, into a pie shell!

Pie Crust Nuts Note: This is a very standard all-purpose pie crust that holds its own quite well. A few thoughts, though: I've tried pulverizing the nuts in a food processor. This works well and is quick! I've tried using pre-ground meals and flours. This is also quite easy to do, but is costlier. Each of these methods results in a nice and even crust, but it tends to be crumbly. For a crust that really seems to "hold its own," oddly, the best method is to take whole nuts, chop them a bit, then place them in a large sturdy bag and whack at them with a rolling pin, mallet, or the bottom of a pan (or shoe). It's just as good for crust making as it is for releasing stress! Just whack the bag until the nuts are evenly pulverized, but not "butter-fied."

Pie Crust Honey Note: Much like the molasses, yacón, or honey used in the streusels in this book, the honey acts as a glue to hold everything together. The crust will stay together without one of these three sticky substances, but it'll be on the crumbly side. The honey helps it to maintain a firmer resolve, lends a bit more sweetness and can help with some waterproofing (decrease the rate at which the crust will sog out, in wetter pies). While the addition of honey does add about 17 net carbs to the whole thing, that's only 2.8 net carbs per Muffpie. It's really up to you to decide if the sturdier crust is worth the 2.8 carbs. Without the honey, these pies come in at less than 7 net carbs per pie.

Pie Crust

1 1/2 cups (360ᵐᴸ)	toasted hazelnuts (or hazelnut flour)
1/4 cup (60ᵐᴸ)	melted butter
1 tbsp (15ᵐᴸ)	honey (optional)
1 tsp (5ᵐᴸ)	vanilla extract
Dash	salt

Pumpkin Muffin

1/2 cup + 2 tbsp (150ᵐᴸ)	hazelnut flour
1/4 cup (60ᵐᴸ)	coconut flour
1/4 cup (60ᵐᴸ)	sugar replacement
2 tbsp (30ᵐᴸ)	ground chia
1/2 tsp (3ᵐᴸ)	baking soda
1/2 tsp (3ᵐᴸ)	salt
1/2 tsp (3ᵐᴸ)	ground cinnamon
1/4 tsp (1ᵐᴸ)	ground nutmeg
1/8 tsp (.5ᵐᴸ)	ground cloves
2 large	eggs
1/2 cup (120ᵐᴸ)	canned or mashed pumpkin
1/2 cup (120ᵐᴸ)	sour cream
1 tsp (5ᵐᴸ)	blackstrap molasses or yacón syrup

- Preheat oven to 350° F (177° C).

- Grease 6 small shallow tart pans (3-inch by 1/2-inch [7.5ᶜᵐ x 1.25ᶜᵐ]). Set aside. Ramekins or small pie pans would work well for this. You could use a large muffin pan, but I'd suggest adding some xanthan gum to the muffin portion of the recipe, to help it carry its weight.

- Using the recipe notes from the previous page as a guide, put 1 1/2 cups (360ᵐᴸ) pulverized hazelnuts into a medium sized mixing bowl.

- Add melted butter, optional honey, vanilla extract, and salt to the hazelnuts. Combine well.

- Distribute the nut crust between the 6 baking vessels. *Firmly* press the crust into the pans, so that a clear crust is formed. I have a small rubber tamper (think pencil with a firm rubber quarter glued onto the end) I use to help really PUSH the nuts tightly together. The bottom of a small glass jar can help, as can the base of a spoon.

- Once the crust is evenly formed around the pans, place the crusts into the oven to help them set. Bake for about 7 minutes.

- For the muffins, in a large bowl, combine the hazelnut flour, coconut flour, sugar replacement, chia, baking soda, salt, cinnamon, nutmeg, and cloves. With a whisk or a fork, combine the dry ingredients so they are evenly mixed and distributed in and amongst one another.

- In a separate smaller bowl, whisk together eggs with the pumpkin mash, sour cream, and molasses or yacón syrup.

- Pour egg mixture into the large bowl of dry ingredients. Whisk together and combine well. Allow the batter to sit for about 2 minutes, to let the chia gel and thicken.

- The batter should be like a thick pancake batter. These ingredients tend to be a bit inconsistent from brand to brand and grind to grind. You may need to add a little water to thin it out (just not too much!).

- Pour the pumpkin batter evenly between the 6 pans.

- Bake for about 18 to 21 minutes, or until the muffins have crowned and the tops are golden and dry.

- Remove from the oven and let rest for 5 minutes before removing from the pan.

- Enjoy!

Strawberry Yogurt Muffins

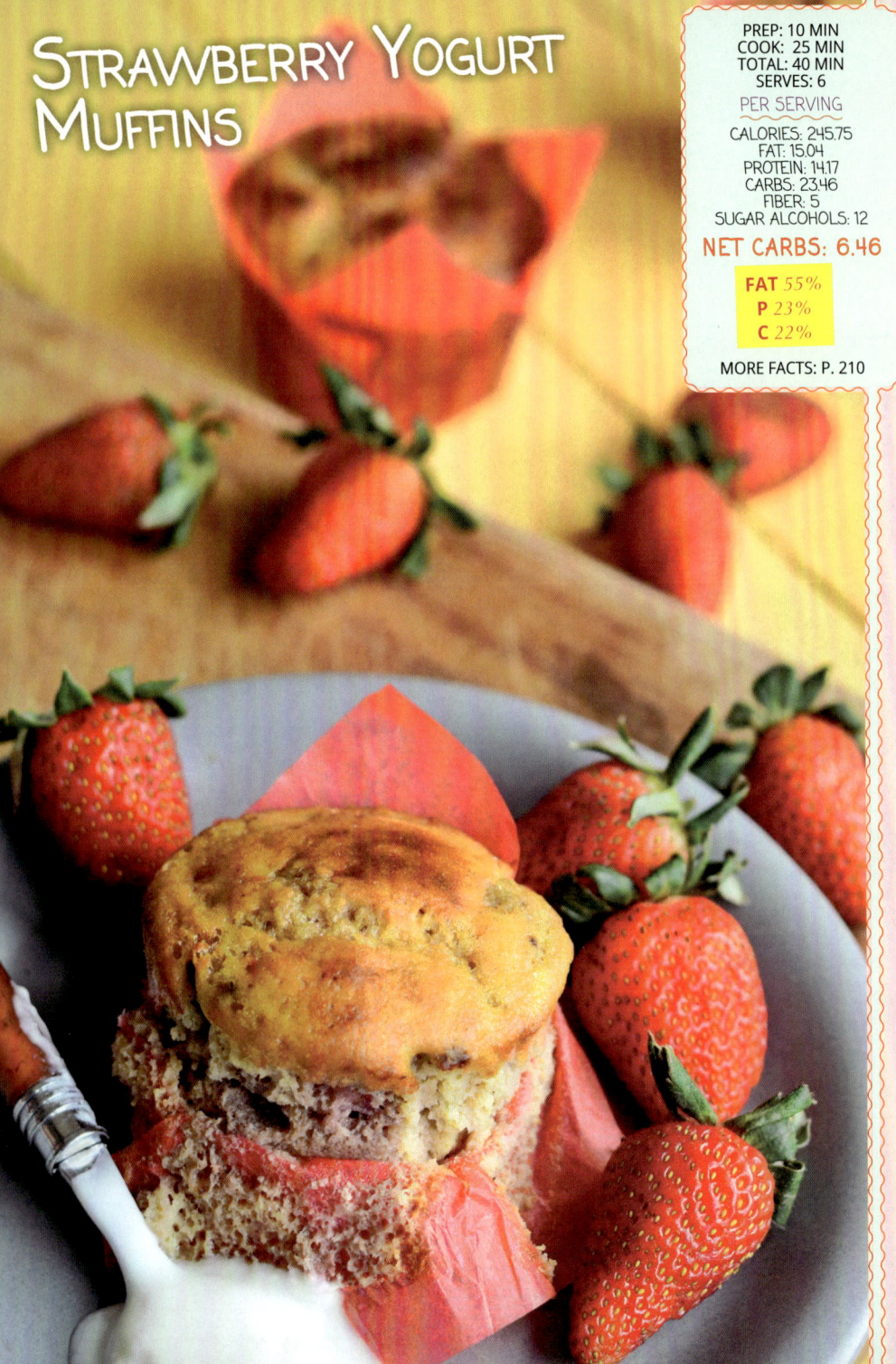

PREP: 10 MIN
COOK: 25 MIN
TOTAL: 40 MIN
SERVES: 6

PER SERVING

CALORIES: 245.75
FAT: 15.04
PROTEIN: 14.17
CARBS: 23.46
FIBER: 5
SUGAR ALCOHOLS: 12

NET CARBS: 6.46

FAT 55%
P 23%
C 22%

MORE FACTS: P. 210

Here's another one that takes advantage of the acidity in one of the ingredients, as well as the fat. Plus, who doesn't love strawberry yogurt?

3/4 cup (180ᵐᴸ)	almond flour
1/4 cup + 2 tbsp (90ᵐᴸ)	sugar-free vanilla whey protein isolate
1/4 cup + 2 tbsp (90ᵐᴸ)	coconut flour
1/4 cup + 2 tbsp (90ᵐᴸ)	sugar replacement
3/4 tsp (4ᵐᴸ)	baking soda
3/4 tsp (4ᵐᴸ)	salt
6 large	eggs
1/2 cup + 2 tbsp (150ᵐᴸ)	plain full-fat Greek yogurt
1 cup (240ᵐᴸ)	coarsely chopped strawberries

- Preheat oven to 350° F (177° C).
- Grease a standard 12-cup muffin pan (or two standard sized 6-cup muffin pans [We're looking for 12 smallish muffins.]). Set aside.
- In a large bowl, combine the almond flour, protein powder, coconut flour, sugar replacement, baking soda, and salt. With a whisk or a fork, combine the dry ingredients so they are evenly mixed and distributed in and amongst one another.
- In a separate smaller bowl, whisk together eggs with the yogurt.
- Pour egg mixture into the dry ingredients. Whisk together to combine.
- Fold in the strawberries.
- The batter should be like a thick pancake batter. These ingredients tend to be a bit inconsistent from brand to brand and grind to grind. You may need to add a little water or almond milk to thin it out (just not too much!).
- Once the batter is well mixed, pour even amounts between the 12 muffin cups.
- Bake for about 18 to 21 minutes, or until the muffins have crowned and the surface is dry, beginning to crisp, and has turned golden.
- Remove from the oven and let rest for 5 minutes before removing from the pan.
- Serve with more yogurt!

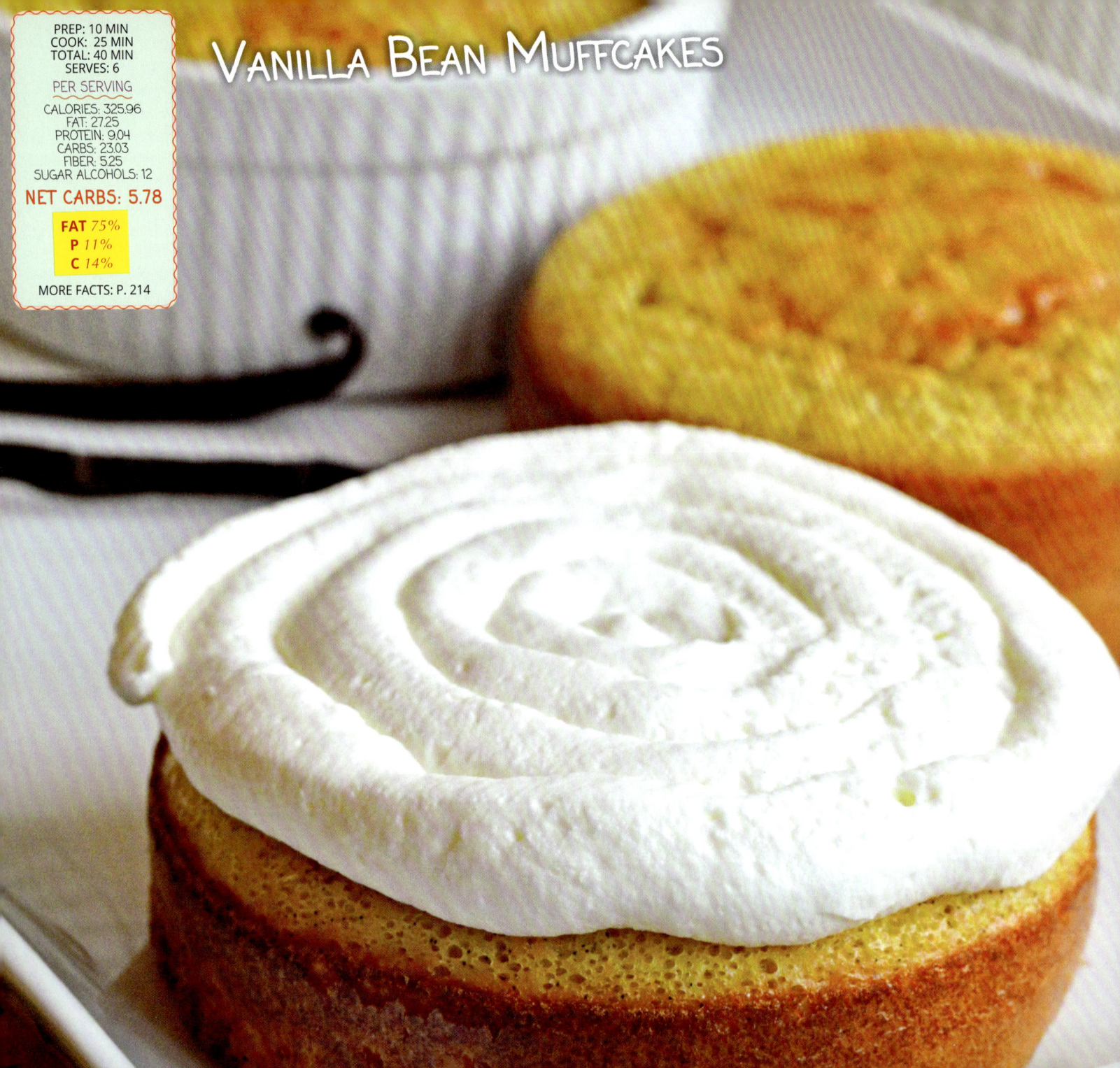

Vanilla Bean Muffcakes

PREP: 10 MIN
COOK: 25 MIN
TOTAL: 40 MIN
SERVES: 6

PER SERVING
CALORIES: 325.96
FAT: 27.25
PROTEIN: 9.04
CARBS: 23.03
FIBER: 5.25
SUGAR ALCOHOLS: 12
NET CARBS: 5.78

FAT 75%
P 11%
C 14%

MORE FACTS: P. 214

Did you know that both chocolate and vanilla come from Mexico? The vanilla pod, from the vanilla orchid, was first cultivated about 600 years ago by the Totonac people in an area currently occupied by the Mexican state of Veracruz. Shortly thereafter, the Aztecs showed the Totonac people who the boss was, developing a taste for vanilla in the process. *They* called it *tlilxochitl*, meaning "black flower."

It was Spanish conquistador Hernán Cortés who is credited with introducing both vanilla and chocolate to Europe in the 1520s.

It's interesting to note that while *vanilla* is a term suggesting that something or someone is very ordinary, standard, or without any special or noteworthy features ("Oh, Patricia and Stan are so vanilla!"), the International Ice Cream Organization credits vanilla as being the single most popular ice cream flavor. Twenty-nine percent of people choose vanilla. In second place, a mere 8.9% choose chocolate. Butter-pecan comes in third, with 5.3%. So, for something so strongly associated with bland or uninteresting... it sure is popular!

(I have a sneaking suspicion that it's because A LOT of people get vanilla, then douse it with their favorite toppings, but I have no proof.)

It is in knowing that plain ol' vanilla is top dog that I conclude this book.

Vanilla.

3/4 cup (180ᵐᴸ)	heavy cream
1/4 cup + 2 tbsp (90ᵐᴸ)	sugar replacement
1	vanilla bean
1 cup + 2 tbsp (270ᵐᴸ)	almond flour
1/4 cup + 2 tbsp (90ᵐᴸ)	coconut flour
1 tbsp (15ᵐᴸ)	baking powder
3/4 tsp (4ᵐᴸ)	salt
6 large	eggs

~~~~~~~~~~~~~~~~~~~~~~~~~

- Add the heavy cream and sugar replacement to a small saucepan and place on the stove over medium heat.

- While waiting for the cream mixture to simmer, split the vanilla bean in half lengthwise.

- With the back of a knife, scrape the beans out of the two halves of the pod and place in the small saucepan. Add the scraped pod halves to the pan, as well.

- Once the cream mixture is *just* starting to simmer, whisk the mixture to make sure the sweetener has fully dissolved. Remove from heat, cover, and set aside to steep for 15 minutes.

- After 15 minutes, mix again, cover, and allow to steep for a final 15 minutes.

- Strain cream mixture, removing and discarding the pods and any fibrous matter that may have broken off of them. Set cream mixture aside.

- Preheat oven to 350° F (177° C).

- Grease six 8 oz (240ᵐᴸ) ceramic ramekins (or any other non-porous, similarly sized, oven-friendly baking vessels).

- In a large bowl, combine the almond flour, coconut flour, baking powder, and salt. With a whisk or a fork, combine the dry ingredients so they are evenly mixed and distributed in and amongst one another.

- In a separate smaller bowl, whisk eggs until lemony in color. While whisking, pour in the warm cream mixture and whisk until well combined.

- Pour egg mixture into the dry ingredients. Whisk together to combine.

- The batter should be like a thick pancake batter. These ingredients tend to be a bit inconsistent from brand to brand and grind to grind. You may need to add a little water to thin it out (just not too much!).

- Once the batter is well mixed, pour even amounts between the 6 cups.

- Bake for about 23 to 28 minutes, or until the muffins have crowned and the surface is dry, beginning to crisp, and has turned golden.

- Remove from the oven and let rest for 5 minutes before removing from the pan.

- Like/unlike the *ever-so-vanilla* Pat and Stan it seems logical to serve with a frumpy whipped cream spiral!

- (I'd TOTALLY smother this with a warm berry goo!... Put some berries in a saucepan and simmer... in a separate bowl, mix some powdered sweetener with a tiny amount of xanthan gum, tapioca starch and/or arrowroot, and a dash of salt. Mix together, then add to berries, while stirring. Let simmer for about 2 more minutes to thicken. Works with apples, too. Goo!)

BONUS

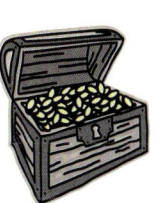

In this next section, I'm going to include the quick-bread recipes that exist on my website. They're already written, they're fully beloved on the social networks, are tried, true, and it just makes a whole lot of sense to keep them all together.

Some break outside the ratios given early in the book, but they were written prior to my having that little epiphany. Additionally, these recipes are all quite flexible, suggesting that "close enough" can also be "good enough."

Enjoy them!

Chocolate OMM

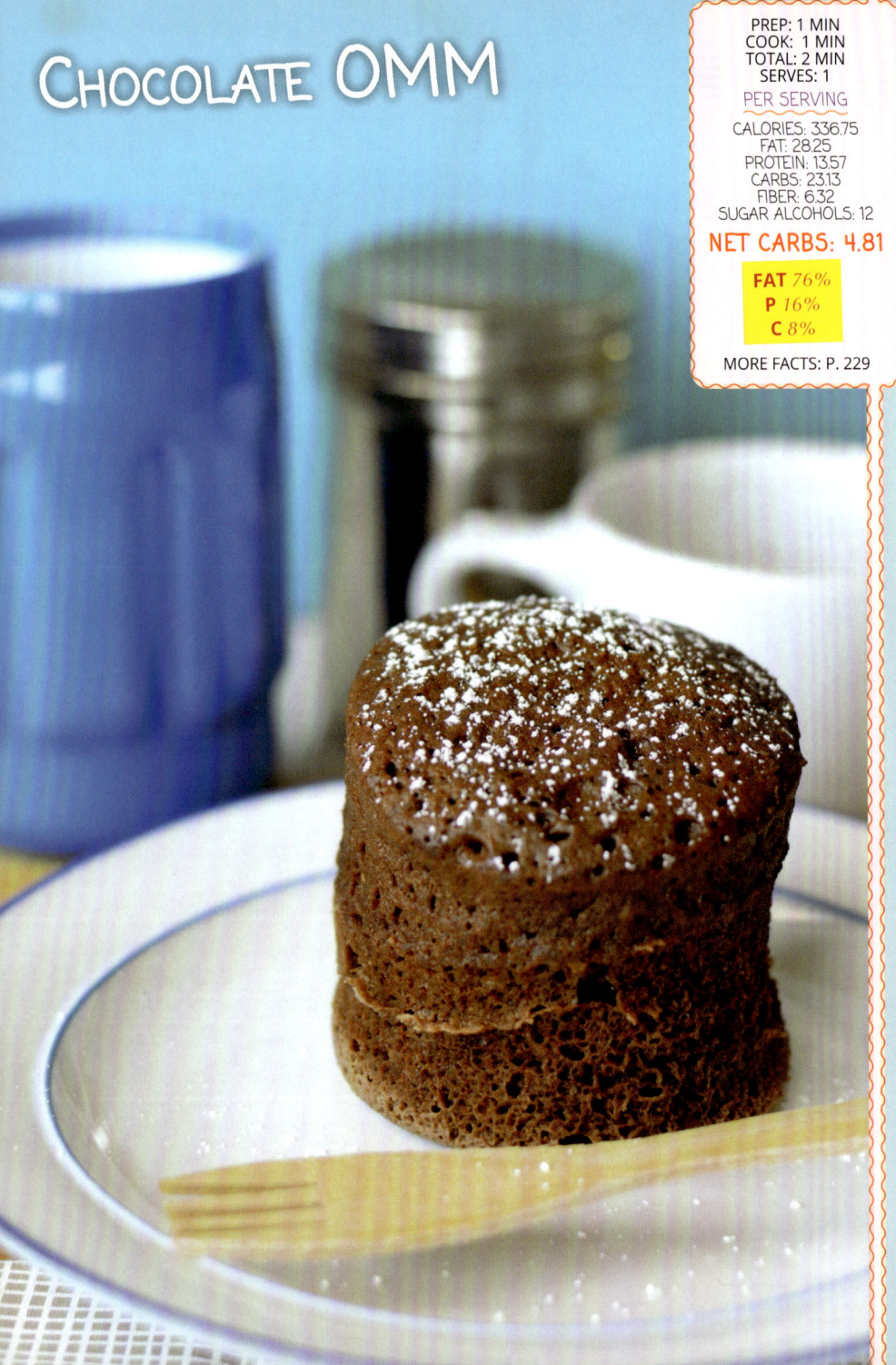

PREP: 1 MIN
COOK: 1 MIN
TOTAL: 2 MIN
SERVES: 1

PER SERVING

CALORIES: 336.75
FAT: 28.25
PROTEIN: 13.57
CARBS: 23.13
FIBER: 6.32
SUGAR ALCOHOLS: 12

NET CARBS: 4.81

FAT 76%
P 16%
C 8%

MORE FACTS: P. 229

Try folding some raspberries and toasted almond slivers into this delicious Chocolate OMM (One-Minute Muffin) for a super tasty treat! Try chopping up some sugar-free chocolate bars and folding the chocolate chunks into the batter. This would become a truly hot, melty, gooey, double-chocolate delight... in 120 seconds! I know that some consider bananas to be the root of all evil, but with a small amount of freshly smooshed banana, maybe some natural banana flavoring, and a few toasted walnuts, a low-primal chocolate banana treat is quickly within reach! Maybe throw some espresso grounds into the batter. Make a Morning Mocha Alert (MMA OMM)! Try putting a nice dollop of almond butter in the center, before nuking it up. Chocolate and almond butter! MMMMmmmm...

2 tbsp (30ᵐᴸ)	flaxseed meal
2 tbsp (30ᵐᴸ)	almond meal
1 tbsp (15ᵐᴸ)	sugar replacement
1 tbsp (15ᵐᴸ)	unsweetened cocoa powder
1/2 tsp (3ᵐᴸ)	baking powder
Dash	salt
1 large	egg
1 tbsp (15ᵐᴸ)	melted butter

- Combine your flax, almond meal, sugar replacement, cocoa powder, baking powder, and salt in a coffee mug or other microwaveable safe mold of some kind. (I like to grease my mug first, but I don't think it's necessary.)
- Mix in your egg and melted butter.
- Microwave on high for 60 seconds (90 seconds if using a weaker microwave, or if you've added lots of other ingredients, like nuts, frozen berries, etc.).
- Enjoy!

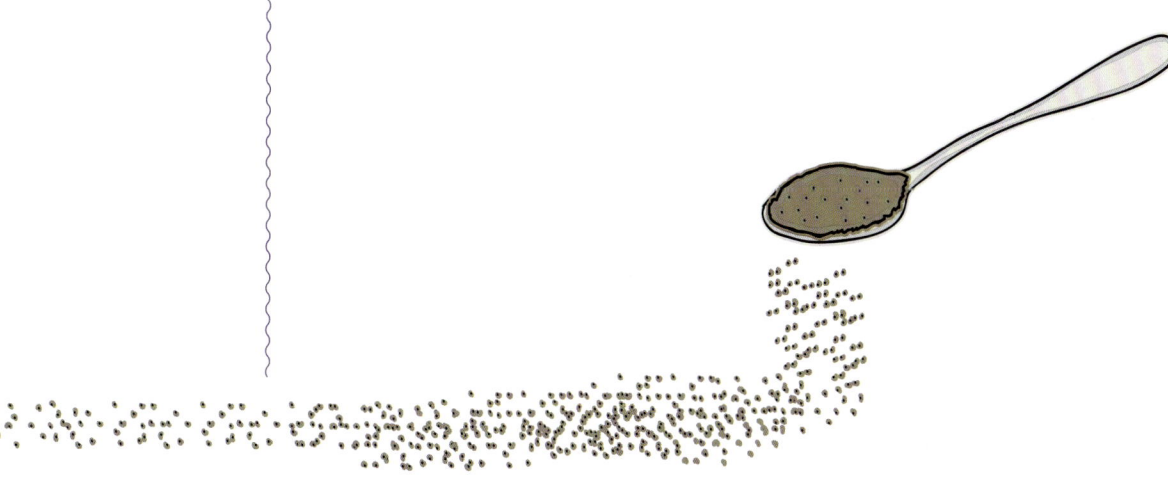

Cinnamon Roll OMM

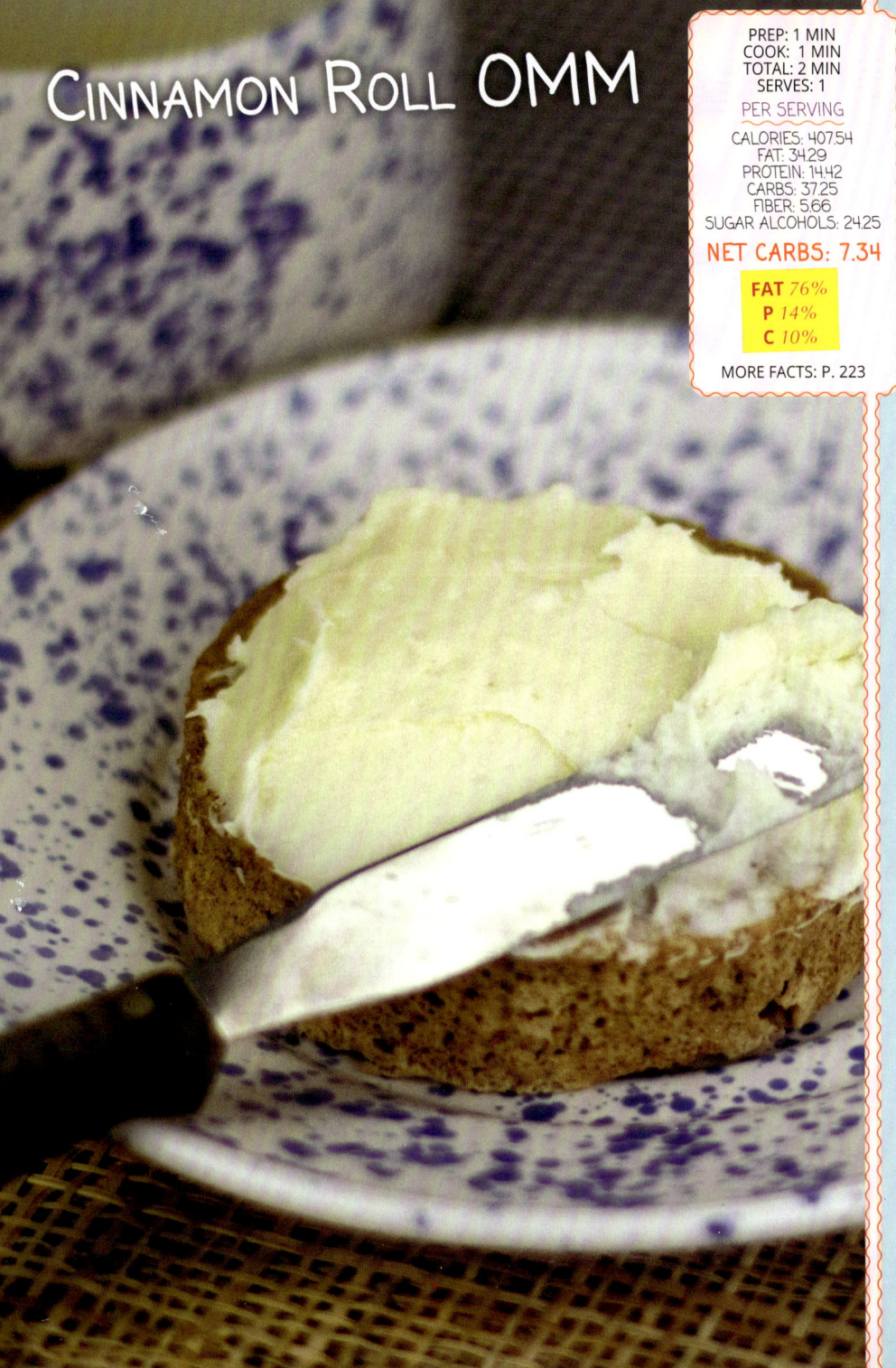

PREP: 1 MIN
COOK: 1 MIN
TOTAL: 2 MIN
SERVES: 1

PER SERVING

CALORIES: 407.54
FAT: 34.29
PROTEIN: 14.42
CARBS: 37.25
FIBER: 5.66
SUGAR ALCOHOLS: 24.25

NET CARBS: 7.34

FAT 76%
P 14%
C 10%

MORE FACTS: P. 223

As a kid, I fell in love with cinnamon rolls at a Fresno farmers' market. The market had sweet, hot, fresh, steaming, aromatic cinnamon rolls. These rolls became almost something like a part of my own DNA. Without them, I couldn't function. Years later, I owned a catering company outside of Cabo San Lucas, in Mexico. To promote the catering business, I set up camp on the weekend at a local farmers' market. Onsite, I baked fresh cinnamon rolls, for all the world to sniff out and eat. I LOVE cinnamon rolls!

2 tbsp (30 mL)	flaxseed meal
2 tbsp (30 mL)	almond meal
2 tsp (10 mL)	sugar replacement
1/2 tsp (3 mL)	ground cinnamon
1/2 tsp (3 mL)	baking powder
Dash	salt
1 tbsp (15 mL)	chopped walnuts
1 tsp (5 mL)	quartered raisins
1 large	egg
1 tsp (5 mL)	melted butter
3 tbsp (45 mL)	cream cheese frosting (p. 196)

- Combine the flax, almond meal, sugar replacement, cinnamon, baking powder, and salt in a coffee mug or other microwaveable safe mold of some kind. (I like to grease my mug first, but I don't think it's necessary.)
- Mix in your raisins, walnuts, egg, and melted butter.
- Microwave on high for 60 seconds (90 seconds if using a weaker microwave).
- Once your muffin is done, slather with frosting and smile, smile, smile!

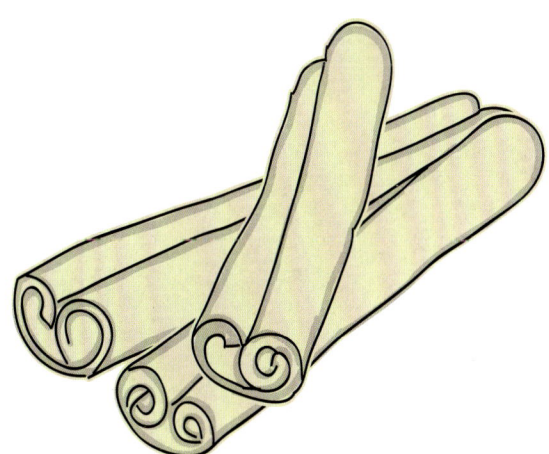

OMM French Toast

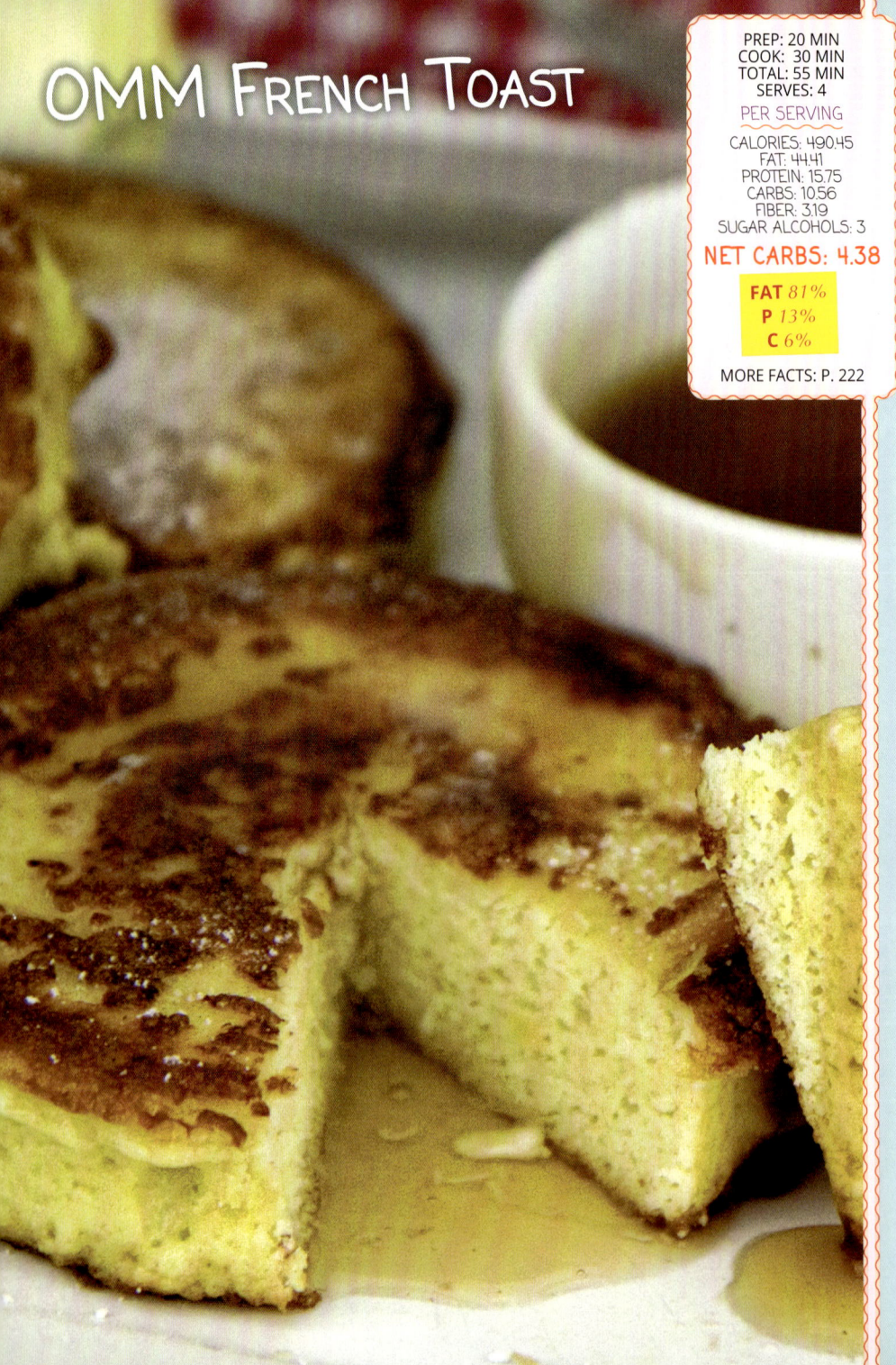

PREP: 20 MIN
COOK: 30 MIN
TOTAL: 55 MIN
SERVES: 4

PER SERVING
CALORIES: 490.45
FAT: 44.41
PROTEIN: 15.75
CARBS: 10.56
FIBER: 3.19
SUGAR ALCOHOLS: 3

NET CARBS: 4.38

FAT 81%
P 13%
C 6%

MORE FACTS: P. 222

I was lurking on a Paleo Facebook page (called Chowstalker) and noticed a post about "Paleo-friendly English muffin in a hurry." In the comments, Sve Ta suggested "you can french toust, too." Immediately, I knew I wanted that!

This whole recipe came about because Chowstalker shared an English muffin recipe and someone else commented that French toast could be a way to go.

Note: It should be noted that this is a great use of a microwave. Because these *fake* evenly and don't crown like they would in an oven, they toast perfectly and evenly in the pan!

1/4 cup (60 mL)	coconut flour
1 tbsp (15 mL)	sugar replacement
2 tsp (10 mL)	baking powder
1 hearty dash (1 mL)	salt
8 large	whole eggs, divided
3/4 cup (180 mL)	unsweetened almond milk, divided
1 tsp (5 mL)	vanilla extract
1/4 cup (60 mL)	melted butter
1/2 cup (120 mL)	heavy cream
1/4 cup (60 mL)	fresh whole butter

- Mix together your coconut flour, sugar replacement (if it's powdered; if it's a liquid, add with the liquids), baking powder, and a dash of salt.

- In a separate bowl, whisk together 4 of the 8 eggs. Add only 1/4 cup (60 mL) of the almond milk and your vanilla. Whisk.

- Add your dry ingredients to your wet ingredients and whisk, while pouring in your melted butter.

- Grease 12 microwave-safe containers that are fairly wide. I used 8 oz (240 mL) ramekins, but you could also use flat-bottomed soup bowls, wide coffee mugs, etc. You could even use tall coffee cups and simply cut your muffins in half.

- Microwave your muffins. For each muffin, add a minute to the microwave. I did 3 batches of 4, with 4 minutes on the timer for each batch. Total: 12 minutes.

- While your muffins are nuking, in a large and wide mixing bowl, whisk together your remaining 4 eggs, 1/2 cup (120 mL) of almond milk, and 1/2 cup (120 mL) of heavy cream.

- As your muffins come out of the nuker, pop them out of their containers and let them cool for about 1 minute—just long enough to keep them from cooking the egg mixture. When they are cool enough, add them to the egg mixture and allow to sit for a few minutes, flipping them occasionally. They are somewhat fragile, but not too bad. You can fairly easily grab and flip them around. They will absorb the egg mixture.

- When they have absorbed some of the egg mixture, heat a large skillet, sauté pan, or flat-top griddle over medium-low heat. Add some of your fresh butter and melt it. Everyone has their own method for doing this. So, I'm just going to say... Fry like you're making French toast!

- Keep warm in the oven until they are all ready. Serve!

- **Baking Note:** It makes some sense to simply grease a 12-cup muffin pan and bake these for about 12 minutes at 400°F (204°C). Then, pop them out of their cups and slice them in half, so they can cool and will absorb the egg mixture more quickly and fry more evenly. Again, the downside is that the muffins will crown, making half of them semi-spheres and tougher to fry. For those looking to avoid the nuker, this is a way to go. It will result in 24 discs instead of 12.

One-Minute Cheddar Bread and Buns

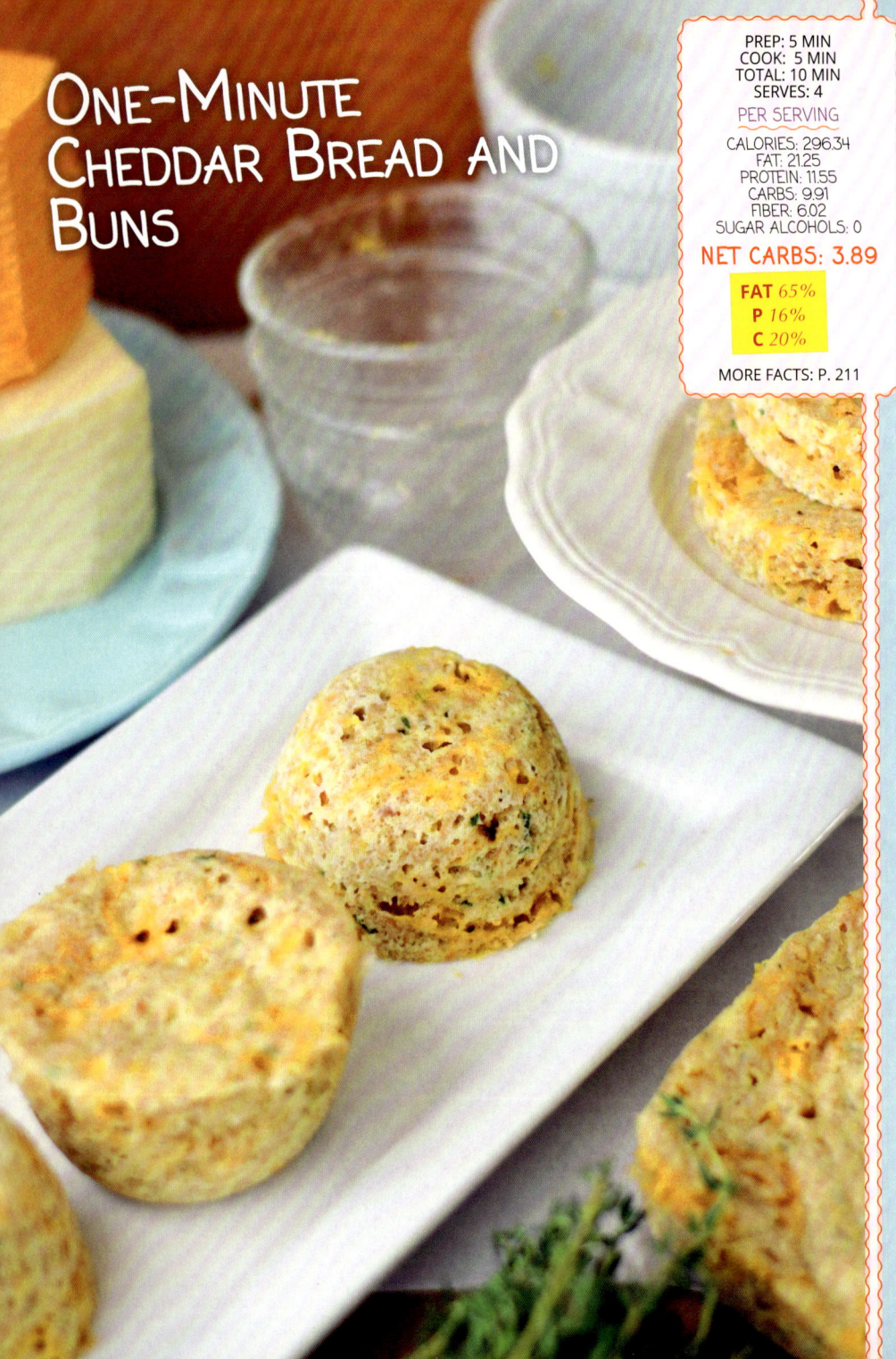

PREP: 5 MIN
COOK: 5 MIN
TOTAL: 10 MIN
SERVES: 4

PER SERVING

CALORIES: 296.34
FAT: 21.25
PROTEIN: 11.55
CARBS: 9.91
FIBER: 6.02
SUGAR ALCOHOLS: 0

NET CARBS: 3.89

FAT 65%
P 16%
C 20%

MORE FACTS: P. 211

OMMs also take the shape of anything you put the batter in. In the photo, you'll see that I have little round ones and bigger square ones. The smaller ones were nuked in little 6.5 ounce glass cups that I stash homemade ice cream in. The bigger ones were nuked in microwaveable plastic sandwich containers.

Once you make the blob, you can spray the container with some spray (or butter it up!), then pour the batter into it. You can expect it to rise about double the height of the batter.

1 cup (240ᵐᴸ)	flaxseed meal
2 tsp (10ᵐᴸ)	baking powder
4 large	eggs
1 tbsp (15ᵐᴸ)	melted butter
1/2 cup (120ᵐᴸ)	grated cheddar/ colby blend
2 cloves	garlic, minced
1/2 tsp (3ᵐᴸ)	fresh chopped thyme
To taste	salt, fresh-cracked pepper, and chili flakes

≶ Grease your microwaveable containers.

≶ Combine all ingredients, then distribute evenly between your chosen nuking vessels.

≶ Microwave on high for 60 to 90 seconds (I had better luck at 90 seconds). Let the containers sit in the microwave for 1 more minute.

≶ **Note:** This recipe makes 4 large coffee cup-sized buns, 4 sandwich squares or about 6 small buns. Also note that I used golden flaxseed meal in this to get the lighter color, but it would work with the darker shade, as well.

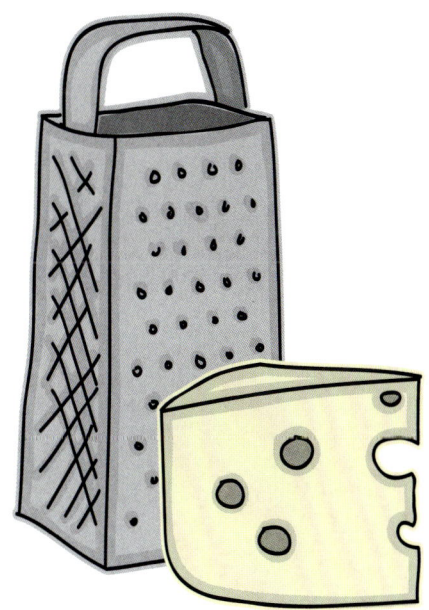

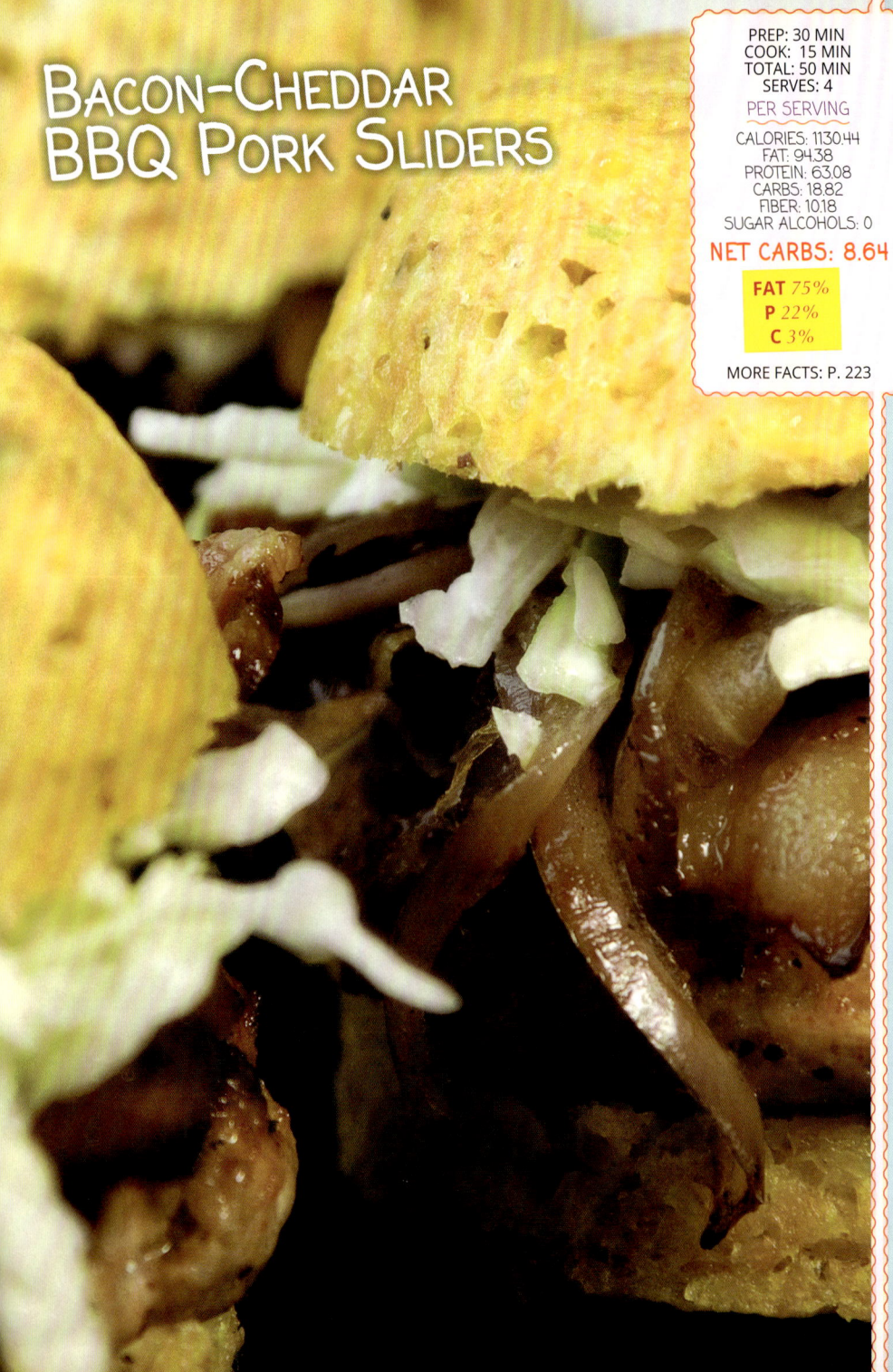

Bacon-Cheddar BBQ Pork Sliders

PREP: 30 MIN
COOK: 15 MIN
TOTAL: 50 MIN
SERVES: 4

PER SERVING

CALORIES: 1130.44
FAT: 94.38
PROTEIN: 63.08
CARBS: 18.82
FIBER: 10.18
SUGAR ALCOHOLS: 0

NET CARBS: 8.64

FAT 75%
P 22%
C 3%

MORE FACTS: P. 223

I'm not completely sure where this idea came from. I'm a massive fan of anything BBQ'd, and had just made my first batch of one-minute bread, ever. I wanted to try something small, tasty and... to use my own slangy vernacular... *grubbin'*.

This starts with ground pork from the butcher. I added all the spices and flavorings I'd add to a dry rub for a smoked pork butt. The flavor profile is about the same. Then I added coleslaw, which is a traditional fixin' for a BBQ pork sandwich. Then, to make it more "slider-y," I topped it with some caramelized onions and crispy bacon!

This was all placed within small one-minute cheddar buns and... well... I'm not sure what happened after that. They disappeared so quickly! "Where did they go?", he says guiltily with a spot of sauce on his cheek and forehead.

These little guys are perfect for a summer day, Super Bowl party, Fourth of July BBQ, or any meal of the day: breakfast, lunch, or dinner.

1 1/2 lb (681g)	ground pork
2 tbsp (30mL)	Dijon mustard
3 cloves	garlic, minced
1 tbsp (15mL)	paprika (preferably smoked)
1 tsp (5mL)	ground cayenne pepper
1 tsp (5mL)	fresh chopped thyme
12 slices	raw bacon
1 small	onion, sliced into strips
3/4 cup (180mL)	low-sugar BBQ sauce
12	mini one-minute cheddar buns (p. 172)
1 cup (240mL)	Sweet 'n' Creamy Coleslaw (p. 176)
To taste	salt and fresh-cracked pepper

- **Note:** This recipe assumes you've already got coleslaw, BBQ sauce, and one-minute buns all ready to go.
- In a mixing bowl, blend together your pork, mustard, garlic, paprika, cayenne, thyme, and a little salt and pepper. Mix well and then divide into twelve 2-oz (56 g) balls.
- Press each ball into a small pork patty. Set aside.
- Fry up 12 slices of bacon, saving the bacon fat. When the bacon is ready, dry on paper towels. Tear each slice in half.
- Place a sauté pan over medium-high heat. Add about 2 tablespoons (30mL) of the bacon grease to the pan.
- Quickly add your onions to the pan with a little salt and pepper. Cook the onions until they have caramelized and have turned a nice shade of brown. Lower and slower is better (yields a softer and more charismatic onion), but high heat is fine, as well. Keep the onions warm, but set aside.
- Season your pork patties with a little salt and pepper. Cook them like you'd cook a hamburger (everyone has their way of doing this... in a pan, over a grill, in a George Foreman grill, etc. I recommend high heat and don't overcook them). Baste them with a little BBQ sauce as they cook.
- Split your buns in half. Spread a small amount of BBQ sauce on the tops and bottoms.
- Assemble 12 small sliders with the bun bottoms, a pork patty, 2 half-slices of bacon, caramelized onions, coleslaw, and a lid. Call your friends!

Sweet 'n' Creamy Coleslaw

PREP: 10 MIN
COOK: 20 MIN
TOTAL: 30 MIN
SERVES: 8

PER SERVING

CALORIES: 113.17
FAT: 10.43
PROTEIN: 1.34
CARBS: 5.57
FIBER: 2.38
SUGAR ALCOHOLS: 0.28

NET CARBS: 2.9

FAT 83%
P 5%
C 12%

MORE FACTS: P. 224

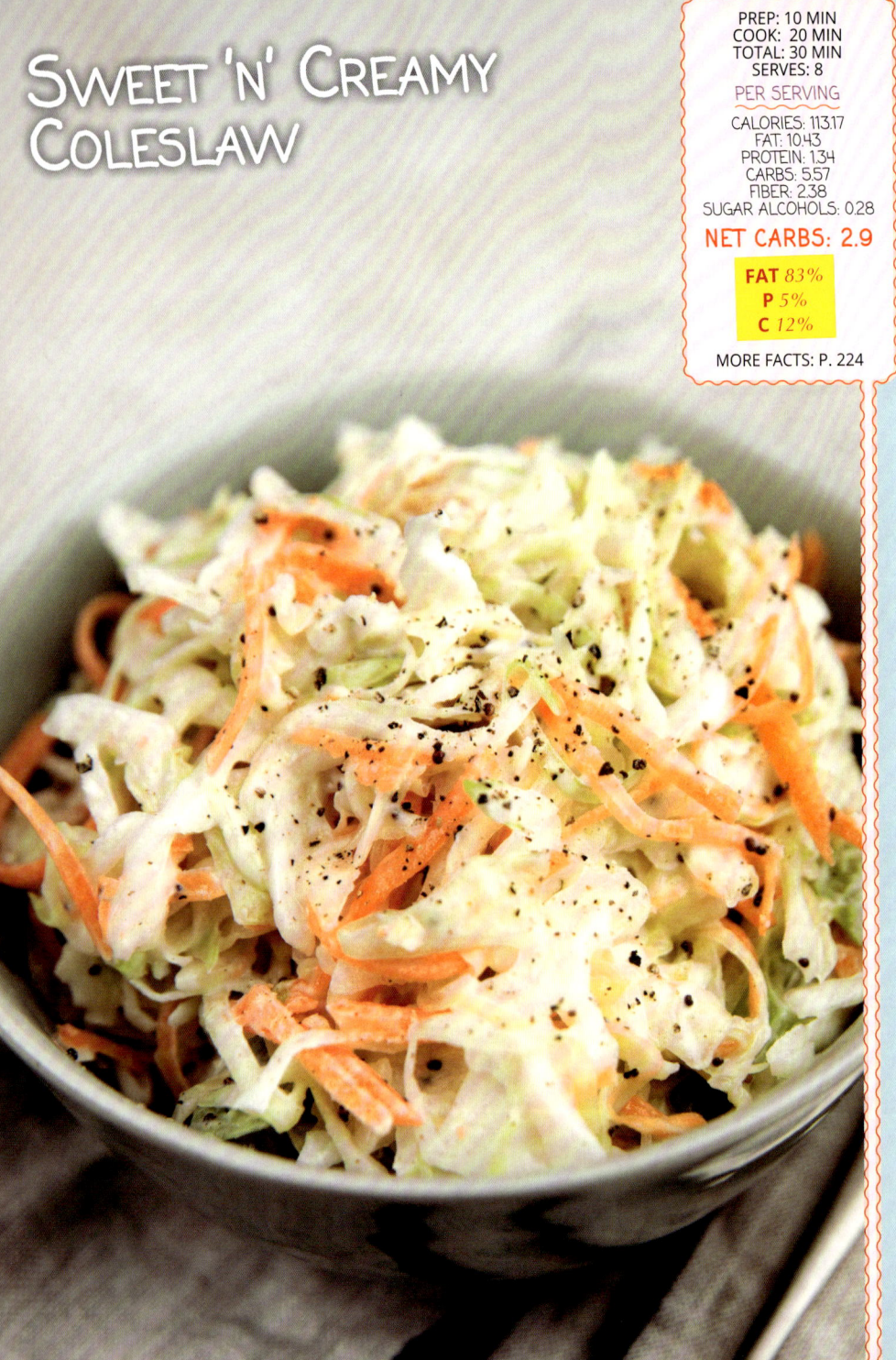

Coleslaw is a relative newcomer in my life. I would NEVER eat it growing up. The idea of cabbage was just foul to me. Mayo wasn't a favorite, and a sweetened creamy cabbage salad just sounded... yuck. As I aged and learned about foods, I started to gain an appreciation for coleslaw. Now, it's... *YUM*!

At its core, it's a really basic salad. It's literally mayonnaise with a little sugar, tossed with shredded cabbage and carrots. That's it! I've seen all kinds of variations over the years, though. Shredded raw broccoli (and stems) with cabbage, carrots, raisins, and almonds, for example. Raw sliced onions are another common addition. Just about anything is improved with the addition of bacon! Poppy seeds, celery seeds, sesame seeds, and pecans. Dried cranberries. Apples, orange juice, and orange zest. My suggestion is... start with a good base and toss the stuff you love into it!

All this said, I'm generally pretty simple and straightforward. Sometimes I like to get zany, but streamlined is also a fantastic approach. It's a purist's minimalist coleslaw. Great on BBQ Sliders *(p. 174)*!

8 cups (1.9ᴸ)	shredded cabbage (about 1/2 head)
1/4 cup (60ᵐᴸ)	grated carrot
1/2 cup (120ᵐᴸ)	mayonnaise
2 tbsp (30ᵐᴸ)	fresh lemon juice
2 tbsp (30ᵐᴸ)	sugar replacement
To taste	salt and fresh-cracked pepper

- Combine all the ingredients.
- Let sit for 20 minutes before eating.
- Enjoy!

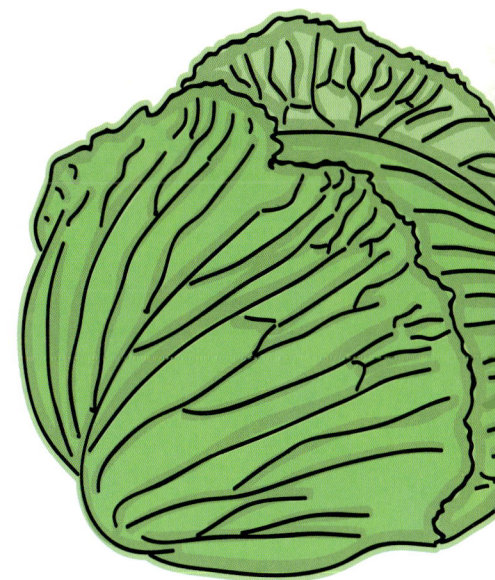

Blue Cheese Lamburgers with Poppy Seed OMMs

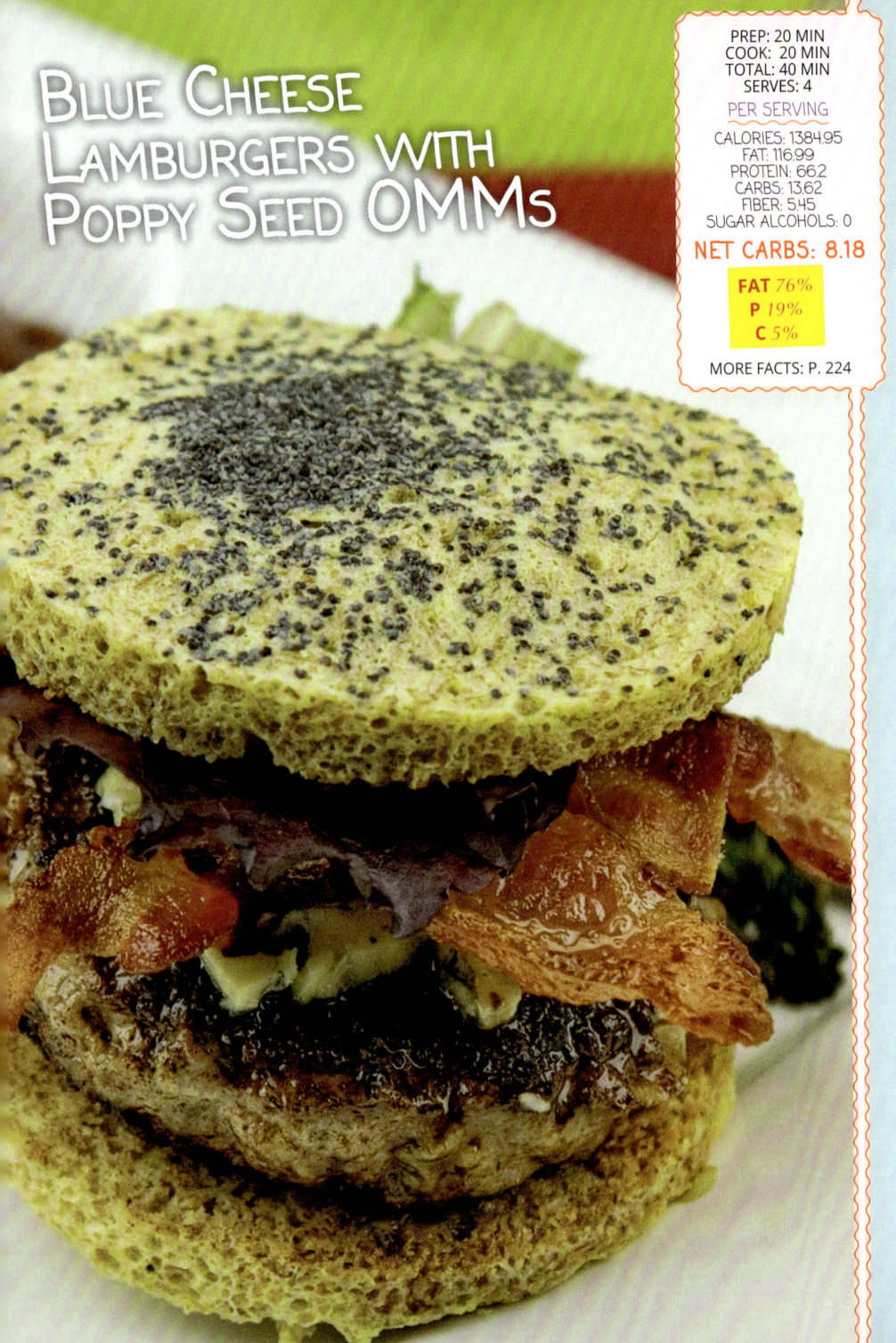

PREP: 20 MIN
COOK: 20 MIN
TOTAL: 40 MIN
SERVES: 4

PER SERVING
CALORIES: 1384.95
FAT: 116.99
PROTEIN: 66.2
CARBS: 13.62
FIBER: 5.45
SUGAR ALCOHOLS: 0

NET CARBS: 8.18

FAT 76%
P 19%
C 5%

MORE FACTS: P. 224

I like hamburgers. They're delicious! While they're not technically, historically "American" food, I feel pretty strongly that the US has appropriated the burger as its own (for better or worse).

While I *do* enjoy a good piece of ground beef, I also like to play with the idea. A "burger," in my opinion, doesn't necessarily need to be beef. There are those who make them with pork, turkey, chicken, a combination of ground meats, sausage patties, etc. There are also burgers served with buns, open faced, packed in lettuce leaves and so on. I've also seen burgers made from fish and seafood blends. Of course, there are also a whole range of veggie burgers, including the common Portobello burger, where the patty is a giant, tasty mushroom cap. In this case, I'm playing with the idea and throwing some lamb at the burger: Lamburgers! YUM!

I'm using ground lamb and adding a few goodies to the raw meat, just to add a little more flavor and charm. I'm also using a very simple One-Minute Muffin as the bun, but split in the middle, brushed with butter, and toasted. Then I'm topping it all with little more than baby greens, bacon, and... blue cheese. If I haven't said it yet (I have)... I'll say it again: *YUM!*

Poppy Seed Omms

1/2 cup (120mL)	flaxseed meal
1/2 cup (120mL)	almond flour
2 tsp (10mL)	baking powder
4 large	eggs
1/2 tsp (3mL)	salt
1 tbsp (15mL)	melted butter
1 tbsp (15mL)	poppy seeds

Lamburgers

8 slices	raw bacon
1 small	onion, diced
4 cloves	garlic, minced
2 tsp (10mL)	fresh chopped thyme, divided
2 lb (908g)	ground lamb
1 large	egg
1/4 cup (60mL)	fresh whole butter, softened
1 cup (240mL)	loosely crumbled blue cheese
1 cup (240mL)	washed and dried mixed greens
To taste	salt and fresh-cracked pepper

- Combine your flax, almond meal, baking powder, and salt in a mixing bowl.
- Mix in your eggs and butter.
- Evenly distribute your batter into 4 individual bowls (each with a base about as wide as a hamburger patty) or other microwave-safe mold of some kind. (In my case, I used 8 oz (240mL) ramekins, which I like to grease first, but I'm not convinced it's necessary.)
- Sprinkle a small amount of poppy seeds onto the top of each bowl of dough.
- Place all 4 buns in the microwave and nuke on high for 4 to 6 minutes. When they are done, remove them from the microwave and pop them from their bowls. Let them cool.
- Fry up 8 slices of bacon. Tear each one in half. Save the bacon fat.
- Heat a sauté pan over medium heat. When it is hot, add about 1 tbsp (15mL) of bacon fat, onions, garlic, and half of your chopped thyme, with a little bit of salt and pepper. Stir until the onions and garlic turn a light shade of brown. Once the onions are lightly caramelized, place into a mixing bowl and spread them around the bowl into a thin layer, so that they may cool more quickly.
- Add your ground lamb and egg to the onions, with a little salt and pepper. Blend together the lamb, egg, and onion mixture.
- Form 4 nice patties that are a little a little wider than your buns and a little thinner in the center than the rim. As they cook, they will shrink and the center will thicken.
- Turn your oven on to broil.
- Split each bun into two halves.
- Spread your softened butter on the inside of each bun-half. Sprinkle your remaining fresh thyme and a bit of salt and pepper on your buns. Place them, butter side up, on a baking tray.
- Heat a large sauté pan or skillet over high heat. While the pan is heating, season the surface of your patties with a little salt and pepper.
- Add a bit more bacon fat to the hot pan. Swirl it around and then add your burgers to the pan. Do not crowd them. Assuming your pan was hot, they should sear.
- Once your burgers are nicely seared on one side, flip them over and sear the other side.
- When your lamb burgers are close to done, place your buns on the top rack of the oven to toast. When they are toasted, remove them.
- Place 4 bun bottoms on 4 trays. Place a fresh burger on each base, then add crumbled blue cheese, 4 bacon half-slices, and a handful of mixed greens. Add bun lids. Enjoy!

Greasy Fried Pork Sandwich

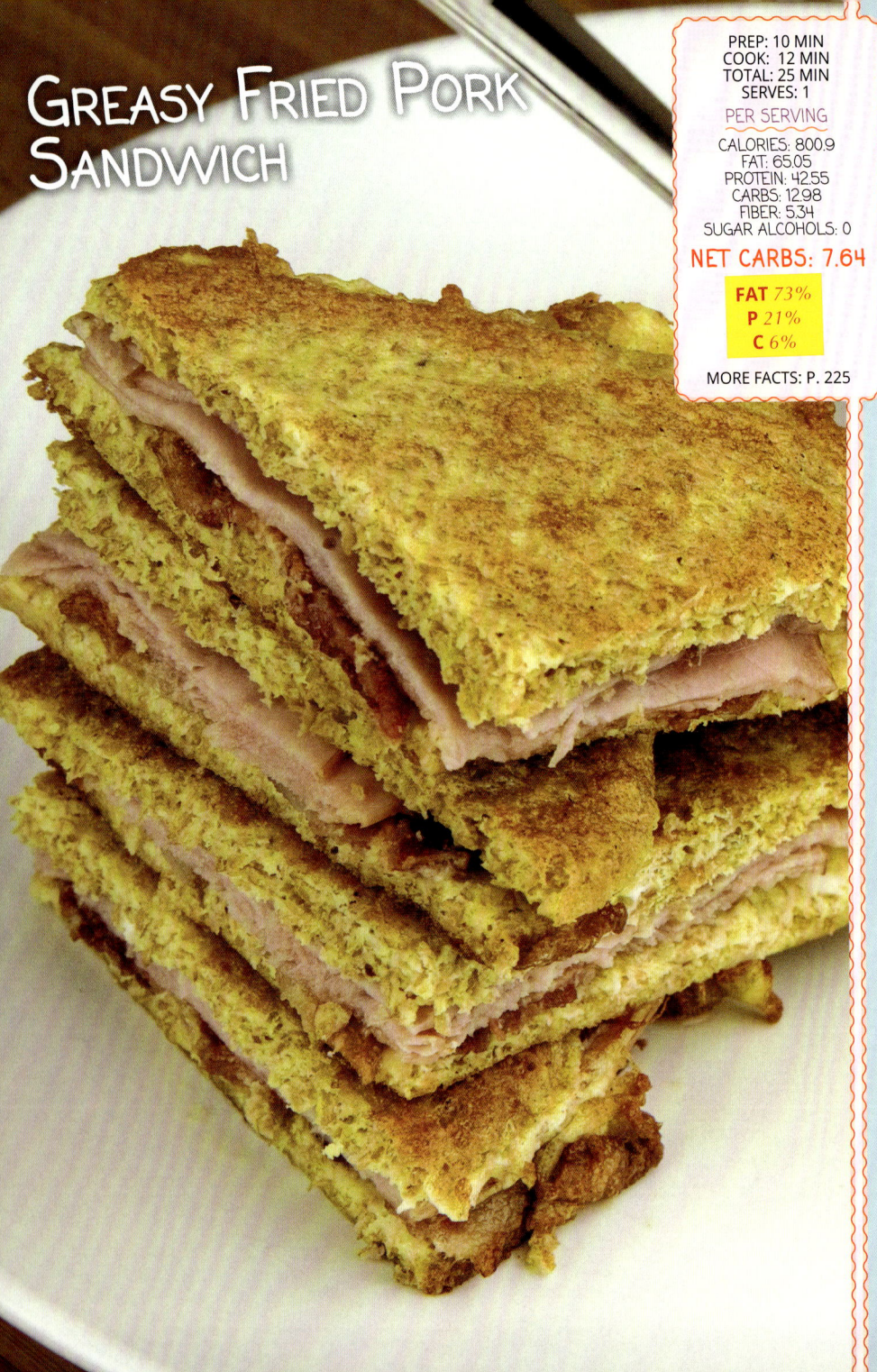

PREP: 10 MIN
COOK: 12 MIN
TOTAL: 25 MIN
SERVES: 1

PER SERVING
CALORIES: 800.9
FAT: 65.05
PROTEIN: 42.55
CARBS: 12.98
FIBER: 5.34
SUGAR ALCOHOLS: 0

NET CARBS: 7.64

FAT *73%*
P *21%*
C *6%*

MORE FACTS: P. 225

This one kind of makes me chuckle.

One day, just sort of playing around, I had this desire for a deep and greasy fried pork sandwich. I don't know why. I think I'd just watched *Weird Science*. I just wanted something greasy, wonderful and amazing, but that felt bad... dirty... *wrong*. To stave off a cheat, what I came up with is nothing short of spectacular! It's little more than a blend of a basic square one-minute muffin, which is then split in half, loaded with a bit of ham and crispy bacon, and then dipped into an egg bath. From there, it's fried like French toast. Kind of like a greasy-spoon version of a Monte Cristo. Oh, I was so happy!

Bread/Muffin

2 tbsp (30 mL)	flaxseed meal
2 tbsp (30 mL)	almond meal
1 large	egg
1 tsp (5 mL)	melted bacon fat or butter
1/2 tsp (3 mL)	baking powder
Dash	salt

The Rest of the Fixin's

3 slices	deli ham
3 slices	pre-cooked and crispy bacon
1 large	egg
2 tbsp (30 mL)	heavy cream
1 tbsp (15 mL)	bacon fat or butter
To taste	salt and pepper

- In a flat-bottomed glass or china bowl (preferably square and about the surface area of sandwich bread), mix the ingredients for your muffin. Microwave this for 60 to 90 seconds on high. Let the bread sit for a further 60 seconds. Remove from the microwave and slice into two halves (a top and a bottom).
- Line the bottom with ham and bacon. Place the top on the sandwich.
- In a separate bowl (I used a pie tin), whisk your egg and cream with a little salt and pepper.
- Add your sandwich to the egg mixture and coat it evenly, flipping it over and pushing it into the egg mixture, so that the bread absorbs the egg like a sponge. This may take a few minutes, but just keep flipping it. Eventually, most of it gets absorbed and you have a nice egg-coated sandwich.
- Heat a skillet or sauté pan over medium-low heat.
- Add your bacon fat or butter and swirl it around. Add your sandwich to the pan and allow it to turn golden brown on one side. Flip it and cook the other side. Turn the heat down to low and cook for about 4 to 6 minutes on either side, until it's cooked through.
- Cut into tasty pieces and eat!

Frosted Carrot Cake OMM with Pecans

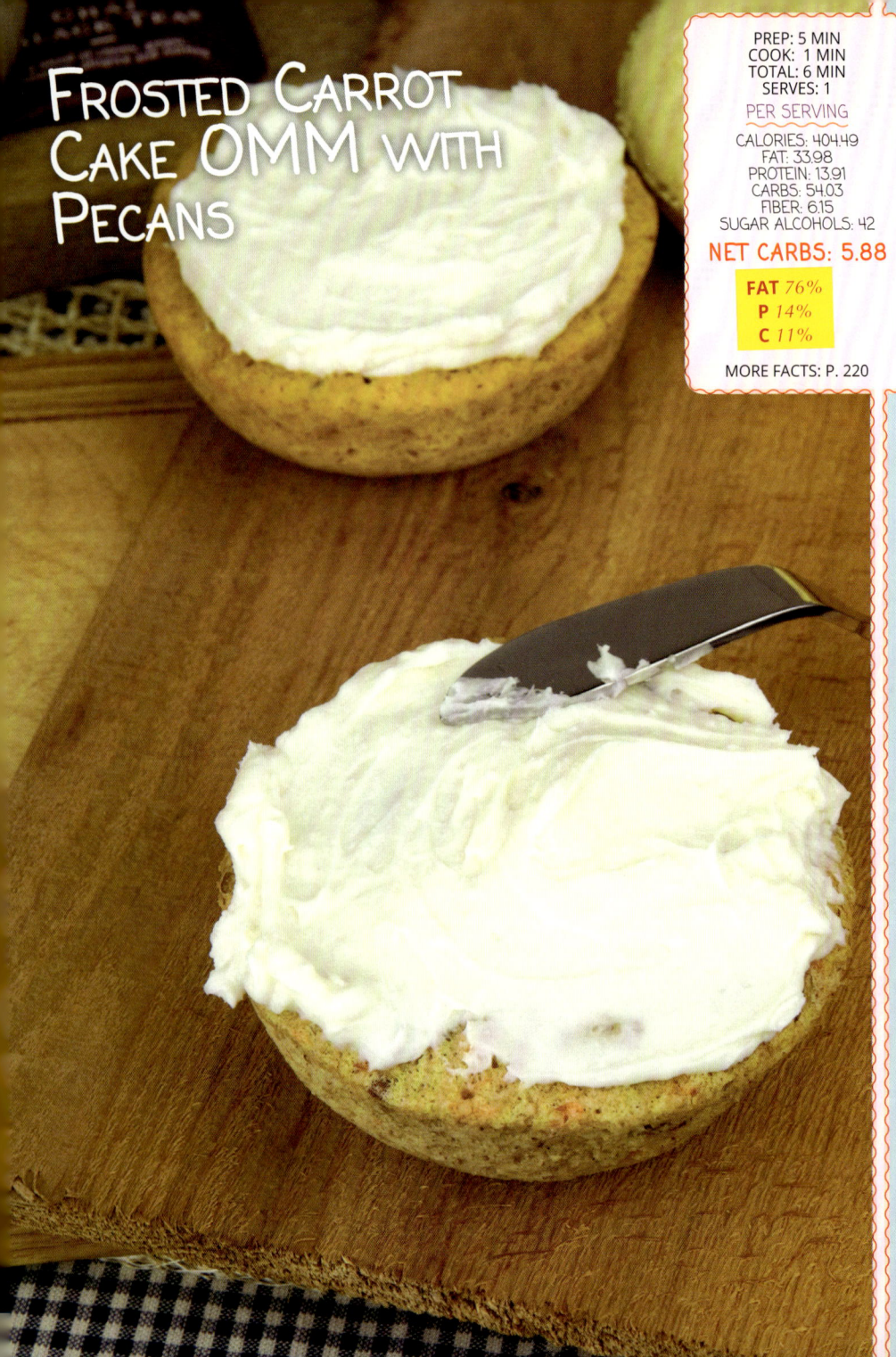

PREP: 5 MIN
COOK: 1 MIN
TOTAL: 6 MIN
SERVES: 1

PER SERVING
CALORIES: 404.49
FAT: 33.98
PROTEIN: 13.91
CARBS: 54.03
FIBER: 6.15
SUGAR ALCOHOLS: 42
NET CARBS: 5.88

FAT 76%
P 14%
C 11%

MORE FACTS: P. 220

Someone, somewhere, at some point in time decided to conduct a poorly run test on cooked carrots, deeming them to be INCREDIBLY high glycemic, converting to glucose in the blood MUCH FASTER than regular ol' table sugar! As a result, these fairly low-carb underground orange sticks have been passed over, time and time again, by folks looking to maintain a stable level of blood sugar.

I'm here to tell you... lies. ALL LIES!!

Carrots are fine! They are, in fact, good for you! Cooked, raw, peeled or unpeeled, carrots are NOT going to hurt you. When I really stop and think about it, it's silly to think that someone, somewhere, at some point in time became obese by a carrot-heavy diet. I just don't believe that to be true.

Carrots were once thought to have a GI of 90+ (pure glucose is 100, while table sugar is merely 65!). Current reports clock cooked carrots in at closer to 30 or 40, which is fairly low glycemic (lower than sweet potatoes).

THESE sweet carrot and pecan muffins attempt to capture the spirit of a fresh carrot cake, smeared with a bit of cream cheese frosting! It's pretty amazing what can be done in 60 seconds!

1/6th recipe

2 tbsp (30ᵐᴸ) flaxseed meal
2 tbsp (30ᵐᴸ) almond meal
2 tbsp (30ᵐᴸ) sugar replacement
1/2 tsp (3ᵐᴸ) baking powder
1/2 tsp (3ᵐᴸ) ground cinnamon
1/4 tsp (1ᵐᴸ) ground nutmeg
Dash salt
2 tbsp (30ᵐᴸ) grated raw carrot
1 tbsp (15ᵐᴸ) chopped pecans
1 large egg
1 tsp (5ᵐᴸ) melted butter
1/2 tsp (3ᵐᴸ) vanilla extract

Cream Cheese Frosting (p. 196)

- **Note:** Make sure you have your Cream Cheese Frosting (p.196) made and ready to go for this recipe.
- In a wide-mouthed coffee mug, combine your flax, almond meal, sugar replacement, baking powder, cinnamon, nutmeg, and salt. (I like to grease my mug first, but I don't think it's necessary.)
- Mix in your carrots, pecans, egg, butter, and vanilla.
- Microwave on high for 60 seconds (90 seconds if using a weaker microwave).
- While the muffin is nuking, beat together your cream cheese, butter, powdered sugar replacement, vanilla, and salt. Make sure your cream cheese and butter are soft (leave out at room temperature for a while) before whipping, or else mixing will be difficult at best.
- Slather some frosting on top. Eat and enjoy!

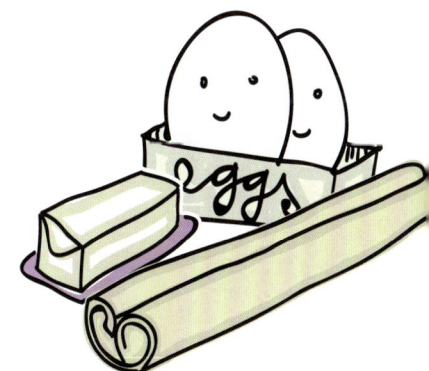

Pumpkin-Spice OMM with Maple Butter

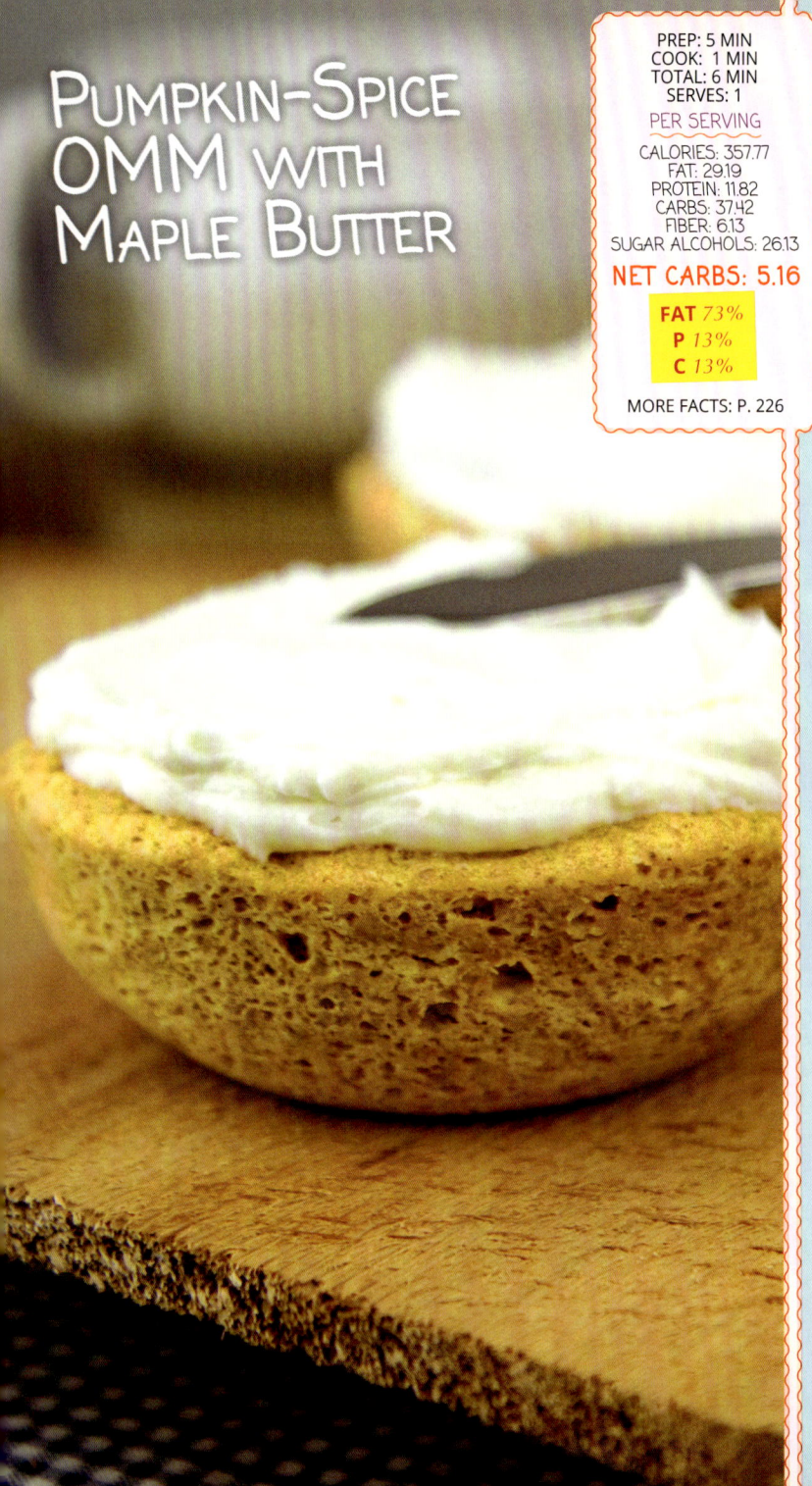

PREP: 5 MIN
COOK: 1 MIN
TOTAL: 6 MIN
SERVES: 1

PER SERVING
CALORIES: 357.77
FAT: 29.19
PROTEIN: 11.82
CARBS: 37.42
FIBER: 6.13
SUGAR ALCOHOLS: 26.13

NET CARBS: 5.16

FAT 73%
P 13%
C 13%

MORE FACTS: P. 226

Here we have a very simple pumpkin One-Minute Muffin. It's little more than a basic OMM recipe, but with the addition of some spices and a healthy spoonful of pumpkin puree! The result is little more than a quick pumpkin yum, perfect for any time of the day!

The one thing that I personally feel makes this a bit on the special side is the partner in crime: maple butter! The reality is, this is something I should have probably made its own recipe, rather than hiding it here, but... that's not the road I chose. Only you reading the Pumpkin OMM recipe will be privy to the maple butter, which is *awesome* slathered on a pork chop! It's *amazing* on a fresh, hot pumpkin OMM straight from the nuker. It's perfect melted on top of a thick stack of pancakes in the morning. Make a batch of this splendid butter and stash it in the freezer, in one big plastic-wrapped log. Just slice off a disk when you need some. You'll find it won't last long!

Maple Butter: The recipe for the maple butter is: 1/2 cup (120^{mL}) butter (softened), 1/4 cup (60^{mL}) sugar-free maple syrup (I prefer a xylitol-based pancake syrup), and a dash of salt. With a mixer, whip the butter until it's light in color and airy. Then pour in the syrup with a dash of salt, and whip until combined. Lay a sheet of plastic wrap on the counter, then spread your butter into a small log. Roll the log in the plastic wrap and refrigerate or freeze. This will make enough butter for about 6 to 8 OMMs. Note that the recipes that follow are for a single serving.

Maple Butter

1 tbsp (15 mL)	butter
1/2 tbsp (8 mL)	sugar-free maple syrup
Dash	salt

Pumpkin-Spice OMM

2 tbsp (30 mL)	flaxseed meal
2 tbsp (30 mL)	hazelnut flour
2 tbsp (30 mL)	sugar replacement
1/2 tsp (3 mL)	baking powder
1/2 tsp (3 mL)	ground cinnamon
1/4 tsp (1 mL)	ground nutmeg
Dash	ground cloves
Dash	powdered ginger
Dash	salt
2 tbsp (30 mL)	mashed pumpkin
1 large	egg

- Read the notes about the Maple Butter, above. The best method for this is to make a large batch in advance.
- In a wide-mouthed coffee mug, combine your flax (or chia), hazelnut (or almond) meal, sugar replacement, baking powder, cinnamon, nutmeg, cloves, ginger, and salt. I like to grease my mug first, but I don't think it's necessary.
- Mix in your egg and pumpkin puree.
- Microwave on high for 60 seconds (90 seconds if using a weaker microwave).
- Alternatively, bake in a muffin tin at 350°F (177°C) for 13 to 15 minutes, or until golden.
- Slather some maple butter on top. Eat and enjoy!

Savory Zucchini, Bacon and Herb OMM

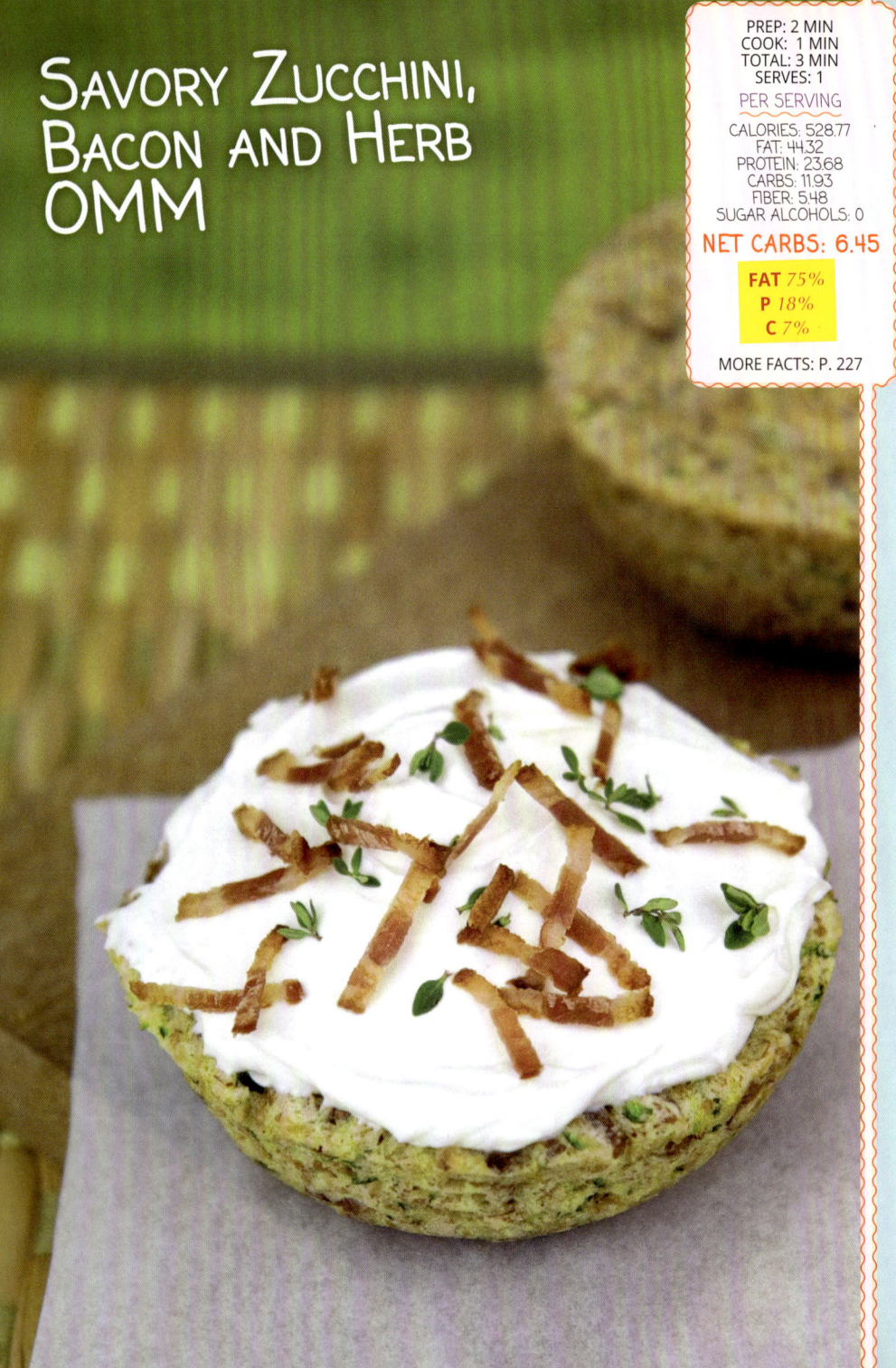

PREP: 2 MIN
COOK: 1 MIN
TOTAL: 3 MIN
SERVES: 1

PER SERVING
CALORIES: 528.77
FAT: 44.32
PROTEIN: 23.68
CARBS: 11.93
FIBER: 5.48
SUGAR ALCOHOLS: 0

NET CARBS: 6.45

FAT 75%
P 18%
C 7%

MORE FACTS: P. 227

Since making my first OMM, I've been tinkering with all sorts of flavors.

I sought to try something different. No more *sweet* flavors, and no simple plain breads, either. I wanted something interesting, unique, and special! The kind of thing you could serve in place of a bread basket during a nice meal and NO ONE would question you about the lack of "bread"... they'd just gobble THESE tasty things down and beg for more!

I chose to go savory this time by starting with a zucchini base. I then incorporated bacon, parmesan, fresh herbs, and a simple topping of cream cheese!

Pretty, tasty, and... pretty tasty, too!

2 tbsp (30mL)	flaxseed meal
2 tbsp (30mL)	almond meal
2 tbsp (30mL)	grated parmesan cheese
1/2 tsp (3mL)	baking powder
Dash	salt
2 tbsp (30mL)	grated zucchini
1 tbsp (15mL)	chopped toasted pecans
1 large	egg
1 tsp (5mL)	melted bacon fat
1 tbsp (15mL)	real bacon bits, divided
1/2 tsp (3mL)	chopped fresh thyme, divided
3 tbsp (45mL)	full fat cream cheese, warmed

- In a wide-mouthed coffee mug, combine your flax, almond meal, parmesan, baking powder, and salt. (I like to grease my mug first, but I don't think it's necessary.)
- Squeeze the water out of your zucchini by squeezing it within your fist, over the sink. Un-clump the zucchini so it is back in strand form.
- Mix in your zucchini, pecans, egg, bacon fat, half of the bacon bits, and half of the thyme.
- Microwave on high for 60 seconds (90 seconds if using a weaker microwave).
- Garnish with a nice layer of cream cheese and then sprinkle the remaining bacon bits and thyme onto the top!

Spiced Zucchini Bread OMM

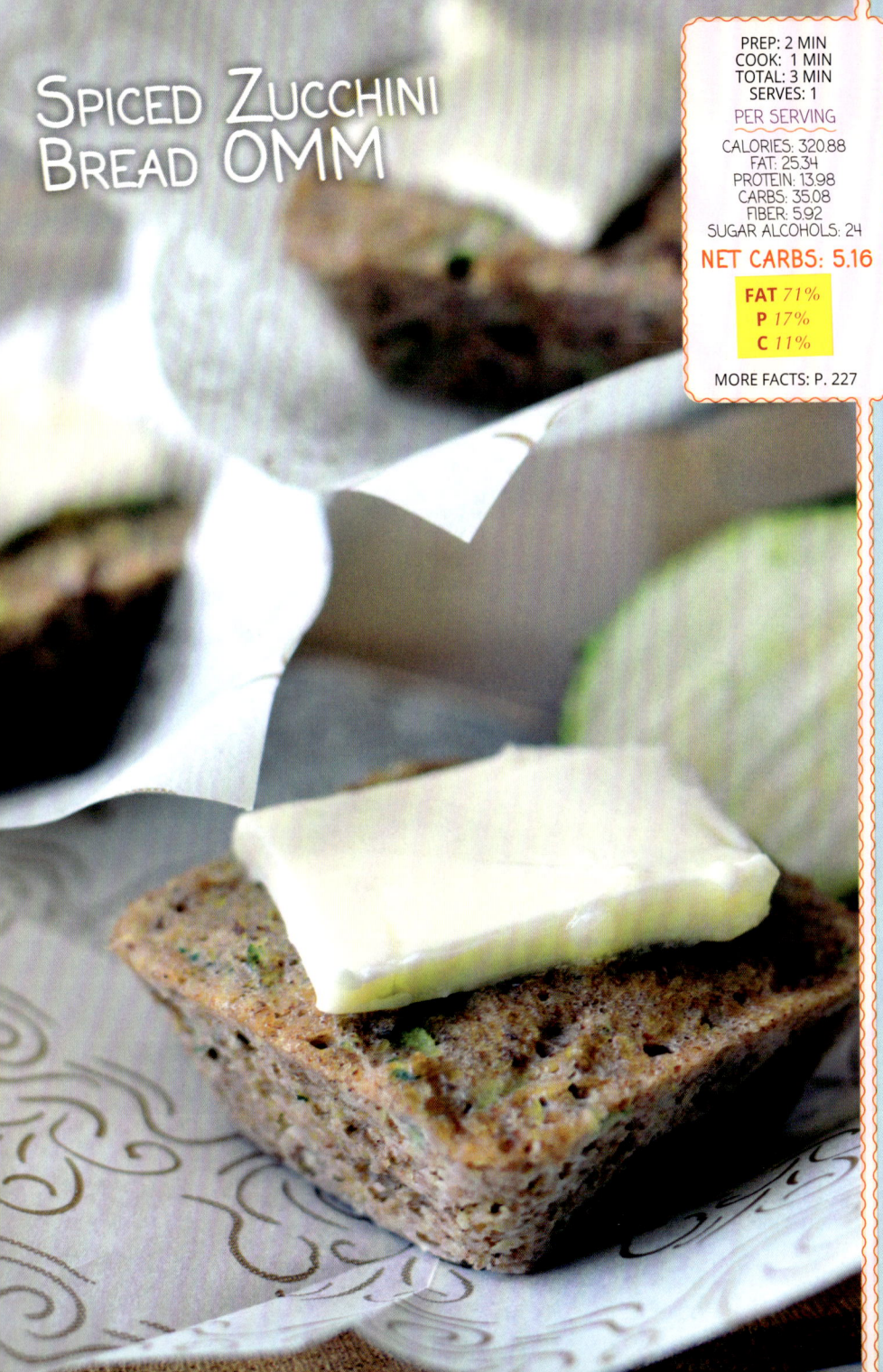

PREP: 2 MIN
COOK: 1 MIN
TOTAL: 3 MIN
SERVES: 1

PER SERVING

CALORIES: 320.88
FAT: 25.34
PROTEIN: 13.98
CARBS: 35.08
FIBER: 5.92
SUGAR ALCOHOLS: 24

NET CARBS: 5.16

FAT *71%*
P *17%*
C *11%*

MORE FACTS: P. 227

I thought about coming up with some kind of exotic frosting for this muffin, but then decided to keep it simple. Fresh from the microwave, this hearty treat is MORE than complemented by a simple, inviting smear of softened, salted butter. Its particular blend of ingredients, including fiber-rich flax, comes across as quite earthy, a bit coarse, and not entirely unlike a zucchini bread made with whole grains.

2 tbsp (30mL)	flaxseed meal
2 tbsp (30mL)	almond meal
2 tbsp (30mL)	sugar replacement
1/2 tsp (3mL)	baking powder
1/2 tsp (3mL)	ground cinnamon
1/4 tsp (1mL)	ground nutmeg
Dash	ground cloves
Dash	salt
2 tbsp (30mL)	grated zucchini
1 tbsp (15mL)	chopped and toasted walnut halves
1 large	egg
1 tsp (5mL)	melted butter
1/2 tsp (3mL)	vanilla extract

- In a wide-mouthed coffee mug, combine your flax, almond meal, sugar replacement, baking powder, cinnamon, nutmeg, cloves, and salt. (I like to grease my mug first, but I don't think it's necessary.)
- Squeeze the water out of your zucchini by squeezing it within your fist, over the sink. Un-clump the zucchini so it is back in strand form. Mix in your zucchini, walnuts, egg, butter, and vanilla.
- Microwave on high for 60 seconds (90 seconds if using a weaker microwave). Try it with butter. Eat and enjoy!

Herby Sandwich Bread (Focaccia)

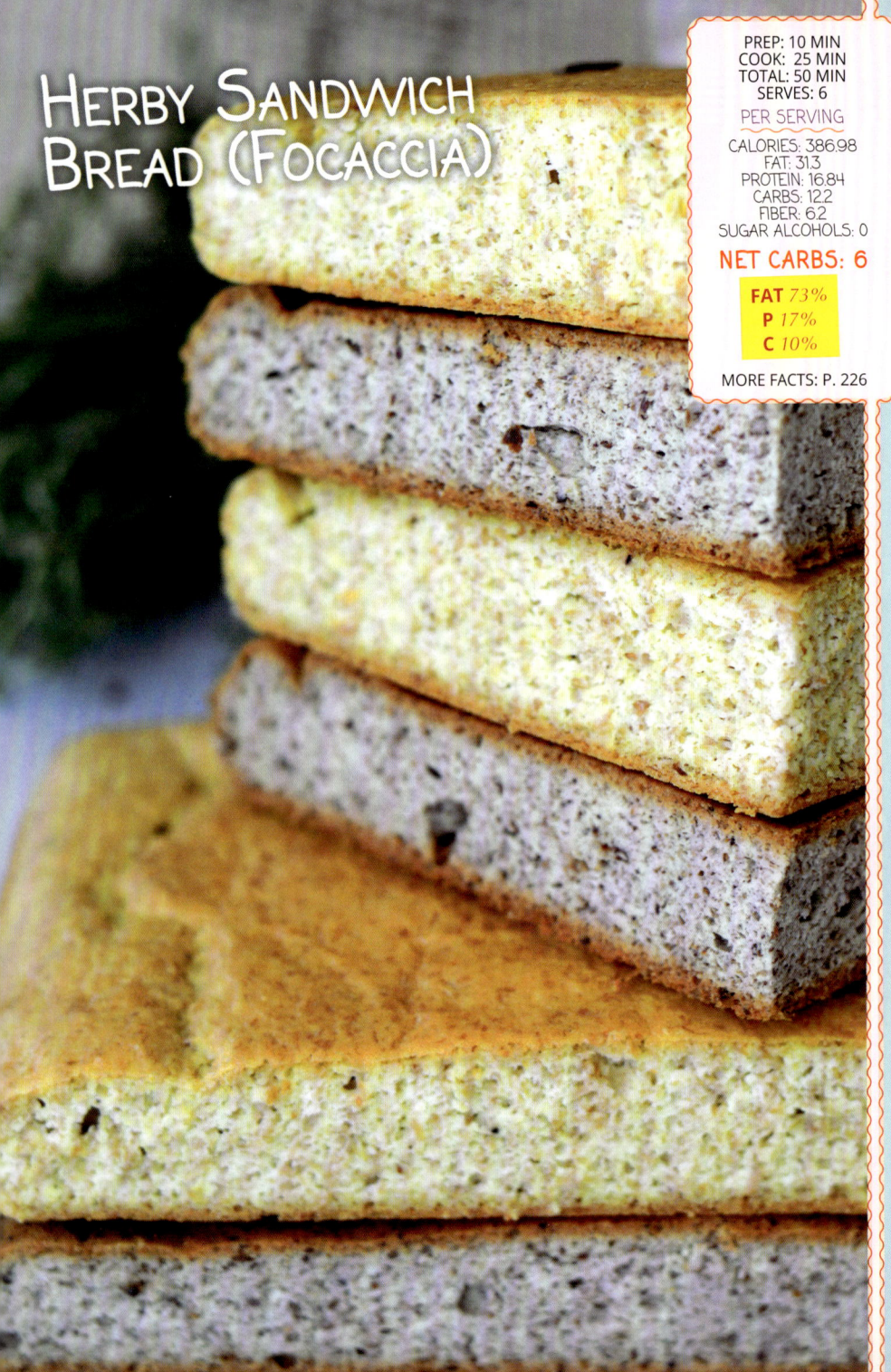

PREP: 10 MIN
COOK: 25 MIN
TOTAL: 50 MIN
SERVES: 6

PER SERVING

CALORIES: 386.98
FAT: 31.3
PROTEIN: 16.84
CARBS: 12.2
FIBER: 6.2
SUGAR ALCOHOLS: 0

NET CARBS: 6

FAT 73%
P 17%
C 10%

MORE FACTS: P. 226

This recipe was unearthed by experimentation. I wanted to conduct a test by making a big batch of basic, unsweetened OMM batter, infused with a few herbs and some garlic. I wanted something resembling a focaccia, but without yeast or wheat. I wanted it "quick-bread" style.

This recipe makes too much batter for the microwave, but the leftover batter can be popped into the microwave for little savory herb muffins.

Let's just say... it worked! IT WORKED WONDERS!! Delicious! Try some with dinner, or... slice it for AMAZING sandwiches!

Note: The "Why Bother?" variation of this recipe can be found on *p. 106*.

1 cup (240 mL)	golden flaxseed meal
1 cup (240 mL)	almond flour
1 1/2 tbsp (23 mL)	baking powder
1 tbsp (15 mL)	fresh chopped rosemary
1/2 tsp (3 mL)	crushed red chili flakes (or to taste)
1 tsp (5 mL)	salt, divided
8 large	eggs, beaten
1/4 cup (60 mL)	extra-virgin olive oil
6 cloves	garlic, minced

- Preheat oven to 350°F (177°C).
- In a medium bowl, combine the flax, almond flour, baking powder, rosemary, chili flakes, and half of the salt. Mix well.
- Add the eggs, olive oil, and garlic to the mix. Mix well.
- Grease a 9" x 9" (23cm x 23cm) square baking pan. Pour the batter into the pan. With a spatula, smooth it out so that it is evenly distributed throughout the pan. Sprinkle the remaining salt over the top of the batter.
- Bake for about 20 to 25 minutes, or until lightly golden brown and nicely puffed.
- Place on a rack and cool for at least 10 minutes before slicing. Serve!

Italian Turkey Club Sandwich

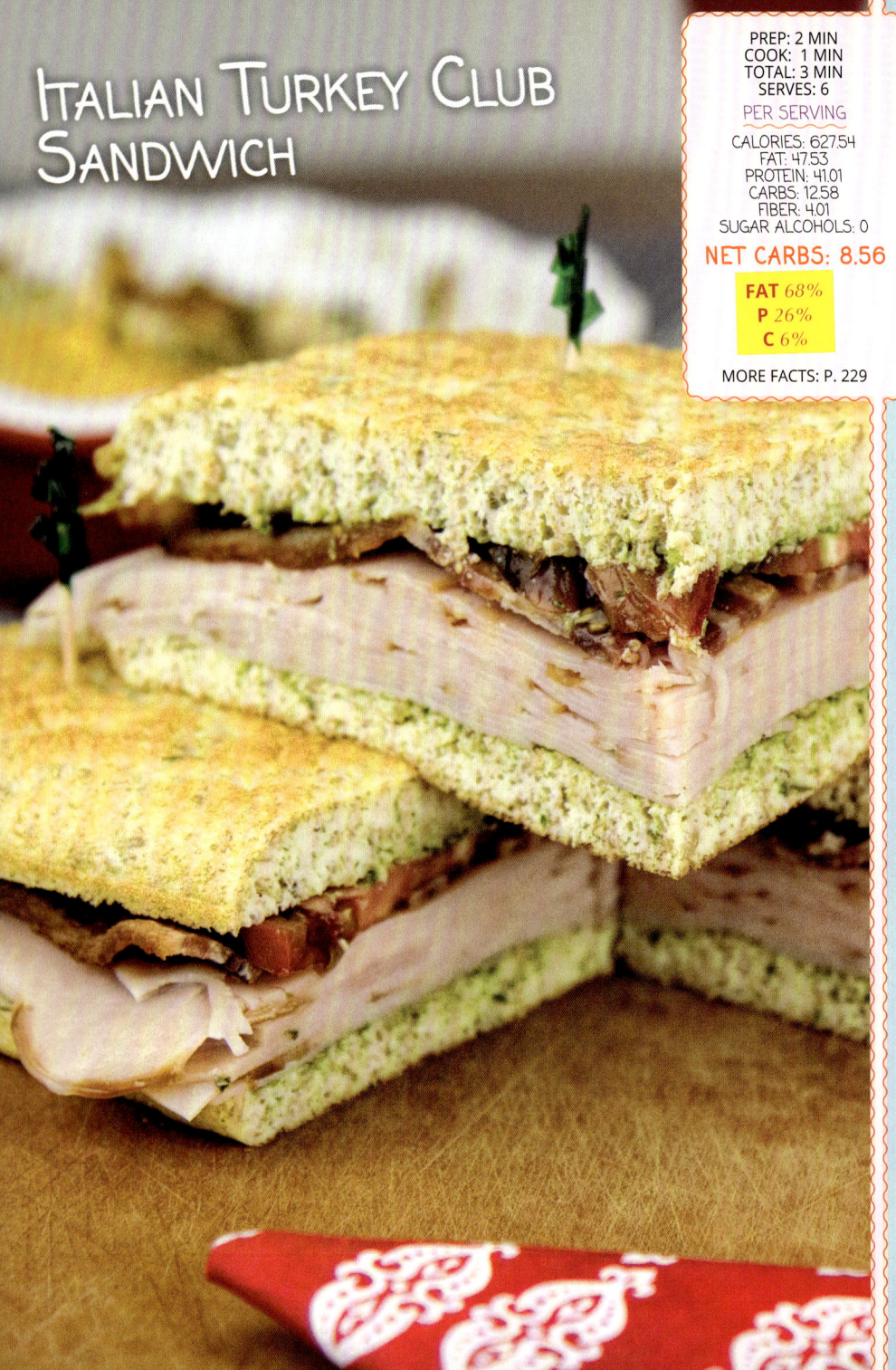

PREP: 2 MIN
COOK: 1 MIN
TOTAL: 3 MIN
SERVES: 6

PER SERVING
CALORIES: 627.54
FAT: 47.53
PROTEIN: 41.01
CARBS: 12.58
FIBER: 4.01
SUGAR ALCOHOLS: 0

NET CARBS: 8.56

FAT 68%
P 26%
C 6%

MORE FACTS: P. 229

When I was younger, I worked in a high-end deli in West Seattle. We made all manner of sandwiches, on a wide variety of breads. Hot, cold, custom style, etc. It didn't matter.

There was one sandwich concept that I LOVED and always thought was so cool, but never really made in my real life until recently! One day I made a sort of Super Low-Carb Focaccia. It's a big sheet of slightly spicy and herby bread, loaded with garlic and topped with salt. It's just FANTASTIC and SOOO easy to make! With this perfect homemade sheet of goodness, I was able to start making this sandwich again!

This is where the idea becomes less a specific recipe (even though it is one) and more a general concept for a larger sandwich idea.

The idea is, take the large sheet of focaccia and split it evenly through the center, creating thin sheets representing the top and bottom. Imagine a GIGANTIC sandwich! Once you've got the two halves, you can spread your condiments into it, layer in your fillings, put the top on and...

then CUT OUT the sandwiches in any size and shape you'd like! Imagine you're making sandwiches for the whole family. By doing this, you can cut out a big sandwich for Papa Bear, a medium sandwich for Mama Bear, and 3 little sandwiches for the cubs. This will likely leave a small sandwich or two for a midnight snack!

At the deli, we would cut different sizes and just sell them by the pound. Oh, I loved that idea!

1 sheet (624g)

1/2 cup (120mL)

1 1/2 lb (681g)
12 slices
1 medium
To taste

Grain-Free Fauxcaccia (p. 106)

Pesto alla Genovese (p. 194)

sliced turkey
cooked bacon
tomato, sliced thin
salt and pepper

- Cutting this bread works best using a long, sharp serrated knife. Hold your knife directly in the middle of one corner of the focaccia sheet, with the knife blade parallel to the countertop. Slice in about 6 inches (15cm). Continue slicing, while slowly rotating the sheet in a circle. Be very careful not to break through the top or the bottom as you gently saw away and rotate. The key is keeping the knife at precisely the midpoint between the top and bottom and making sure that it's ALWAYS perfectly parallel to your cutting surface. If it tilts, then it will begin to slice upwards or downwards. Ultimately, you want two equal thicknesses to the top and bottom halves.
- Once the bread has been split, spread an equal amount of pesto on the inside of both the top and the bottom.
- On the bottom, evenly lay out the turkey, followed by the bacon and finally the tomatoes. Sprinkle a little salt and pepper on the tomatoes and then place the top on the whole thing, with the pesto side facing the tomatoes.
- Cut out sandwiches! This is designed for 6 substantial sandwiches, but any number is possible. Use fun-colored toothpicks and cut out 48 little mini sandwiches for a party!
- Enjoy!

Pesto alla Genovese

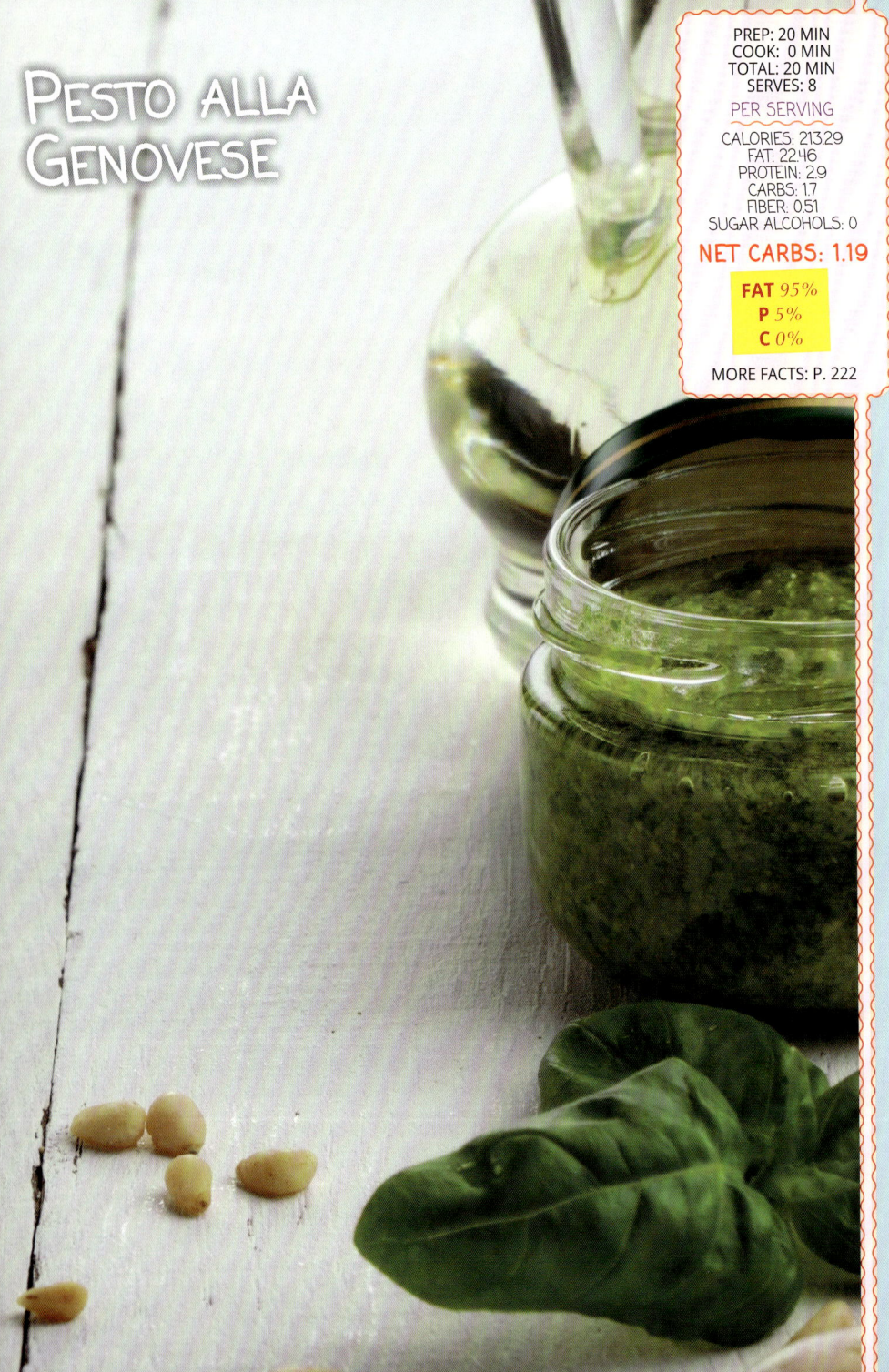

PREP: 20 MIN
COOK: 0 MIN
TOTAL: 20 MIN
SERVES: 8

PER SERVING
CALORIES: 213.29
FAT: 22.46
PROTEIN: 2.9
CARBS: 1.7
FIBER: 0.51
SUGAR ALCOHOLS: 0

NET CARBS: 1.19

FAT 95%
P 5%
C 0%

MORE FACTS: P. 222

Pesto (a word stemming from the Italian word for *pounded*) is that bright-green, paste-like stuff that tastes great on pretty much everything. It's up there with bacon and Heinz Ketchup, in terms of a perfect flavor. It's a very traditional sauce originating in Northern Italy. It's basically a mixture of basil, pine nuts, and cheese, but the combination is OH so much more than the sum of its parts!

I'm counting each serving as 2 tablespoons (30^{mL}), for a total of 8 servings. This particular recipe makes about a cup's (240^{mL}) worth of bright, vibrant, garlicky goodness. It's not uncommon for me to throw a few chili flakes in there... I like that little bit of zippity-zang!

I add pesto to A LOT of things, from spreads on sandwiches, to using as a dip, to a pesto cream sauce, or as layers within a green lasagna. Try carefully rubbing it under the skin of a brined and spatchcocked whole chicken, then roast the dickens out of it. Talk about a flavorful bird!

This sauce is traditionally made with a mortar and pestle, but this recipe uses a food processor ('cause it's what I have). To do it the old-school way, start with the salt and garlic in a large mortar and move the pestle around in a circular fashion. After a paste has been formed, add the basil and lemon juice. Pound. Then add the oil and continue pounding. Finally, add the cheese and toasted pine nuts! Pound to consistency and adjust seasoning. It really is one of those perfect foods.

3 cloves	garlic, coarsely chopped
2/3 cup (160mL)	extra-virgin olive oil
2 cups (480mL)	packed, cleaned and dried fresh basil leaves (about a large bunch's worth)
2 tsp (10mL)	lemon juice
1/4 cup (60mL)	toasted pine nuts
1/4 cup (60mL)	grated parmesan cheese
1/4 cup (60mL)	grated pecorino cheese
To taste	salt and pepper

- Add the garlic, salt, and half of the olive oil to a food processor with a sharp blade.
- Pulse the processor and blend for 30 seconds.
- Add the basil and lemon juice, then pulse for a further 30 seconds.
- Add the pine nuts and cheeses and then pulse to your desired consistency. If it's too thick, add more olive oil to adjust the consistency. I tend to like mine a bit on the pasty, rough side, but some like it smooth and saucy.
- Use immediately or store covered with a thin layer of extra-virgin olive oil. This top floating layer will help keep oxygen out of the wetter ingredients below, preventing the pesto from turning brown and allowing it to last longer in the fridge.

Cream Cheese Frosting

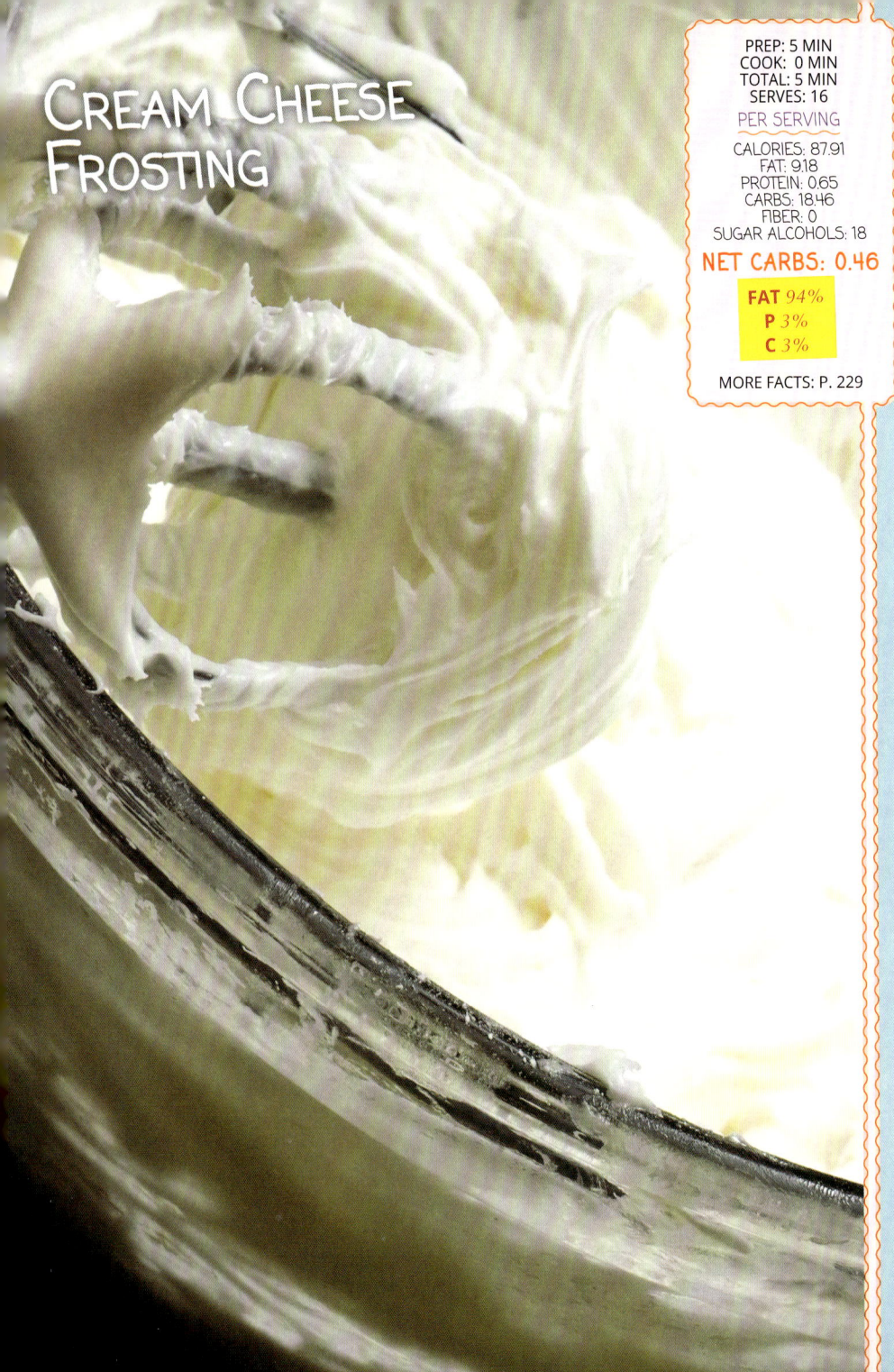

PREP: 5 MIN
COOK: 0 MIN
TOTAL: 5 MIN
SERVES: 16

PER SERVING

CALORIES: 87.91
FAT: 9.18
PROTEIN: 0.65
CARBS: 18.46
FIBER: 0
SUGAR ALCOHOLS: 18

NET CARBS: 0.46

FAT 94%
P 3%
C 3%

MORE FACTS: P. 229

I LOVE this recipe! It's one of those *perfect* flavors, like bacon or Heinz Ketchup. I'm honestly not sure where I originally got it from. I've had this recipe in my arsenal for a good 20 years. It originated as the topping for the fresh, piping hot cinnamon rolls I'd later turn into a business venture. The only variation is switching out the sugar for sugar replacement.

This is a fantastic topping on just about any warm baked good. I've even made batches of it that I then split into little cups and simply enjoyed as fat bombs. You can even pipe it or form little candy-sized blobs and freeze them. Wonderful!

The heart of the recipe, though... is as an icing or frosting. You can use it anywhere you'd want to use a frosting.

Note: Recipe makes just short of 1 cup (240^{mL}) of frosting.

1/4 cup + 1 1/2 tsp (67mL)	full-fat cream cheese, room temperature
3 tbsp (45mL)	whole butter, room temperature
1/2 cup + 1 tbsp (135mL)	powdered sugar replacement
1/2 tsp (3mL)	vanilla extract
Dash	salt

- With a mixer, beat the cream cheese and butter until light and airy. This goes a lot faster if the two ingredients are room temperature.

- Add the powdered sugar replacement, vanilla, and a healthy dash of salt. Be VERY careful when turning the mixer back on, as a massive cloud of sweetener smoke will erupt if the mixer is allowed to run willy-nilly. Manually fold in the sweetener, or toggle the mixer on and off until the sweetener is more or less absorbed. Continue mixing until the frosting is smooth.

- Spread on stuff!

Notella

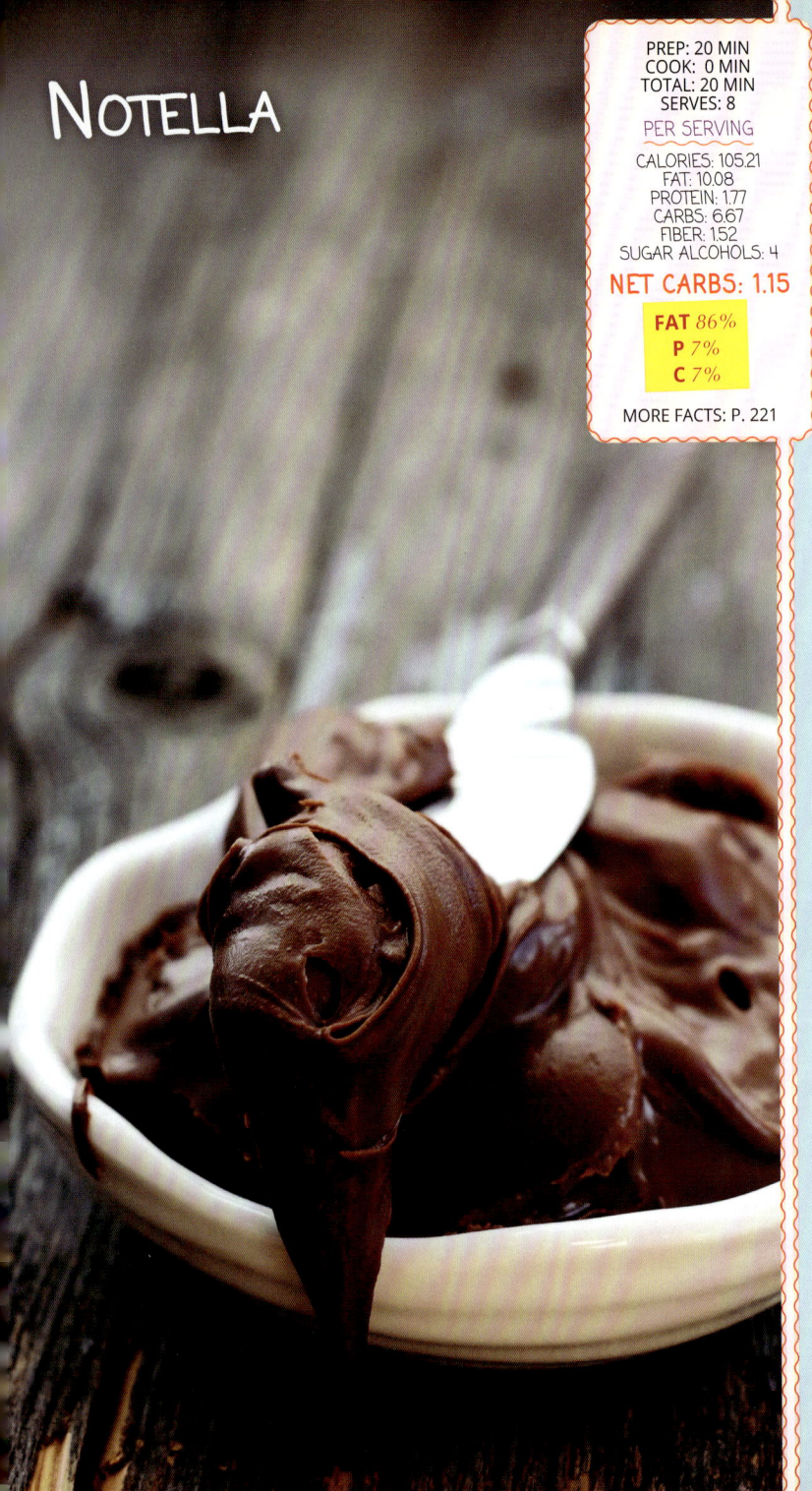

PREP: 20 MIN
COOK: 0 MIN
TOTAL: 20 MIN
SERVES: 8

PER SERVING

CALORIES: 105.21
FAT: 10.08
PROTEIN: 1.77
CARBS: 6.67
FIBER: 1.52
SUGAR ALCOHOLS: 4

NET CARBS: 1.15

FAT 86%
P 7%
C 7%

MORE FACTS: P. 221

Here, like the previous cream cheese frosting, we find another perfect flavor. There's something so incredibly satiating about this combination of ingredients. It brings a certain calm and comfort that is difficult to match with other blends. Maybe it's the spoonable peanut-butter texture? Or, the complex character, so harmoniously balanced with a final note of salt? Whatever it is, it's amazing!

I remember the first time I made this, I used it but had overtoasted the hazelnuts (don't do that). The end result was just bitter enough to turn my nose up. Unable to throw it away, I put the jar in the fridge; I was frustrated enough with it to want it out of my sight. Over the coming weeks, it slowly migrated to the back of the fridge, forgotten with the tamarind and that furry lump I call Griselda.

One day I was kneeling way down, looking for something *way* in the back of the fridge. I spotted the Notella. Surprisingly, it was still in good shape. Bitter, but very much edible.

I don't know what it was, the fact that my emotional investment in this jar had dissipated, or that the bitterness had simply mellowed with time, but I took a big spoonful out, put it in my mouth, and savored every loving second of it as I swirled it around my mouth. I continued that trend until I heard the clank of the spoon against the bottom of the jar. #NoRegrets

Note: Recipe makes about 3/4 cup (180^{mL}) of Notella.

1/2 cup (120mL)	peeled and lightly toasted hazelnuts
2 tbsp (30mL)	unsweetened cocoa powder
2 tbsp (30mL)	powdered sugar replacement
2 tbsp (30mL)	sustainable red palm or coconut oil
1/2 tsp (3mL)	vanilla extract
1/2 tsp (3mL)	salt

- Add the lightly toasted and peeled hazelnuts to a food processor. Turn the processor on and allow it to turn your nuts into butter. This can take some time, so be sure you've got the time. A very perfectly smooth nut butter can take upwards of 10 minutes as the nuts are chopped, then pulverized, then slowly converted into ever smoother nut butter.
- Once a smooth nut butter has developed, add the cocoa powder, powdered sugar replacement, oil, vanilla, and salt to the food processor.
- Process these ingredients until a smooth Notella has formed.
- Notella is spoonable and a bit viscous at room temperature. It hardens to something like a thickish peanut butter when refrigerated. There are no wrong answers.

Chocolate Ganache

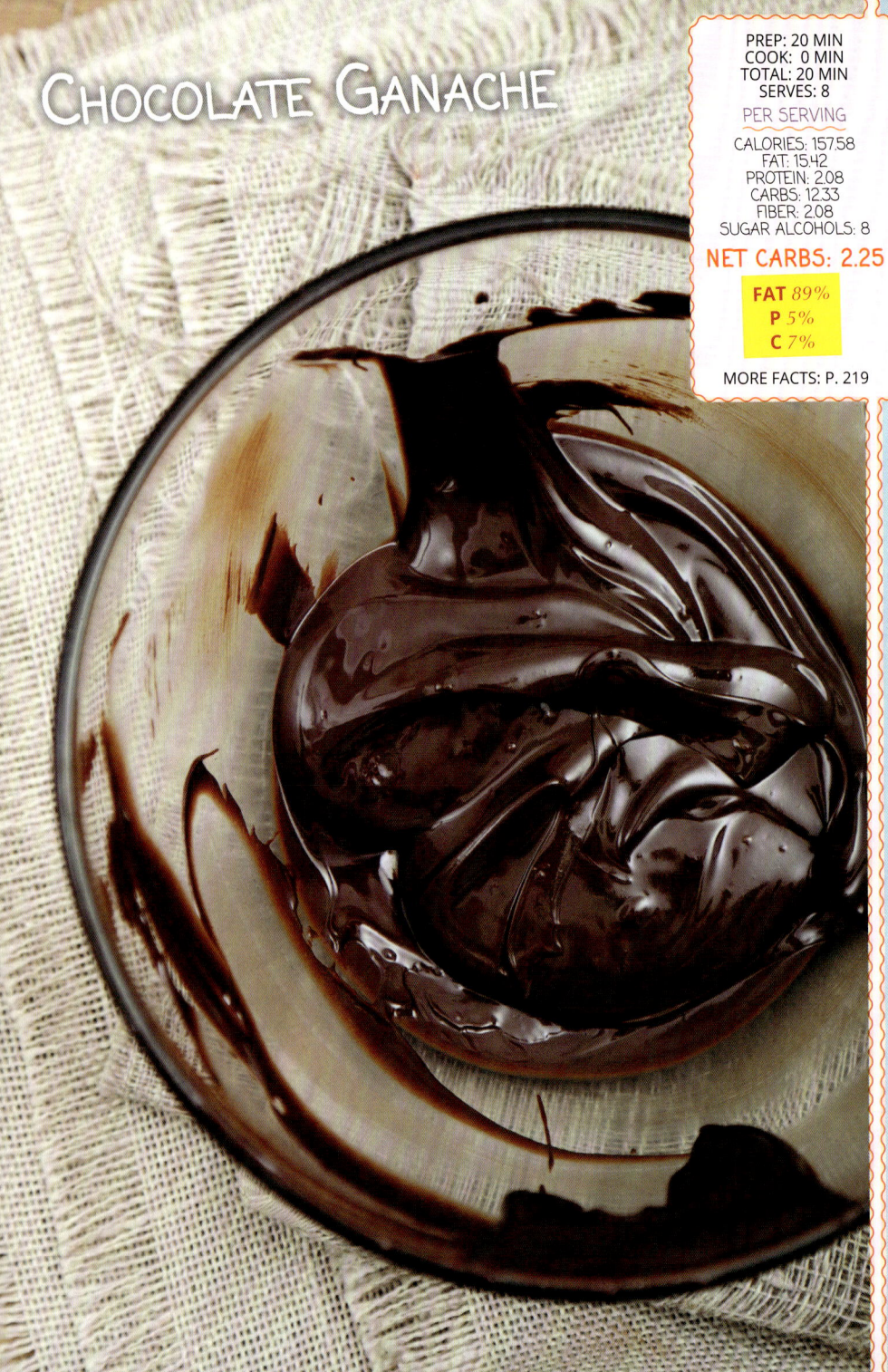

PREP: 20 MIN
COOK: 0 MIN
TOTAL: 20 MIN
SERVES: 8

PER SERVING

CALORIES: 157.58
FAT: 15.42
PROTEIN: 2.08
CARBS: 12.33
FIBER: 2.08
SUGAR ALCOHOLS: 8

NET CARBS: 2.25

FAT 89%
P 5%
C 7%

MORE FACTS: P. 219

If you're in the need for a simple chocolate ganache, look no further! This stuff is easy to make and absolutely wonderful. It's a bit on the bittersweet side. Feel free to add a bit more sweetener if you'd like. Don't tell anyone, but I've been known to plop a few liquid sucralose droplets in there from time to time. (I usually use an erythritol-based sweetener, but it tends to crystalize at too high a concentration. So I extend the sweetness with a concentrated sweetener, like sucralose. Stevia is another concentrated sweetener and can work to extend the sweetness for the stevia fans. I personally find the bitter in stevia to be amplified by the bitter notes in chocolate.)

All this said, I typically use the ganache with something else that is super sweet, to compensate. Or I just embrace the bittersweet nature of it.

The ease and texture of this ganache is amazing. Perfectly malleable while warm, it chills into something resembling the texture of a smooth fudge. AMAZING for the inside of a truffle, or the base of a mud pie. Also? Great with muffins!

1/2 cup (120ᵐᴸ)	heavy cream
1/4 cup (60ᵐᴸ)	sugar replacement
Dash	salt
2 1/2 oz (70ᵍ)	unsweetened baking chocolate squares, chopped
1 tbsp (15ᵐᴸ)	butter, cubed

- Heat up your cream on the stove, but don't let it boil.
- Once your cream is hot and is *just* about to simmer, whisk in the sugar replacement and salt until they have dissolved.
- Place your chopped chocolate pieces and butter cubes into a small mixing bowl. Pour your hot cream mixture over the chocolate and quickly whisk it in the bowl until the chocolate is fully melted and incorporated.
- Add to other recipes to increase the chocolatiness of them!

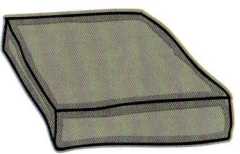
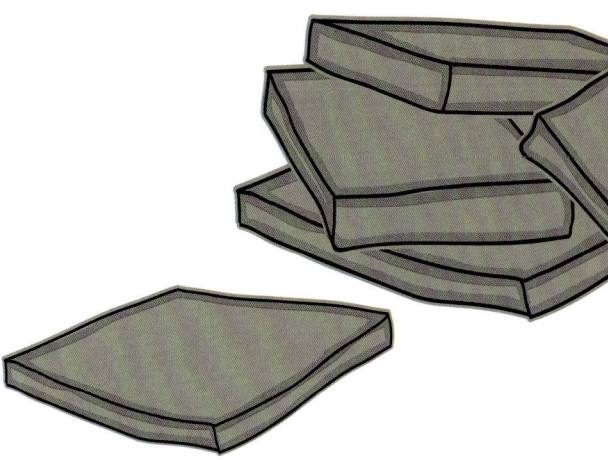

Luxurious Eggnog

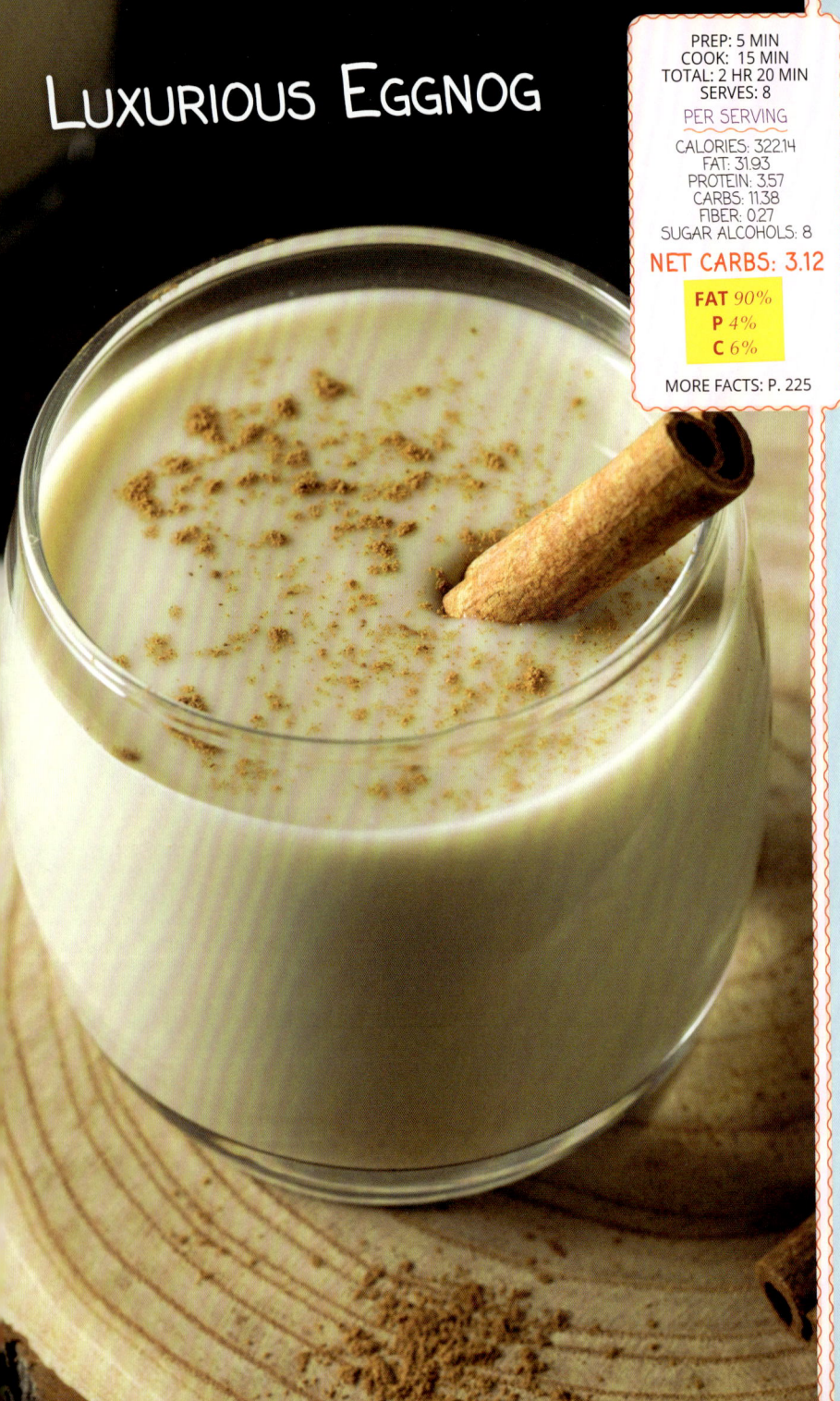

PREP: 5 MIN
COOK: 15 MIN
TOTAL: 2 HR 20 MIN
SERVES: 8

PER SERVING
CALORIES: 322.14
FAT: 31.93
PROTEIN: 3.57
CARBS: 11.38
FIBER: 0.27
SUGAR ALCOHOLS: 8

NET CARBS: 3.12

FAT 90%
P 4%
C 6%

MORE FACTS: P. 225

Eggnog is one word. Did you know that? I didn't! I've always spelled it as two words! Wacky stuff!

When eating a low-primal and sugar-free way of life, sometimes it becomes reasonable to adapt to meals, snacks, beverages, or desserts that are outside the norm. Eggnog is something that I view as being a part of the winter season. However, it's actually quite delicious at any time of year! It's a good way to get some healthy fats. It's also great as a base in protein shakes. Whisk some into your morning coffee or tea for a different kind of taste sensation!

Most eggnog recipes use raw eggs. However, the store-bought stuff is at least pasteurized. I'm picky, I suppose. I balk at raw eggs. Even my normal eggs that I eat for breakfast are famously overcooked. So, because I'm fussy... and I don't mind making a custard base... this thick and luxurious eggnog recipe is cooked!

I made it quite regularly when I was focused on a zero-carb way of eating and wanted something different. I drank a lot of eggnog that month!

Try it. Don't wait for winter. It's good... year-round!

Note: Recipe makes a bit less than 6 cups (1.4^L) of eggnog, or roughly eight 6 oz (180^{mL}) portions.

2 1/2 cups (600 mL)	heavy cream
1 1/2 cups (360 mL)	unsweetened almond milk
1 single	vanilla bean, split lengthwise (or 2 tsp [10 mL] vanilla extract)
1/2 tsp (3 mL)	ground cinnamon
1/4 tsp (1 mL)	freshly ground nutmeg
1/3 cup (80 mL)	sugar replacement
Dash	salt
6 large	eggs

⋛ Combine cream and almond milk in a medium saucepan.

⋛ Scrape the seeds from the vanilla bean. Add the bean and seeds to the milk and cream.

⋛ Add the cinnamon and nutmeg. Then bring the milk to a slow simmer.

⋛ Remove the milk from the heat and whisk the sugar replacement and salt into the milk. Make sure it dissolves.

⋛ In a separate bowl, whisk the eggs well.

⋛ Pouring very slowly, whisk the hot milk mixture into the eggs. Whisk quickly, so as to incorporate the hot liquid evenly, without cooking or scrambling the eggs.

⋛ Once the liquid has been incorporated into the eggs, pour the milk-egg mixture back into the saucepan and return to a low heat.

⋛ Stir constantly until the eggnog thickens. The temperature should be between 165°F and 175°F (74°C and 79°C). Whatever you do, do not boil this mixture.

⋛ Strain the eggnog.

⋛ Chill!

CA: Calories | **FAT:** Fat | **P:** Protein | **C:** Carbohydrates | **F:** Fiber | **SA:** Sugar Alcohols | **NC:** Net Carbs
FAT%: Calories from Fat | **P%:** Calories from Protein | **C%:** Calories from Carbohydrates

the back of the book

CA: Calories | **FAT:** Fat | **P:** Protein | **C:** Carbohydrates | **F:** Fiber | **SA:** Sugar Alcohols | **NC:** Net Carbs
FAT%: Calories from Fat | **P%:** Calories from Protein | **C%:** Calories from Carbohydrates

Orange-Blueberry Chia Pudding — P. 38

	CA	FAT	P	C	F	SA	NC	FAT%	P%	C%
3 tbsp (23 g) chia seeds	105	6.75	4.5	10.5	9	0	1.5	58%	17%	25%
1/4 cup (39 g) fresh or frozen unsweetened blueberries	19.75	0.25	0.25	4.75	1	0	3.75	11%	5%	84%
1/2 cup (120 g) unsweetened almond milk	22.5	1.75	1	1.5	0.5	0	1	70%	18%	12%
2 tbsp (24 g) sugar replacement	0	0	0	2	0	2	0	0%	0%	100%
2 tbsp (31 g) fresh orange juice	14	0	0	3	0	0	3	0%	0%	100%
1/2 tsp (2 g) vanilla extract	5.77	0	0	0.25	0	0	0.25	0%	0%	100%
1/2 tsp (1 g) fresh orange zest (peel)	0.97	0	0.01	0.25	0.11	0	0.14	0%	4%	96%
2 tbsp (18 g) blanched and slivered almonds, toasted	105.25	9.13	4	3.63	1.88	0	1.75	78%	15%	7%
Dash salt	0	0	0	0	0	0	0	0%	0%	0%
Totals (of 1 Serving):	273.24	17.88	9.76	25.88	12.49	2	11.39	59%	14%	27%
Per Serving:	273.24	17.88	9.76	25.88	12.49	2	11.39	59%	14%	27%

Deep-Dish Pizza — P. 92

	CA	FAT	P	C	F	SA	NC	FAT%	P%	C%
2 cups (500 g) no-sugar-added pizza sauce	280	20	8	24	8	0	16	64%	11%	24%
1/4 cup (28 g) almond flour	160	14	6	6	3	0	3	79%	15%	6%
1/4 cup (28 g) hazelnut flour	180	17	4	5	3	0	2	85%	9%	6%
1/4 cup (24 g) ground chia	112	7.2	3.2	11.2	9.6	0	1.6	58%	11%	31%
1/4 cup (26 g) flaxseed meal	140	9	6	8	6	0	2	58%	17%	25%
2 1/4 tsp (10 g) baking powder	4.5	0	0	2.93	0	0	2.93	0%	0%	100%
1 tbsp (3 g) chopped herbs, divided	0.9	0.03	0.09	0.12	0.09	0	0.03	30%	40%	30%
1 tsp (4 g) salt	0	0	0	0	0	0	0	0%	0%	0%
Dash chili flakes	0	0	0	0	0	0	0	0%	0%	0%
4 large (200 g) eggs	285.33	20	8.67	2	0	0	2	63%	12%	25%
1/4 cup (60 g) unsweetened almond milk	11.25	0.88	0.5	0.75	0.25	0	0.5	70%	18%	12%
3 tbsp (42 g) extra-virgin olive oil, divided	360	36	0	0	0	0	0	90%	0%	10%
4 (12 g) garlic cloves, chopped	16	0	0	4	0	0	4	0%	0%	100%
1 cup (56 g) grated whole milk, low-moisture mozzarella	175.5	14	12	2	0	0	2	72%	27%	1%
1/2 cup (50 g) grated parmesan cheese	215.5	14.5	19	2	0	0	2	61%	35%	4%
4 oz (114 g) pepperoni slices	560.7	49.94	26.11	0	0	0	0	80%	19%	1%
Totals (of 4 Servings):	2501.6	202.55	93.57	68	29.94	0	38.06	73%	15%	12%
Per Serving:	625.42	50.64	23.39	17.00	7.49	0.00	9.52	73%	15%	12%

CA: Calories | **FAT**: Fat | **P**: Protein | **C**: Carbohydrates | **F**: Fiber | **SA**: Sugar Alcohols | **NC**: Net Carbs
FAT%: Calories from Fat | **P%**: Calories from Protein | **C%**: Calories from Carbohydrates

Cheesy Bacon-Chive Muffins — P. 96

Ingredient	CA	FAT	P	C	F	SA	NC	FAT%	P%	C%
3/4 cup (84 g) almond flour	480	42	18	18	9	0	9	79%	15%	6%
1/2 cup (48 g) white chia seed flour	224	14.4	6.4	22.4	19.2	0	3.2	58%	11%	31%
1/4 cup (30 g) tapioca flour (optional)	100	0	0	26	0	0	26	0%	0%	100%
1/4 cup (26 g) golden flaxseed meal	140	9	6	8	6	0	2	58%	17%	25%
1 tbsp (14 g) baking powder	6	0	0	3.9	0	0	3.9	0%	0%	100%
1 tsp (6 g) xanthan gum (optional)	20	0	0	4.68	4.68	0	0	0%	0%	100%
3/4 tsp (3 g) salt	0	0	0	0	0	0	0	0%	0%	0%
Dash pepper (or to taste)	0	0	0	0	0	0	0	0%	0%	0%
Dash chili flakes (or to taste)	0	0	0	0	0	0	0	0%	0%	0%
6 large (300 g) eggs	428	30	13	3	0	0	3	63%	12%	25%
1/4 cup + 2 tbsp (90 g) unsweetened almond milk	16.88	1.32	0.75	1.13	0.38	0	1.32	70%	18%	12%
3 tbsp (42 g) melted butter	300	33	0	0	0	0	0	99%	0%	1%
8 oz (227 g) cheddar cheese	902.43	74.36	56	2.75	0	0	2.75	74%	25%	1%
1/2 cup (57 g) real bacon bits	200	12	24	0	0	0	0	54%	48%	-2%
1/4 cup (12 g) chopped fresh chives	3.6	0.12	0.36	0.48	0.36	0	0.12	30%	40%	30%
Totals (of 6 Servings):	2820.9	216.2	124.51	90.34	39.62	0	51.29	69%	18%	13%
Per Serving:	470.15	36.03	20.75	15.06	6.60	0.00	**8.55**	69%	18%	13%

Chocolate-Banana Muffcakes — P. 124

Ingredient	CA	FAT	P	C	F	SA	NC	FAT%	P%	C%
1 cup (112 g) almond flour	640	56	24	24	12	0	12	79%	15%	6%
1/4 cup + 2 tbsp (42 g) coconut flour	186	4.5	10.5	27	18	0	9	22%	23%	56%
1/4 cup + 2 tbsp (72 g) sugar replacement	0	0	0	72	0	72	0	0%	0%	100%
1/4 cup + 2 tbsp (32 g) unsweetened cocoa powder	73.5	4.48	6.42	18.78	10.92	0	7.86	55%	35%	10%
1/4 cup (24 g) ground chia	112	7.2	3.2	11.2	9.6	0	1.6	58%	11%	31%
1 tbsp (14 g) baking powder	6	0	0	3.9	0	0	3.9	0%	0%	100%
3/4 tsp (3 g) salt	0	0	0	0	0	0	0	0%	0%	0%
2 small (202 g) bananas	180	0	2	46	6	0	40	0%	4%	96%
4 large (200 g) eggs	285.33	20	8.67	2	0	0	2	63%	12%	25%
2 tbsp (30 g) unsweetened almond milk	5.63	0.44	0.25	0.38	0.13	0	0.25	70%	18%	12%
3 tbsp (42 g) melted butter	300	33	0	0	0	0	0	99%	0%	1%
Totals (of 6 Servings):	1788.4	125.62	55.04	205.26	56.65	72	76.61	63%	12%	24%
Per Serving:	298.08	20.94	9.17	34.21	9.44	12.00	**12.77**	63%	12%	24%

CA: Calories | FAT: Fat | P: Protein | C: Carbohydrates | F: Fiber | SA: Sugar Alcohols | NC: Net Carbs
FAT%: Calories from Fat | P%: Calories from Protein | C%: Calories from Carbohydrates

Muffin aux Fines Herbes — P. 100

	CA	FAT	P	C	F	SA	NC	FAT%	P%	C%
3/4 cup (84 g) almond flour	480	42	18	18	9	0	9	79%	15%	6%
1/2 cup (48 g) white chia seed flour	224	14.4	6.4	22.4	19.2	0	3.2	58%	11%	31%
1/4 cup (26 g) golden flaxseed meal	140	9	6	8	6	0	2	58%	17%	25%
3/4 tsp (3 g) baking soda	0	0	0	0	0	0	0	0%	0%	0%
3/4 tsp (3 g) salt	0	0	0	0	0	0	0	0%	0%	0%
Dash pepper	0	0	0	0	0	0	0	0%	0%	0%
1 lemon (108 g)	108	0	0	12	5	0	7	0%	0%	100%
6 large (300 g) eggs	428	30	13	3	0	0	3	63%	12%	25%
1/4 cup (60 g) unsweetened almond milk	11.25	0.88	0.5	0.75	0.25	0	0.5	70%	18%	12%
3 tbsp (42 g) melted butter	300	33	0	0	0	0	0	99%	0%	1%
1 tbsp (3 g) fresh chopped parsley	1.08	0.03	0.09	0.18	0.09	0	0.09	25%	33%	42%
1 tbsp (3 g) fresh chopped tarragon	1.08	0.03	0.09	0.18	0.09	0	0.09	25%	33%	42%
1 tbsp (3 g) fresh chopped chives	0.9	0.03	0.09	0.12	0.09	0	0.03	30%	40%	30%
1 tbsp (3 g) fresh chopped chervil	1.08	0.03	0.09	0.18	0.09	0	0.09	25%	33%	42%
Totals (of 6 Servings):	1695.4	129.4	44.26	64.81	39.81	0	16	69%	10%	21%
Per Serving:	282.57	21.57	7.38	10.80	6.64	0.00	2.67	69%	10%	21%

Pesto, Sausage and Parmesan Muffins — P. 102

	CA	FAT	P	C	F	SA	NC	FAT%	P%	C%
8 oz (227 g) Italian sausage links (sweet or spicy)	454	32.05	37.39	5.34	0	0	5.34	64%	33%	4%
3/4 cup (84 g) almond flour	480	42	18	18	9	0	9	79%	15%	6%
1/2 cup (48 g) white chia seed flour	224	14.4	6.4	22.4	19.2	0	3.2	58%	11%	31%
1/4 cup (26 g) golden flaxseed meal	140	9	6	8	6	0	2	58%	17%	25%
1 tbsp (14 g) baking powder	6	0	0	3.9	0	0	3.9	0%	0%	100%
Dash chili flakes	0	0	0	0	0	0	0	0%	0%	0%
Dash salt and pepper	0	0	0	0	0	0	0	0%	0%	0%
6 large (300 g) eggs	428	30	13	3	0	0	3	63%	12%	25%
1/4 cup (60 g) unsweetened almond milk	11.25	0.88	0.5	0.75	0.25	0	0.5	70%	18%	12%
1/3 cup (80 g) pesto	568.77	59.89	7.25	4.54	1.37	0	3.17	95%	5%	0%
1/3 cup (33 g) grated parmesan cheese	143.67	9.67	12.67	1.33	0	0	1.33	61%	35%	4%
Totals (of 6 Servings):	2455.7	197.89	101.21	67.26	35.82	0	31.44	73%	16%	11%
Per Serving:	409.28	32.98	16.87	11.21	5.97	0.00	5.24	73%	16%	11%

CA: Calories | **FAT**: Fat | **P**: Protein | **C**: Carbohydrates | **F**: Fiber | **SA**: Sugar Alcohols | **NC**: Net Carbs
FAT%: Calories from Fat | **P%**: Calories from Protein | **C%**: Calories from Carbohydrates

Cream Cheese-Filled Spiced Apple Muffins — P. 110

	CA	FAT	P	C	F	SA	NC	FAT%	P%	C%
1 large (223 g) apple	116	0	1	31	5	0	26	0%	3%	97%
3 tbsp (42 g) butter	300	33	0	0	0	0	0	99%	0%	1%
1 tsp (4 g) salt, divided	0	0	0	0	0	0	0	0%	0%	0%
3/4 cup (174 g) cream cheese	595.5	59.25	10.5	6.75	0	0	6.75	90%	7%	3%
3/4 cup (144 g) sugar replacement	0	0	0	144	0	144	0	0%	0%	100%
3/4 cup (84 g) almond flour	480	42	18	18	9	0	9	79%	15%	6%
1/2 cup (48 g) white chia seed flour	224	14.4	6.4	22.4	19.2	0	3.2	58%	11%	31%
1/4 cup (26 g) golden flaxseed meal	140	9	6	8	6	0	2	58%	17%	25%
1/2 tsp (1 g) ground cinnamon	3.17	0	0	1	0.67	0	0.33	0%	0%	100%
1/4 tsp (.5) ground nutmeg	3.08	0.25	0	0.25	0.08	0	0.17	73%	0%	27%
3/4 tsp (3 g) baking soda	0	0	0	0	0	0	0	0%	0%	0%
6 large (300 g) eggs	428	30	13	3	0	0	3	63%	12%	25%
1/4 cup (60 g) unsweetened almond milk	11.25	0.88	0.5	0.75	0.25	0	0.5	70%	18%	12%
1 tsp (7 g) blackstrap molasses or yacón syrup	19.33	0	0	5	0	0	5	0%	0%	100%
1 tbsp (15 g) apple cider vinegar	3	0	0	0	0	0	0	0%	0%	100%
Totals (of 6 Servings):	2323.3	188.78	55.4	240.15	40.2	144	55.95	73%	10%	17%
Per Serving:	387.22	31.46	9.23	40.03	6.70	24.00	**9.33**	**73%**	10%	17%

Chorizo, Cilantro and Cotija Muffins — P. 98

	CA	FAT	P	C	F	SA	NC	FAT%	P%	C%
8 oz (227 g) chorizo links	480.71	32.05	42.73	5.34	2.67	0	2.67	60%	36%	4%
3/4 cup (84 g) almond flour	480	42	18	18	9	0	9	79%	15%	6%
1/2 cup (48 g) white chia seed flour	224	14.4	6.4	22.4	19.2	0	3.2	58%	11%	31%
1/4 cup (26 g) golden flaxseed meal	140	9	6	8	6	0	2	58%	17%	25%
1 tbsp (14 g) baking powder	6	0	0	3.9	0	0	3.9	0%	0%	100%
Dash salt and pepper	0	0	0	0	0	0	0	0%	0%	0%
6 large (300 g) eggs	428	30	13	3	0	0	3	63%	12%	25%
1/4 cup + 2 tbsp (90 g) unsweetened almond milk	16.88	1.32	0.75	1.13	0.38	0	1.32	70%	18%	12%
2 tbsp (28 g) melted butter or lard	200	22	0	0	0	0	0	99%	0%	1%
8 oz (227 g) crumbled Cotija cheese	808.26	63.63	51.59	6.88	0	0	6.88	71%	26%	4%
1/4 cup (22 g) chopped cilantro	5.06	0.22	0.44	0.88	0.66	0	0.22	39%	35%	26%
Totals (of 6 Servings):	2788.9	214.62	138.91	69.53	37.91	0	32.19	69%	20%	11%
Per Serving:	464.82	35.77	23.15	11.59	6.32	0.00	**5.37**	**69%**	20%	11%

CA: Calories | **FAT:** Fat | **P:** Protein | **C:** Carbohydrates | **F:** Fiber | **SA:** Sugar Alcohols | **NC:** Net Carbs
FAT%: Calories from Fat | **P%:** Calories from Protein | **C%:** Calories from Carbohydrates

Jalapeño Cheddar Muffins — P. 104

	CA	FAT	P	C	F	SA	NC	FAT%	P%	C%
1/2 cup (50 g) pecan halves	345.5	36	4.5	7	5	0	2	94%	5%	1%
1/2 cup (48 g) white chia seed flour	224	14.4	6.4	22.4	19.2	0	3.2	58%	11%	31%
1/4 cup (26 g) golden flaxseed meal	140	9	6	8	6	0	2	58%	17%	25%
1/4 cup (28 g) almond flour	160	14	6	6	3	0	3	79%	15%	6%
3/4 tsp (3 g) baking soda	0	0	0	0	0	0	0	0%	0%	0%
3/4 tsp (3 g) salt	0	0	0	0	0	0	0	0%	0%	0%
Dash pepper	0	0	0	0	0	0	0	0%	0%	0%
1 large (67 g) lime	20	0	0	7	2	0	5	0%	0%	100%
6 large (300 g) eggs	428	30	13	3	0	0	3	63%	12%	25%
1/4 cup (60 g) unsweetened almond milk	11.25	0.88	0.5	0.75	0.25	0	0.5	70%	18%	12%
3 tbsp (42 g) melted butter or lard	300	33	0	0	0	0	0	99%	0%	1%
8 oz (227 g) cheddar cheese	902.43	74.36	56	2.75	0	0	2.75	74%	25%	1%
2 fresh (28 g) jalapeño peppers	8.4	0.28	0.28	1.68	0.84	0	0.84	30%	13%	57%
Totals (of 6 Servings):	2539.6	211.92	92.68	58.58	36.29	0	22.29	75%	15%	10%
Per Serving:	423.26	35.32	15.45	9.76	6.05	0.00	3.72	75%	15%	10%

Grain-Free, Nut-Free Fauxcaccia — P. 106

	CA	FAT	P	C	F	SA	NC	FAT%	P%	C%
1 cup (64 g) sunflower seed flour	395.43	36.57	11.43	13.71	6.86	0	6.85	83%	12%	5%
1/2 cup (52 g) flaxseed meal	280	18	12	16	12	0	4	58%	17%	25%
1/2 cup (48 g) ground chia	224	14.4	6.4	22.4	19.2	0	3.2	58%	11%	31%
1 tbsp (3 g) fresh chopped thyme	3.03	0.06	0.18	0.72	0.36	0	0.36	18%	24%	58%
1 1/8 tsp (4.5 g) baking soda	0	0	0	0	0	0	0	0%	0%	0%
1 tsp (4 g) salt	0	0	0	0	0	0	0	0%	0%	0%
1/2 tsp (1 g) crushed red chili flakes	3.18	0.17	0.12	0.57	0.27	0	0.3	48%	15%	37%
8 large (400 g) eggs, beaten	570.66	40	17.34	4	0	0	4	63%	12%	25%
1/4 cup + 2 tbsp (90 g) unsweetened hempseed milk or water	26.25	1.88	1.13	0.75	0.75	0	0	64%	17%	18%
1/4 cup (56 g) extra-virgin olive oil	480.00	48.00	0	0	0	0	0	90%	0%	10%
1 1/2 tbsp (23 g) white vinegar or lemon juice	4.5	0	0	0	0	0	0	0%	0%	100%
6 each (18 g) garlic cloves	24	0	0	6	0	0	6	0%	0%	100%
Totals (of 6 Servings):	2011	159.08	48.6	64.15	39.44	0	24.71	71%	10%	19%
Per Serving:	335.17	26.51	8.10	10.69	6.57	0.00	4.12	71%	10%	19%

CA: Calories | **FAT:** Fat | **P:** Protein | **C:** Carbohydrates | **F:** Fiber | **SA:** Sugar Alcohols | **NC:** Net Carbs
FAT%: Calories from Fat | **P%:** Calories from Protein | **C%:** Calories from Carbohydrates

Mini Carrot Cakes with Cream Cheese Frosting — P. 116

	CA	FAT	P	C	F	SA	NC	FAT%	P%	C%
1 cup (56 g) grated raw carrot	45.04	0	1.04	11.04	3.04	0	8	0%	9%	91%
1 tsp (4 g) salt	0	0	0	0	0	0	0	0%	0%	0%
1/2 cup + 2 tbsp (84 g) walnut flour	549.5	54.6	12.6	11.2	5.6	0	5.6	89%	9%	1%
1/2 cup (56 g) almond flour	320	28	12	12	6	0	6	79%	15%	6%
1/4 cup + 2 tbsp (42 g) coconut flour	186	4.5	10.5	27	18	0	9	22%	23%	56%
1/4 cup + 2 tbsp (72 g) sugar replacement	0	0	0	72	0	72	0	0%	0%	100%
1 tbsp (14 g) baking powder	6	0	0	3.9	0	0	3.9	0%	0%	100%
1/2 tsp (1 g) ground cinnamon	3.17	0	0	1	0.67	0	0.33	0%	0%	100%
1/4 tsp (.5) ground nutmeg	3.08	0.25	0	0.25	0.08	0	0.17	73%	0%	27%
6 large (300 g) eggs	428	30	13	3	0	0	3	63%	12%	25%
1/4 cup (60 g) unsweetened almond milk	11.25	0.88	0.5	0.75	0.25	0	0.5	70%	18%	12%
1 tsp (7 g) blackstrap molasses or yacón syrup	19.33	0	0	5	0	0	5	0%	0%	100%
2 tbsp (18 g) coarsely chopped raisins	61.63	0.13	0.63	16.38	0.75	0	15.63	2%	4%	94%
3 tbsp (42 g) melted butter	300	33	0	0	0	0	0	99%	0%	1%
1 recipe Cream Cheese Frosting (p. 196)	527.43	55.05	3.91	110.76	0	108	2.76	94%	3%	3%
Totals (of 6 Servings):	2460.4	206.41	54.18	274.28	34.39	180	59.89	76%	9%	16%
Per Serving:	410.07	34.40	9.03	45.71	5.73	30.00	**9.98**	**76%**	9%	16%

Strawberry Yogurt Muffins — P. 106

	CA	FAT	P	C	F	SA	NC	FAT%	P%	C%
3/4 cup (84 g) almond flour	480	42	18	18	9	0	9	79%	15%	6%
1/4 cup + 2 tbsp (45 g) sugar-free vanilla protein powder	165	0	37.5	1.5	0	0	1.5	0%	91%	9%
1/4 cup + 2 tbsp (42 g) coconut flour	186	4.5	10.5	27	18	0	9	22%	23%	56%
1/4 cup + 2 tbsp (72 g) sugar replacement	0	0	0	72	0	72	0	0%	0%	100%
3/4 tsp (3 g) baking soda	0	0	0	0	0	0	0	0%	0%	0%
3/4 tsp (3 g) salt	0	0	0	0	0	0	0	0%	0%	0%
6 large (300 g) eggs	428	30	13	3	0	0	3	63%	12%	25%
1/2 cup + 2 tbsp (141 g) plain full-fat Greek yogurt	162.5	13.75	5	6.25	0	0	6.25	76%	12%	12%
1 cup (166 g) coarsely chopped strawberries	53	0	1	13	3	0	10	0%	8%	92%
Totals (of 6 Servings):	1474.5	90.25	85	140.75	30	72	38.75	55%	23%	22%
Per Serving:	245.75	15.04	14.17	23.46	5.00	12.00	**6.46**	**55%**	23%	22%

CA: Calories | FAT: Fat | P: Protein | C: Carbohydrates | F: Fiber | SA: Sugar Alcohols | NC: Net Carbs
FAT%: Calories from Fat | P%: Calories from Protein | C%: Calories from Carbohydrates

Carrot, Coconut and Macadamia Mega-Muffins — P. 122

	CA	FAT	P	C	F	SA	NC	FAT%	P%	C%
1/2 cup (56 g) grated raw carrot	22.52	0	0.52	5.52	1.52	0	4	0%	9%	91%
1 tsp (4 g) salt	0	0	0	0	0	0	0	0%	0%	0%
1/2 cup + 2 tbsp (84 g) macadamia flour	603.04	63.94	6.9	11.91	7.52	0	4.39	95%	5%	-0%
1/2 cup (56 g) almond flour	320	28	12	12	6	0	6	79%	15%	6%
1/4 cup + 2 tbsp (42 g) coconut flour	186	4.5	10.5	27	18	0	9	22%	23%	56%
1/4 cup + 2 tbsp (72 g) sugar replacement	0	0	0	72	0	72	0	0%	0%	100%
3 tbsp (23 g) tapioca flour (optional)	75	0	0	19.5	0	0	19.5	0%	0%	100%
1 tsp (6 g) xanthan gum (optional)	20	0	0	4.68	4.68	0	0	0%	0%	100%
3/4 tsp (3 g) baking soda	0	0	0	0	0	0	0	0%	0%	0%
1 large (67 g) lime	20	0	0	7	2	0	5	0%	0%	100%
6 large (300 g) eggs	428	30	13	3	0	0	3	63%	12%	25%
1/4 cup (60 g) unsweetened almond milk	11.25	0.88	0.5	0.75	0.25	0	0.5	70%	18%	12%
1 tsp (7 g) blackstrap molasses or yacón syrup	19.33	0	0	5	0	0	5	0%	0%	100%
1/2 cup (36 g) flaked unsweetened coconut	200	20	4	8	8	0	0	90%	8%	2%
1/2 cup (67 g) chopped macadamia nuts	481	51	5.5	9.5	6	0	3.5	95%	5%	0%
2 tbsp (28 g) coconut oil	240	24	0	0	0	0	0	90%	0%	10%
Totals (of 6 Servings):	2626.1	222.32	52.92	185.86	53.97	72	59.89	76%	8%	16%
Per Serving:	437.69	37.05	8.82	30.98	9.00	12.00	9.98	76%	8%	16%

One-Minute Cheddar Bread and Buns — P. 172

	CA	FAT	P	C	F	SA	NC	FAT%	P%	C%
1 cup (104g) golden flaxseed meal	560	36	24	32	24	0	8	58%	17%	25%
2 tsp (9 g) baking powder	10	0	0	2	0	0	2	0%	0%	100%
4 large (200 g) eggs	285.33	20	8.67	2	0	0	2	63%	12%	25%
1 tbsp (14 g) olive oil	100	11	0	0	0	0	0	99%	0%	1%
1/2 cup (57 g) shredded cheddar/colby cheese blend	221.5	18	13.5	1.5	0	0	1.5	73%	24%	2%
2 each (6 g) garlic cloves	8	0	0	2	0	0	2	0%	0%	100%
1/2 tsp (.5g) fresh chopped thyme	0.52	0.01	0.03	0.12	0.08	0	0.04	17%	23%	60%
salt, fresh-cracked pepper, and chili flakes, to taste	0	0	0	0	0	0	0	0%	0%	0%
Totals (of 4 Servings):	1185.3	85.01	46.2	39.62	24.08	0	15.54	65%	16%	20%
Per Serving:	296.34	21.25	11.55	9.91	6.02	0.00	3.89	65%	16%	20%

CA: Calories | **FAT:** Fat | **P:** Protein | **C:** Carbohydrates | **F:** Fiber | **SA:** Sugar Alcohols | **NC:** Net Carbs
FAT%: Calories from Fat | **P%:** Calories from Protein | **C%:** Calories from Carbohydrates

Chocolate-Chocolate Chunk Muffins with Chocolate Ganache — P. 126

	CA	FAT	P	C	F	SA	NC	FAT%	P%	C%
1 cup (112 g) almond flour	640	56	24	24	12	0	12	79%	15%	6%
1/4 cup + 2 tbsp (42 g) coconut flour	186	4.5	10.5	27	18	0	9	22%	23%	56%
1/4 cup + 2 tbsp (72 g) sugar replacement	0	0	0	72	0	72	0	0%	0%	100%
1/4 cup + 2 tbsp (32 g) unsweetened cocoa powder	73.5	4.48	6.42	18.78	10.92	0	7.86	55%	35%	10%
1/4 cup (24 g) ground chia	112	7.2	3.2	11.2	9.6	0	1.6	58%	11%	31%
1 tbsp (14 g) baking powder	6	0	0	3.9	0	0	3.9	0%	0%	100%
3/4 tsp (3 g) salt	0	0	0	0	0	0	0	0%	0%	0%
4 large (200 g) eggs	285.33	20	8.67	2	0	0	2	63%	12%	25%
1/4 cup + 2 tbsp (90 g) unsweetened almond milk	16.89	1.32	0.75	1.14	0.39	0	0.75	70%	18%	12%
3 tbsp (42 g) melted butter	300	33	0	0	0	0	0	99%	0%	1%
1 3.5 oz (100 g) dark chocolate bar	575	45	12.5	37.5	15	0	22.5	70%	9%	21%
1 recipe warm Chocolate Ganache (p. 200)	855	76.5	22	82.5	18.5	48	16	81%	10%	9%
Totals (of 6 Servings):	3049.7	248	88.04	280.02	84.41	120	75.61	73%	12%	15%
Per Serving:	508.29	41.33	14.67	46.67	14.07	20.00	**12.60**	**73%**	12%	15%

Brown Butter Ginger-Spice "Riddles & Games" — P. 118

	CA	FAT	P	C	F	SA	NC	FAT%	P%	C%
1 cup (238 g) heavy cream	821	88	5	7	0	0	7	96%	2%	1%
1 cup + 2 tbsp (126 g) almond flour	720	63	27	27	13.5	0	13.5	79%	15%	6%
1/4 cup + 2 tbsp (42 g) coconut flour	186	4.5	10.5	27	18	0	9	22%	23%	56%
1/4 cup + 2 tbsp (72 g) sugar replacement	0	0	0	72	0	72	0	0%	0%	100%
1 tbsp (14 g) baking powder	6	0	0	3.9	0	0	3.9	0%	0%	100%
3/4 tsp (3 g) salt	0	0	0	0	0	0	0	0%	0%	0%
1/2 tsp (1 g) ground cinnamon	3.17	0	0	1	0.67	0	0.33	0%	0%	100%
1/4 tsp (.5 g) ground nutmeg	3.08	0.25	0	0.25	0.08	0	0.17	73%	0%	27%
1/8 tsp (.25 g) ground cloves	0.58	0.05	0.02	0.15	0.09	0	0.06	78%	14%	9%
6 large (300 g) eggs	428	30	13	3	0	0	3	63%	12%	25%
1/4 cup (60 g) unsweetened almond milk	11.25	0.88	0.5	0.75	0.25	0	0.5	70%	18%	12%
1 tbsp (14 g) freshly grated ginger	11.2	0.14	0.28	2.52	0.28	0	2.24	11%	10%	79%
Totals (of 6 Servings):	2190.3	186.82	56.3	144.57	32.87	72	39.7	77%	10%	13%
Per Serving:	365.05	31.14	9.38	24.10	5.48	12.00	**6.62**	**77%**	10%	13%

CA: Calories | **FAT**: Fat | **P**: Protein | **C**: Carbohydrates | **F**: Fiber | **SA**: Sugar Alcohols | **NC**: Net Carbs
FAT%: Calories from Fat | **P%**: Calories from Protein | **C%**: Calories from Carbohydrates

Mini Coconut Muffaroons — P. 130

	CA	FAT	P	C	F	SA	NC	FAT%	P%	C%
1/2 cup + 2 tbsp (84 g) almond flour	400	35	15	15	7.5	0	7.5	79%	15%	6%
1/2 cup (96 g) sugar replacement	0	0	0	96	0	96	0	0%	0%	100%
1/4 cup + 2 tbsp (45 g) sugar-free vanilla protein powder	165	0	37.5	1.5	0	0	1.5	0%	91%	9%
1/4 cup + 2 tbsp (42 g) coconut flour	186	4.5	10.5	27	18	0	9	22%	23%	56%
1 tbsp (14 g) baking powder	6	0	0	3.9	0	0	3.9	0%	0%	100%
3/4 tsp (3 g) salt	0	0	0	0	0	0	0	0%	0%	0%
1 cup (88 g) unsweetened shredded coconut	480	48	8	24	16	0	8	90%	7%	3%
6 large (300 g) eggs	428	30	13	3	0	0	3	63%	12%	25%
1/4 cup + 2 tbsp (90 g) unsweetened almond milk	16.89	1.32	0.75	1.14	0.39	0	0.75	70%	18%	12%
1 tsp (7 g) blackstrap molasses or yacón syrup	19.33	0	0	5	0	0	5	0%	0%	100%
3 tbsp (42 g) melted butter	300	33	0	0	0	0	0	99%	0%	1%
1 recipe Chocolate Ganache (optional - p. 200)	855	76.5	22	82.5	18.5	48	16	81%	10%	9%
Totals (of 6 Servings):	2856.2	228.32	106.75	259.04	60.39	144	54.65	72%	15%	13%
Per Serving:	476.04	38.05	17.79	43.17	10.07	24.00	**9.11**	**72%**	15%	13%

Fried Blob — P. 140

	CA	FAT	P	C	F	SA	NC	FAT%	P%	C%
Refined coconut oil or ghee, for frying	0	0	0	0	0	0	0	0%	0%	0%
3/4 cup (84 g) almond flour	480	42	18	18	9	0	9	79%	15%	6%
1/4 cup + 2 tbsp (45 g) sugar-free vanilla protein powder	165	0	37.5	1.5	0	0	1.5	0%	91%	9%
1/4 cup + 2 tbsp (42 g) coconut flour	186	4.5	10.5	27	18	0	9	22%	23%	56%
1/4 cup + 2 tbsp (72 g) sugar replacement	0	0	0	72	0	72	0	0%	0%	100%
1 tbsp (14 g) baking powder	6	0	0	3.9	0	0	3.9	0%	0%	100%
3/4 tsp (3 g) salt	0	0	0	0	0	0	0	0%	0%	0%
6 large (300 g) eggs	428	30	13	3	0	0	3	63%	12%	25%
1/4 cup (60 g) heavy whipping cream	205.25	22	1.25	1.75	0	0	1.75	96%	2%	1%
1/2 cup (96 g) powdered sugar replacement	0	0	0	96	0	96	0	0%	0%	100%
1/2 tsp (1 g) ground cinnamon	3.17	0	0	1	0.67	0	0.33	0%	0%	100%
1/4 tsp (.5 g) ground nutmeg	3.08	0.25	0	0.25	0.08	0	0.17	73%	0%	27%
Totals (of 6 Servings):	1476.5	98.75	80.25	224.4	27.75	168	28.65	60%	22%	18%
Per Serving:	246.08	16.46	13.38	37.40	4.63	28.00	**4.78**	**60%**	22%	18%

CA: Calories | **FAT:** Fat | **P:** Protein | **C:** Carbohydrates | **F:** Fiber | **SA:** Sugar Alcohols | **NC:** Net Carbs
FAT%: Calories from Fat | **P%:** Calories from Protein | **C%:** Calories from Carbohydrates

Sour Cream Coffee Cake with Hazelnut Struesel — P. 132

	CA	FAT	P	C	F	SA	NC	FAT%	P%	C%
Sour Cream Coffee Cake										
1 cup + 2 tbsp (126 g) hazelnut flour	810	76.5	18	22.5	13.5	0	9	85%	9%	6%
1/4 cup + 2 tbsp (42 g) coconut flour	186	4.5	10.5	27	18	0	9	22%	23%	56%
1/4 cup + 2 tbsp (72 g) sugar replacement	0	0	0	72	0	72	0	0%	0%	100%
3/4 tsp (3 g) baking soda	0	0	0	0	0	0	0	0%	0%	0%
3/4 tsp (3 g) salt	0	0	0	0	0	0	0	0%	0%	0%
6 large (300 g) eggs	428	30	13	3	0	0	3	63%	12%	25%
1 (4 g) tsp vanilla extract	11.54	0	0	0.5	0	0	0.5	0%	0%	100%
3/4 cup (173 g) sour cream	333	33.75	3.75	6	0	0	6	91%	5%	4%
Hazelnut Struesel										
1/2 cup (56 g) hazelnut flour	360	34	8	10	6	0	4	85%	9%	6%
1/2 cup (56 g) chopped hazelnuts	361	35	8.5	9.5	5.5	0	4	87%	9%	3%
2 tbsp (24 g) sugar replacement	0	0	0	24	0	24	0	0%	0%	100%
1 tbsp (14 g) melted butter	100	10	0	0	0	0	0	90%	0%	10%
1 tsp (7 g) blackstrap molasses or yacón syrup	19.33	0	0	5	0	0	5	0%	0%	100%
1/2 tsp (1 g) ground cinnamon	3.17	0	0	1	0.67	0	0.33	0%	0%	100%
Dash salt	0	0	0	0	0	0	0	0%	0%	0%
Totals (of 6 Servings):	2612	223.75	61.75	180.5	43.67	96	40.83	77%	9%	13%
Per Serving:	435.34	37.29	10.29	30.08	7.28	16.00	**6.81**	**77%**	9%	13%

Vanilla Bean Muffcakes — P. 162

	CA	FAT	P	C	F	SA	NC	FAT%	P%	C%
3/4 cup (180 g) heavy cream	615.75	66	3.75	5.25	0	0	5.25	96%	2%	1%
1/4 cup + 2 tbsp (72 g) sugar replacement	0	0	0	72	0	72	0	0%	0%	100%
1 vanilla bean	0	0	0	0	0	0	0	0%	0%	0%
1 cup + 2 tbsp (126 g) almond flour	720	63	27	27	13.5	0	13.5	79%	15%	6%
1/4 cup + 2 tbsp (42 g) coconut flour	186	4.5	10.5	27	18	0	9	22%	23%	56%
1 tbsp (14 g) baking powder	6	0	0	3.9	0	0	3.9	0%	0%	100%
3/4 tsp (3 g) salt	0	0	0	0	0	0	0	0%	0%	0%
6 large (300 g) eggs	428	30	13	3	0	0	3	63%	12%	25%
Totals (of 6 Servings):	1955.7	163.5	54.25	138.15	31.5	72	34.65	75%	11%	14%
Per Serving:	325.96	27.25	9.04	23.03	5.25	12.00	**5.78**	**75%**	11%	14%

Mini Gingerbread Loaves

P. 138

	CA	FAT	P	C	F	SA	NC	FAT%	P%	C%
1 cup + 2 tbsp (126 g) almond flour	720	63	27	27	13.5	0	13.5	79%	15%	6%
1/4 cup + 2 tbsp (42 g) coconut flour	186	4.5	10.5	27	18	0	9	22%	23%	56%
1/4 cup + 2 tbsp (72 g) sugar replacement	0	0	0	72	0	72	0	0%	0%	100%
1 tsp (2 g) ground cinnamon	6.34	0	0	2	1.34	0	0.66	0%	0%	100%
3/4 tsp (3 g) baking soda	0	0	0	0	0	0	0	0%	0%	0%
3/4 tsp (3 g) salt	0	0	0	0	0	0	0	0%	0%	0%
1/2 tsp (1 g) ground nutmeg	6.16	0.5	0	0.5	0.16	0	0.34	73%	0%	27%
1/8 tsp (.25 g) ground cloves	0.58	0.05	0.02	0.15	0.09	0	0.06	78%	14%	9%
6 large (300 g) eggs	428	30	13	3	0	0	3	63%	12%	25%
1/2 cup (119 g) heavy whipping cream	410.5	44	2.5	3.5	0	0	3.5	96%	2%	1%
2 tbsp (42 g) blackstrap molasses or yacón syrup	115.98	0	0	30	0	0	30	0%	0%	100%
2 tbsp (30 g) apple cider vinegar	6	0	0	0	0	0	0	0%	0%	100%
1 tbsp (15 g) freshly grated ginger	11.2	0.14	0.28	2.52	0.28	0	2.24	11%	10%	79%
1 recipe Cream Cheese Frosting (optional - p. 196)	855	76.5	22	82.5	18.5	48	16	81%	10%	9%
Totals (of 6 Servings):	2745.7	218.69	75.3	250.17	51.87	120	78.3	72%	11%	17%
Per Serving:	457.63	36.45	12.55	41.70	8.65	20.00	13.05	72%	11%	17%

Layered Eggnog Discs with Eggnog Chantilly and Eggnog

P. 134

	CA	FAT	P	C	F	SA	NC	FAT%	P%	C%
1 cup + 2 tbsp (126 g) almond flour	720	63	27	27	13.5	0	13.5	79%	15%	6%
1/2 cup (96 g) sugar replacement	0	0	0	96	0	96	0	0%	0%	100%
1/4 cup + 2 tbsp (42 g) coconut flour	186	4.5	10.5	27	18	0	9	22%	23%	56%
1 tbsp (14 g) baking powder	6	0	0	3.9	0	0	3.9	0%	0%	100%
3/4 tsp (3 g) salt	0	0	0	0	0	0	0	0%	0%	0%
1/2 tsp (1 g) ground cinnamon	3.17	0	0	1	0.67	0	0.33	0%	0%	100%
1/4 tsp (.5) ground nutmeg	3.08	0.25	0	0.25	0.08	0	0.17	73%	0%	27%
6 large (300 g) eggs	428	30	13	3	0	0	3	63%	12%	25%
1 1/4 cups (298 g) heavy whipping cream	1026.2	110	6.25	8.75	0	0	8.75	96%	2%	1%
1 tsp (4 g) vanilla extract	11.54	0	0	0.5	0	0	0.5	0%	0%	100%
2 cups (480 g) Eggnog (p. 202)	887.04	87.92	9.83	31.34	0.74	22.03	8.57	89%	4%	6%
Totals (of 6 Servings):	3271	295.67	66.58	198.74	32.99	118.03	47.72	81%	8%	11%
Per Serving:	545.18	49.28	11.10	33.12	5.50	19.67	7.95	81%	8%	11%

CA: Calories | **FAT:** Fat | **P:** Protein | **C:** Carbohydrates | **F:** Fiber | **SA:** Sugar Alcohols | **NC:** Net Carbs
FAT%: Calories from Fat | **P%:** Calories from Protein | **C%:** Calories from Carbohydrates

Mexican Chocolate Muffins — P. 142

	CA	FAT	P	C	F	SA	NC	FAT%	P%	C%
1 cup (112 g) almond flour	640	56	24	24	12	0	12	79%	15%	6%
1/4 cup + 2 tbsp (42 g) coconut flour	186	4.5	10.5	27	18	0	9	22%	23%	56%
1/4 cup + 2 tbsp (72 g) sugar replacement	0	0	0	72	0	72	0	0%	0%	100%
1/4 cup + 2 tbsp (32 g) unsweetened cocoa powder	73.5	4.48	6.42	18.78	10.92	0	7.86	55%	35%	10%
1/4 cup (24 g) ground chia	112	7.2	3.2	11.2	9.6	0	1.6	58%	11%	31%
1 tbsp (14 g) baking powder	6	0	0	3.9	0	0	3.9	0%	0%	100%
1 tsp (2 g) ground cinnamon	6.34	0	0	2	1.34	0	0.66	0%	0%	100%
3/4 tsp (3 g) salt	0	0	0	0	0	0	0	0%	0%	0%
1/2 tsp (1 g) grated nutmeg	6.16	0.5	0	0.5	0.16	0	0.34	73%	0%	27%
1/2 tsp (1 g) ground allspice	2.63	0.09	0.06	0.72	0.22	0	0.5	31%	9%	60%
1/2 tsp (1 g) powdered cayenne or ancho chili pepper	2.84	0.17	0.17	0.5	0.17	0	0.33	54%	24%	22%
4 large (200 g) eggs	285.33	20	8.67	2	0	0	2	63%	12%	25%
1/4 cup + 2 tbsp (90 g) unsweetened almond milk	16.89	1.32	0.75	1.14	0.39	0	0.75	70%	18%	12%
1 (4 g) tsp vanilla extract	11.54	0	0	0.5	0	0	0.5	0%	0%	100%
3 tbsp (42 g) melted butter	300	33	0	0	0	0	0	99%	0%	1%
Totals (of 6 Servings):	1649.2	127.26	53.77	164.24	52.8	72	39.44	69%	13%	18%
Per Serving:	274.87	21.21	8.96	27.37	8.80	12.00	**6.57**	**69%**	13%	18%

Mocha Mint Muffins — P. 144

	CA	FAT	P	C	F	SA	NC	FAT%	P%	C%
1 1/4 cups (300 g) heavy cream	1026.2	110	6.25	8.75	0	0	8.75	96%	2%	1%
1 bunch (about 3.5 oz [100 g]) fresh mint	0	0	0	0	0	0	0	0%	0%	0%
1 cup (112 g) almond flour	640	56	24	24	12	0	12	79%	15%	6%
1/2 cup (96 g) powdered sugar replacement	0	0	0	96	0	96	0	0%	0%	100%
1/4 cup + 2 tbsp (42 g) coconut flour	186	4.5	10.5	27	18	0	9	22%	23%	56%
1/4 cup + 2 tbsp (32 g) unsweetened cocoa powder	73.5	4.48	6.42	18.78	10.92	0	7.86	55%	35%	10%
1/4 cup (24 g) ground chia	112	7.2	3.2	11.2	9.6	0	1.6	58%	11%	31%
1 tbsp (14 g) baking powder	6	0	0	3.9	0	0	3.9	0%	0%	100%
3/4 tsp (3 g) salt	0	0	0	0	0	0	0	0%	0%	0%
4 large (200 g) eggs	285.33	20	8.67	2	0	0	2	63%	12%	25%
Totals (of 6 Servings):	2329.1	202.18	59.04	191.63	50.52	96	45.11	78%	10%	12%
Per Serving:	388.18	33.70	9.84	31.94	8.42	16.00	**7.52**	**78%**	10%	12%

CA: Calories | **FAT:** Fat | **P:** Protein | **C:** Carbohydrates | **F:** Fiber | **SA:** Sugar Alcohols | **NC:** Net Carbs
FAT%: Calories from Fat | **P%:** Calories from Protein | **C%:** Calories from Carbohydrates

Bacon & Orange Muffins with Pecan Streusel & Sour Cream Glaze — P. 148

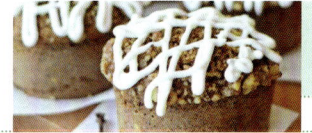

	CA	FAT	P	C	F	SA	NC	FAT%	P%	C%
Bacon & Orange Muffins										
1/2 cup + 2 tbsp (84 g) pecan flour	580.44	60.48	7.56	11.76	8.4	0	3.36	94%	5%	1%
1/4 cup + 2 tbsp (45 g) sugar-free vanilla protein powder	165	0	37.5	1.5	0	0	1.5	0%	91%	9%
1/4 cup + 2 tbsp (42 g) coconut flour	186	4.5	10.5	27	18	0	9	22%	23%	56%
1/4 cup + 2 tbsp (72 g) sugar replacement	0	0	0	72	0	72	0	0%	0%	100%
3/4 tsp (3 g) baking soda	0	0	0	0	0	0	0	0%	0%	0%
3/4 tsp (3 g) salt	0	0	0	0	0	0	0	0%	0%	0%
1 (159 g) orange	100	0	2	25	7	0	18	0%	8%	92%
6 large (300 g) eggs	428	30	13	3	0	0	3	63%	12%	25%
1/2 cup + 2 tbsp (144 g) sour cream	277.5	28.13	3.13	5	0	0	5	91%	5%	4%
1/4 cup + 2 tbsp (43 g) bacon bits	150	9	18	0	0	0	0	54%	48%	-2%
1 tbsp (2 g) fresh chopped rosemary	2.62	0.12	0.06	0.42	0.28	0	0.14	41%	9%	50%
Pecan Struesel										
1/2 cup (56 g) pecan flour	386.96	40.32	5.04	7.84	5.6	0	2.24	94%	5%	1%
1/2 cup (55 g) chopped pecans	380.05	39.6	4.95	7.7	5.5	0	2.2	94%	5%	1%
2 tbsp (24 g) sugar replacement	0	0	0	24	0	24	0	0%	0%	100%
1 tbsp (14 g) melted butter	100	11	0	0	0	0	0	99%	0%	1%
1/4 tsp (.5 g) ground cloves	0.58	0.05	0.02	0.15	0.09	0	0.06	78%	14%	9%
Dash salt	0	0	0	0	0	0	0	0%	0%	0%
Sour Cream Glaze										
1/2 cup (115 g) sour cream	222	22.5	2.5	4	0	0	4	91%	5%	4%
1/4 cup (48 g) powdered sugar replacement	0	0	0	48	0	48	0	0%	0%	100%
1 tsp (2 g) orange zest	0	0	0	0	0	0	0	0%	0%	0%
1 tsp (4 g) vanilla extract	11.54	0	0	0.5	0	0	0.5	0%	0%	100%
Dash orange juice	0	0	0	0	0	0	0	0%	0%	0%
Dash salt	0	0	0	0	0	0	0	0%	0%	0%
Totals (of 6 Servings):	2990.7	245.7	104.26	237.87	44.87	144	49	74%	14%	12%
Per Serving:	498.45	40.95	17.38	39.65	7.48	24.00	8.17	74%	14%	12%

CA: Calories | **FAT:** Fat | **P:** Protein | **C:** Carbohydrates | **F:** Fiber | **SA:** Sugar Alcohols | **NC:** Net Carbs
FAT%: Calories from Fat | **P%:** Calories from Protein | **C%:** Calories from Carbohydrates

Orange-Cranberry Muffins — P. 152

	CA	FAT	P	C	F	SA	NC	FAT%	P%	C%
1/2 cup (48 g) chia seed flour	224	14.4	6.4	22.4	19.2	0	3.2	58%	11%	31%
1/2 cup (56 g) pecan flour	386.96	40.32	5.04	7.84	5.6	0	2.24	94%	5%	1%
1/2 cup (96 g) sugar replacement	0	0	0	96	0	96	0	0%	0%	100%
1/4 cup (26 g) flaxseed meal	140	9	6	8	6	0	2	58%	17%	25%
1/4 cup (28 g) almond flour	160	14	6	6	3	0	3	79%	15%	6%
3/4 tsp (3 g) baking soda	0	0	0	0	0	0	0	0%	0%	0%
3/4 tsp (3 g) salt	0	0	0	0	0	0	0	0%	0%	0%
1 (159 g) orange	100	0	2	25	7	0	18	0%	8%	92%
6 large (300 g) eggs	428	30	13	3	0	0	3	63%	12%	25%
3 tbsp (42 g) melted butter	300	33	0	0	0	0	0	99%	0%	1%
1 tsp (7 g) blackstrap molasses or yacón syrup	19.33	0	0	5	0	0	5	0%	0%	100%
1 cup (110 g) coarsely chopped cranberries	51	0	0	13	5	0	8	0%	0%	100%
2 tbsp (4 g) chopped fresh sage	1.31	0.06	0.03	0.24	0.14	0	0.1	41%	9%	50%
1/4 cup (28 g) chopped pecans	190.03	19.8	2.48	3.85	2.75	0	1.1	94%	5%	1%
Totals (of 6 Servings):	2000.6	160.58	40.95	190.33	48.69	96	45.64	72%	8%	20%
Per Serving:	333.44	26.76	6.83	31.72	8.12	16.00	7.61	72%	8%	20%

Mini Notella Muffnuts — P. 146

	CA	FAT	P	C	F	SA	NC	FAT%	P%	C%
1 cup (112 g) hazelnut flour	720	68	16	20	12	0	8	85%	9%	6%
1/4 cup + 2 tbsp (42 g) coconut flour	186	4.5	10.5	27	18	0	9	22%	23%	56%
1/4 cup + 2 tbsp (72 g) sugar replacement	0	0	0	72	0	72	0	0%	0%	100%
1/4 cup + 2 tbsp (32 g) unsweetened cocoa powder	73.5	4.48	6.42	18.78	10.92	0	7.86	55%	35%	10%
1/4 cup (24 g) ground chia	112	7.2	3.2	11.2	9.6	0	1.6	58%	11%	31%
1 tbsp (14 g) baking powder	6	0	0	3.9	0	0	3.9	0%	0%	100%
1 tsp (6 g) xanthan gum (optional)	20	0	0	4.68	4.68	0	0	0%	0%	100%
3/4 tsp (3 g) salt	0	0	0	0	0	0	0	0%	0%	0%
4 large (200 g) eggs	285.33	20	8.67	2	0	0	2	63%	12%	25%
1/2 cup + 2 tbsp (150 g) heavy cream	513.13	55	3.13	4.38	0	0	4.38	96%	2%	1%
1 recipe Notella (p. 198)	631.27	60.49	10.64	40.01	9.14	24	6.87	86%	7%	7%
Totals (of 6 Servings):	2547.2	219.67	58.56	203.95	64.34	96	43.61	78%	9%	13%
Per Serving:	424.54	36.61	9.76	33.99	10.72	16.00	7.27	78%	9%	13%

CA: Calories | **FAT:** Fat | **P:** Protein | **C:** Carbohydrates | **F:** Fiber | **SA:** Sugar Alcohols | **NC:** Net Carbs
FAT%: Calories from Fat | **P%:** Calories from Protein | **C%:** Calories from Carbohydrates

Pumpkin Cheesecake Swirl Muffin — P. 156

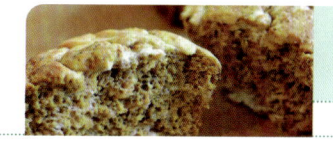

	CA	FAT	P	C	F	SA	NC	FAT%	P%	C%
Pumpkin Muffin										
3/4 cup (84 g) hazelnut flour	540	51	12	15	9	0	6	85%	9%	6%
1/4 cup (28 g) coconut flour	124	3	7	18	12	0	6	22%	23%	56%
1/4 cup (48 g) sugar replacement	0	0	0	48	0	48	0	0%	0%	100%
2 tsp (10 g) baking powder	4	0	0	2.6	0	0	2.6	0%	0%	100%
1/2 tsp (2 g) salt	0	0	0	0	0	0	0	0%	0%	0%
1/2 tsp (1 g) ground cinnamon	3.17	0	0	1	0.67	0	0.33	0%	0%	100%
1/4 tsp (.5) ground nutmeg	3.08	0.25	0	0.25	0.08	0	0.17	73%	0%	27%
1/8 tsp (.25 g) ground cloves	0.58	0.05	0.02	0.15	0.09	0	0.06	78%	14%	9%
4 large (200 g) eggs	285.33	20	8.67	2	0	0	2	63%	12%	25%
1/2 cup (122 g) canned or mashed pumpkin	49.68	0	1	9.92	3.96	0	5.96	0%	8%	92%
2 tbsp (28 g) melted butter	200	22	0	0	0	0	0	99%	0%	1%
1 tsp (7 g) blackstrap molasses or yacón syrup	19.33	0	0	5	0	0	5	0%	0%	100%
Cheesecake										
6 oz (170 g) full fat cream cheese	852.75	57.98	10.28	6.6	0	0	6.6	61%	5%	34%
1 large (50 g) egg	71.33	5	2.17	0.5	0	0	0.5	63%	12%	25%
1/2 tsp (2 g) vanilla extract	5.77	0	0	0.25	0	0	0.25	0%	0%	100%
Dash salt	0	0	0	0	0	0	0	0%	0%	0%
1/4 cup (48 g) powdered sugar replacement	0	0	0	48	0	48	0	0%	0%	100%
1/2 tsp (3 g) lemon juice	0.64	0	0	0.22	0.01	0	0.21	0%	0%	100%
1/4 cup (58 g) sour cream	111	11.25	1.25	2	0	0	2	91%	5%	4%
Totals (of 6 Servings):	2270.6	170.53	42.39	159.49	25.81	96	37.68	68%	7%	25%
Per Serving:	378.44	28.42	7.07	26.58	4.30	16.00	**6.28**	**68%**	7%	25%

Chocolate Ganache — P. 200

	CA	FAT	P	C	F	SA	NC	FAT%	P%	C%
1/2 cup (119 g) heavy whipping cream	410.5	44	2.5	3.5	0	0	3.5	96%	2%	1%
1/4 cup (48 g) sugar replacement	0	0	0	48	0	48	0	0%	0%	100%
2 1/2 oz (70 g) unsweetened baking chocolate squares	435	37.5	10	22.5	12.5	0	10	78%	9%	13%
1 tbsp (14 g) butter	100	11	0	0	0	0	0	99%	0%	1%
Totals (of 6 Servings):	945.5	92.5	12.5	74	12.5	48	13.5	88%	5%	7%
Per Serving:	157.58	15.42	2.08	12.33	2.08	8.00	**2.25**	**88%**	5%	7%

CA: Calories | **FAT:** Fat | **P:** Protein | **C:** Carbohydrates | **F:** Fiber | **SA:** Sugar Alcohols | **NC:** Net Carbs
FAT%: Calories from Fat | **P%:** Calories from Protein | **C%:** Calories from Carbohydrates

Frosted Carrot Cake OMM with Pecans — P. 182

	CA	FAT	P	C	F	SA	NC	FAT%	P%	C%
2 tbsp (13g) golden flaxseed meal	70	4.5	3	4	3	0	1	58%	17%	25%
2 tbsp (14 g) almond meal	80	7	3	3	1.5	0	1.5	79%	15%	6%
2 tbsp (24 g) sugar replacement	0	0	0	24	0	24	0	0%	0%	100%
1/2 tsp (2 g) baking powder	2.5	0	0	0.5	0	0	0.5	0%	0%	100%
1/2 tsp (1 g) ground cinnamon	2.47	0.01	0.04	0.81	0.53	0	0.28	4%	6%	90%
1/4 tsp (.5 g) freshly ground nutmeg	2.63	0.18	0.03	0.25	0.11	0	0.14	62%	5%	34%
Dash salt	0	0	0	0	0	0	0	0%	0%	0%
2 tbsp (14 g) grated raw carrot	5.63	0	0.13	1.38	0.38	0	1	0%	9%	91%
1 tbsp (6 g) chopped toasted pecans	42.75	4.44	0.56	0.88	0.63	0	0.25	93%	5%	1%
1 large (50g) whole egg	71.5	5	6.5	0.5	0	0	0.5	63%	36%	1%
1 tsp (5 g) melted butter	33.33	3.67	0	0	0	0	0	99%	0%	1%
1/2 tsp (2 g) vanilla extract	5.77	0	0	0.25	0	0	0.25	0%	0%	100%
3 tbsp (37 g) Cream Cheese Frosting (p. 196)	87.91	9.18	0.65	18.46	0.00	18.00	0.46	94%	3%	3%
Totals (of 1 Servings):	404.49	33.98	13.91	54.03	6.15	42	5.88	76%	14%	11%
Per Serving:	404.49	33.98	13.91	54.03	6.15	42.00	**5.88**	**76%**	14%	11%

Pear, Walnut and Blue Cheese Tart Fauxtan — P. 154

	CA	FAT	P	C	F	SA	NC	FAT%	P%	C%
1/4 cup (24 g) chia seed flour	112	7.2	3.2	11.2	9.6	0	1.6	58%	11%	31%
1/4 cup (34 g) walnut flour	222.42	22.1	5.1	4.53	2.27	0	2.26	89%	9%	1%
1/4 cup (48 g) sugar replacement	0	0	0	48	0	48	0	0%	0%	100%
2 tbsp (13 g) flaxseed meal	70	4.5	3	4	3	0	1	58%	17%	25%
2 tbsp (14 g) almond flour	80	7	3	3	1.5	0	1.5	79%	15%	6%
1 tsp (5 g) baking powder	2	0	0	1.3	0	0	1.3	0%	0%	100%
Dash salt	0	0	0	0	0	0	0	0%	0%	0%
3 large (150 g) eggs	214	15	6.5	1.5	0	0	1.5	63%	12%	25%
1/4 cup (60 g) heavy cream	205.25	22	1.25	1.75	0	0	1.75	96%	2%	1%
1 large (230 g) pear	133	0	1	36	7	0	29	0%	3%	97%
1/4 cup (34 g) crumbled blue cheese	119.25	9.75	7.25	0.75	0	0	0.75	74%	24%	2%
2 tbsp (16 g) chopped walnuts	98.94	9.47	3.84	1.54	1.15	0	0.39	86%	16%	-2%
Totals (of 6 Servings):	1256.8	97.02	34.14	113.57	24.52	48	41.05	69%	11%	20%
Per Serving:	209.48	16.17	5.69	18.93	4.09	8.00	**6.84**	**69%**	11%	20%

CA: Calories | FAT: Fat | P: Protein | C: Carbohydrates | F: Fiber | SA: Sugar Alcohols | NC: Net Carbs
FAT%: Calories from Fat | P%: Calories from Protein | C%: Calories from Carbohydrates

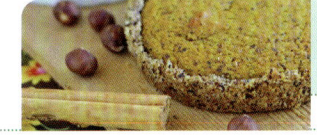

Spiced Pumpkin-Sour Cream Muffin Pies — P. 158

	CA	FAT	P	C	F	SA	NC	FAT%	P%	C%
Pie Crust										
1 1/2 cups (168 g) toasted hazelnuts (or hazelnut flour)	1080	102	24	30	18	0	12	85%	9%	6%
1/4 cup (56 g) melted butter	400	44	0	0	0	0	0	99%	0%	1%
1 tbsp (21 g) honey (optional)	64	0	0	17	0	0	17	0%	0%	100%
1 (4 g) tsp vanilla extract	11.54	0	0	0.5	0	0	0.5	0%	0%	100%
Dash salt	0	0	0	0	0	0	0	0%	0%	0%
Pumpkin Muffin										
1/2 cup + 2 tbsp (70 g) hazelnut flour	450	42.5	10	12.5	7.5	0	5	85%	9%	6%
1/4 cup (28 g) coconut flour	124	3	7	18	12	0	6	22%	23%	56%
1/4 cup (48 g) sugar replacement	0	0	0	48	0	48	0	0%	0%	100%
2 tbsp (12 g) ground chia	56	3.6	1.6	5.6	4.8	0	0.8	58%	11%	31%
1/2 tsp (2 g) baking soda	0	0	0	0	0	0	0	0%	0%	0%
1/2 tsp (2 g) salt	0	0	0	0	0	0	0	0%	0%	0%
1/2 tsp (1 g) ground cinnamon	3.17	0	0	1	0.67	0	0.33	0%	0%	100%
1/4 tsp (.5) ground nutmeg	3.08	0.25	0	0.25	0.08	0	0.17	73%	0%	27%
1/8 tsp (.25 g) ground cloves	0.58	0.05	0.02	0.15	0.09	0	0.06	78%	14%	9%
2 large (100 g) eggs	142.67	10	4.34	1	0	0	1	63%	12%	25%
1/2 cup (122 g) canned or mashed pumpkin	49.68	0	1	9.92	3.96	0	5.96	0%	8%	92%
1/2 cup (116 g) sour cream	222	22.5	2.5	4	0	0	4	91%	5%	4%
1 tsp (7 g) blackstrap molasses or yacón syrup	19.33	0	0	5	0	0	5	0%	0%	100%
Totals (of 6 Servings):	2626	227.9	50.46	152.92	47.1	48	57.82	78%	8%	14%
Per Serving:	437.68	37.98	8.41	25.49	7.85	8.00	**9.64**	**78%**	8%	14%

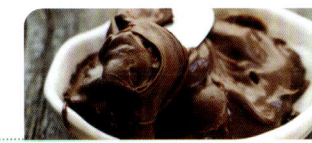

Notella — P. 198

	CA	FAT	P	C	F	SA	NC	FAT%	P%	C%
1/2 cup (55 g) peeled and toasted hazelnuts	361	35	8.5	9.5	5.5	0	4	87%	9%	3%
2 tbsp (11 g) unsweetened cocoa powder	24.5	1.49	2.14	6.26	3.64	0	2.62	55%	35%	10%
2 tbsp (24 g) powdered sugar replacement	0	0	0	24	0	24	0	0%	0%	100%
2 tbsp (28 g) palm or coconut oil	240	24	0	0	0	0	0	90%	0%	10%
1/2 tsp (2 g) vanilla extract	5.77	0	0	0.25	0	0	0.25	0%	0%	100%
1/2 tsp (2 g) salt	0	0	0	0	0	0	0	0%	0%	0%
Totals (of 6 Servings):	631.27	60.49	10.64	40.01	9.14	24	6.87	86%	7%	7%
Per Serving:	105.21	10.08	1.77	6.67	1.52	4.00	**1.15**	**86%**	7%	7%

CA: Calories | **FAT**: Fat | **P**: Protein | **C**: Carbohydrates | **F**: Fiber | **SA**: Sugar Alcohols | **NC**: Net Carbs
FAT%: Calories from Fat | **P%**: Calories from Protein | **C%**: Calories from Carbohydrates

OMM French Toast

P. 170

	CA	FAT	P	C	F	SA	NC	FAT%	P%	C%
1/4 cup (28 g) coconut flour	124	3	7	18	12	0	6	22%	23%	56%
1 tbsp (12 g) sugar replacement	0	0	0	12	0	12	0	0%	0%	100%
2 tsp (9 g) baking powder	10	0	0	2	0	0	2	0%	0%	100%
Dash salt	0	0	0	0	0	0	0	0%	0%	0%
8 large (400g) whole eggs	572	40	52	4	0	0	4	63%	36%	1%
3/4 cup (180 g) unsweetened almond milk	33.75	2.63	1.5	2.25	0.75	0	1.5	70%	18%	12%
1 tsp (4 g) vanilla extract	11.54	0	0	0.5	0	0	0.5	0%	0%	100%
1/4 cup (56 g) melted butter	400	44	0	0	0	0	0	99%	0%	1%
1/2 cup (119 g) heavy cream	410.5	44	2.5	3.5	0	0	3.5	96%	2%	1%
1/4 cup (56 g) fresh whole butter	400	44	0	0	0	0	0	99%	0%	1%
Totals (of 4 Servings):	1961.8	177.63	63	42.25	12.75	12	17.5	81%	13%	6%
Per Serving:	490.45	44.41	15.75	10.56	3.19	3.00	**4.38**	**81%**	13%	6%

Pesto alla Genovese

P. 194

	CA	FAT	P	C	F	SA	NC	FAT%	P%	C%
3 each (9 g) garlic cloves	13	0	1	3	0	0	3	0%	31%	69%
2/3 cup (144 g) extra-virgin olive oil	1273.3	144	0	0	0	0	0	102%	0%	-2%
2 cups (141 g) packed, cleaned, and dried fresh basil leaves (about a large bunch's worth)	32.43	1.41	4.23	4.23	2.82	0	1.41	39%	52%	9%
2 tsp (10 g) lemon juice	2.54	0	0	0.88	0.04	0	0.84	0%	0%	100%
1/4 cup (33 g) pine nuts	227.25	23	4.5	4.5	1.25	0	3.25	91%	8%	1%
1/4 cup (25 g) grated parmesan (reggiano) cheese	107.75	7.25	9.5	1	0	0	1	61%	35%	4%
1/4 cup (25 g) grated pecorino (romano) cheese	50	4	4	0	0	0	0	72%	32%	-4%
Salt and pepper, to taste	0	0	0	0	0	0	0	0%	0%	0%
Totals (of 4 Servings):	1706.3	179.66	23.23	13.61	4.11	0	9.5	95%	5%	-0%
Per Serving:	213.29	22.46	2.90	1.70	0.51	0.00	**1.19**	**95%**	5%	-0%

CA: Calories | FAT: Fat | P: Protein | C: Carbohydrates | F: Fiber | SA: Sugar Alcohols | NC: Net Carbs
FAT%: Calories from Fat | P%: Calories from Protein | C%: Calories from Carbohydrates

Bacon-Cheddar BBQ Pork Sliders — P. 174

	CA	FAT	P	C	F	SA	NC	FAT%	P%	C%
1 1/2 lb (681 g) ground pork	1789.9	144.64	144.5	0	0	0	0	73%	32%	-5%
2 tbsp (30 g) Dijon mustard	24.75	1.17	1.48	2.92	1.2	0	1.72	43%	24%	34%
3 each (9 g) garlic cloves	13	0	1	3	0	0	3	0%	31%	69%
1 tbsp (7 g) paprika (preferably smoked)	20.23	0.91	1.05	3.92	2.59	0	1.33	40%	21%	39%
1 tsp (2 g) ground cayenne pepper	5.68	0.34	0.34	1	0.34	0	0.66	54%	24%	22%
1 tsp (1 g) fresh chopped thyme	1.01	0.02	0.06	0.24	0.14	0	0.1	18%	24%	58%
12 slices (300 g) raw bacon	1374	135	36	3	0	0	3	88%	10%	1%
1 small (110 g) onion	44	0	1	10	2	0	8	0%	9%	91%
3/4 cup (114 g) low-sugar BBQ sauce	30	0	0	6	0	0	6	0%	0%	100%
12 each (389 g) mini One-Minute Cheddar Buns (p. 172)	1106	85.01	65.53	39.62	32.08	0	7.54	69%	24%	7%
1 cup (95 g) prepared Sweet 'n' Creamy Coleslaw (p. 176)	113.18	10.44	1.34	5.58	2.38	0	3.2	83%	5%	12%
Salt and fresh-cracked pepper, to taste	0	0	0	0	0	0	0	0%	0%	0%
Totals (of 4 Servings):	4521.7	377.53	252.3	75.28	40.73	0	34.55	75%	22%	3%
Per Serving:	1130.4	94.38	63.08	18.82	10.18	0.00	8.64	75%	22%	3%

Cinnamon Roll OMM — P. 168

	CA	FAT	P	C	F	SA	NC	FAT%	P%	C%
2 tbsp (13g) flaxseed meal	70	4.5	3	4	3	0	1	58%	17%	25%
2 tbsp (14g) almond meal	80	7	3	3	1.5	0	1.5	79%	15%	6%
2 tsp (8 g) sugar replacement	0	0	0	6.25	0	6.25	0	0%	0%	100%
1/2 tsp (1g) ground cinnamon	2.47	0.01	0.04	0.81	0.53	0	0.28	4%	6%	90%
1/2 tsp (2g) baking powder	2.5	0	0	0.5	0	0	0.5	0%	0%	100%
Dash salt	0	0	0	0	0	0	0	0%	0%	0%
1 tbsp (8 g) chopped walnuts	49.06	4.91	1.13	1	0.5	0	0.5	90%	9%	1%
1 tsp (3 g) coarsely chopped raisins	10.27	0.02	0.1	2.73	0.13	0	2.6	2%	4%	94%
1 large (50g) egg	72	5	6.5	0	0	0	0.5	63%	36%	1%
1 tsp (5 g) melted butter	33.33	3.67	0	0	0	0	0	99%	0%	1%
3 tbsp (37 g) Cream Cheese Frosting (p. 196)	87.91	9.18	0.65	18.46	0.00	18.00	0.46	94%	3%	3%
Totals (of 1 Servings):	407.54	34.29	14.42	37.25	5.66	24.25	7.34	76%	14%	10%
Per Serving:	407.54	34.29	14.42	37.25	5.66	24.25	7.34	76%	14%	10%

THE FAKERY ~ NUTRITIONAL GRIDS

CA: Calories | **FAT:** Fat | **P:** Protein | **C:** Carbohydrates | **F:** Fiber | **SA:** Sugar Alcohols | **NC:** Net Carbs
FAT%: Calories from Fat | **P%:** Calories from Protein | **C%:** Calories from Carbohydrates

Blue Cheese Lamburgers with Poppy Seed Omms — P. 178

	CA	FAT	P	C	F	SA	NC	FAT%	P%	C%
Poppy Seed OMMs										
1/2 cup (52 g) golden flaxseed meal	280	18	12	16	12	0	4	58%	17%	25%
1/2 cup (56 g) almond flour	320	28	12	12	6	0	6	79%	15%	6%
2 tsp (9 g) baking powder	10	0	0	2	0	0	2	0%	0%	100%
4 large (200g) whole eggs	286	20	26	2	0	0	2	63%	36%	1%
1/2 tsp (1 g) salt	0	0	0	0	0	0	0	0%	0%	0%
1 tbsp (14g) melted butter	100	11	0	0	0	0	0	99%	0%	1%
1 tbsp (9 g) poppy seeds	46	4	1	1	1	0	0	78%	9%	13%
Lamburgers										
8 slices (200 g) raw bacon	916	90	24	2	0	0	2	88%	10%	1%
1 small (110 g) onion	44	0	1	10	2	0	8	0%	9%	91%
4 each (12 g) garlic cloves	16	0	0	4	0	0	4	0%	0%	100%
2 tsp (2g) fresh chopped thyme	2.02	0.04	0.12	0.48	0.28	0	0.2	18%	24%	58%
2 lb (908 g) ground lamb	2563.3	208.92	152.67	0	0	0	0	73%	24%	3%
1 large (50 g) egg	72	5	6.5	0.5	0	0	0.5	63%	36%	1%
1/4 cup (56 g) fresh whole butter	400	44	0	0	0	0	0	99%	0%	1%
1 cup (135 g) blue cheese, crumbled but not packed	477	39	29	3	0	0	3	74%	24%	2%
1 cup (71 g) mixed greens, washed and dried	7.5	0	0.5	1.5	0.5	0	0	0%	27%	73%
Salt and fresh-cracked pepper, to taste	0	0	0	0	0	0	0	0%	0%	0%
Totals (of 4 Servings):	5539.8	467.96	264.79	54.48	21.78	0	32.7	76%	19%	5%
Per Serving:	1384.9	116.99	66.20	13.62	5.45	0.00	**8.18**	**76%**	19%	5%

Sweet 'n' Creamy Coleslaw — P. 176

	CA	FAT	P	C	F	SA	NC	FAT%	P%	C%
8 cups (560 g) shredded cabbage (about 1/2 head)	136	0	8	36	18	0	18	0%	24%	76%
1/4 cup (28 g) grated carrot	11.17	0	0.21	2.58	0.86	0	1.72	0%	8%	92%
1/2 cup (110 g) mayonnaise	750.54	83.45	2.4	1.33	0.08	0.25	1	100%	1%	-1%
2 tbsp (31 g) lemon juice, freshly squeezed	7.63	0	0.13	2.63	0.13	0	2.5	0%	7%	93%
2 tbsp (24 g) sugar replacement	0	0	0	2	0	2	0	0%	0%	100%
Salt and fresh-cracked pepper, to taste	0	0	0	0	0	0	0	0%	0%	0%
Totals (of 8 Servings):	905.34	83.45	10.74	44.54	19.07	2.25	23.22	83%	5%	12%
Per Serving:	113.17	10.43	1.34	5.57	2.38	0.28	**2.90**	**83%**	5%	12%

CA: Calories | FAT: Fat | P: Protein | C: Carbohydrates | F: Fiber | SA: Sugar Alcohols | NC: Net Carbs
FAT%: Calories from Fat | P%: Calories from Protein | C%: Calories from Carbohydrates

Luxurious Eggnog — P. 202

	CA	FAT	P	C	F	SA	NC	FAT%	P%	C%
2 1/2 cups (595 g) heavy cream	2052.5	220	12.5	17.5	0	0	17.5	97%	2%	1%
1 1/2 cups (360 g) unsweetened almond milk	67.5	5.25	3	4.5	1.5	0	3	70%	18%	12%
1/3 cup (64 g) sugar replacement	0	0	0	64	0	64	0	0%	0%	100%
1 each (12 g) vanilla bean (or 2 tsp vanilla extract)	23	0	0	1	0	0	1	0%	0%	100%
1/2 tsp (1 g) ground cinnamon	2.47	0.01	0.04	0.81	0.53	0	0.28	4%	6%	90%
1/4 tsp (.5 g) ground nutmeg	2.63	0.18	0.03	0.25	0.11	0	0.14	62%	5%	34%
Dash salt	0	0	0	0	0	0	0	0%	0%	0%
6 large (300 g) eggs	429	30	13	3	0	0	3	63%	12%	25%
Totals (of 8 Servings):	2577.1	255.44	28.57	91.06	2.14	64	24.92	89%	4%	6%
Per Serving:	322.14	31.93	3.57	11.38	0.27	8.00	3.12	89%	4%	6%

Greasy Fried Pork Sandwich — P. 180

	CA	FAT	P	C	F	SA	NC	FAT%	P%	C%
Bread/Muffin										
2 tbsp (13 g) flaxseed meal	70	4.5	3	4	3	0	1	58%	17%	25%
2 tbsp (14 g) almond meal	80	7	3	3	1.5	0	1.5	79%	15%	6%
1 large (50 g) egg	72	5	6.5	0.5	0	0	0.5	63%	36%	1%
1 tsp (5 g) bacon fat or butter, melted	33.33	3.67	0	0	0	0	0	99%	0%	1%
1/2 tsp (2 g) baking powder	2.5	0	0	0.5	0	0	0.5	0%	0%	100%
Dash salt	0	0	0	0	0	0	0	0%	0%	0%
The Rest of the Fixin's										
3 slices (84 g) deli ham	136.92	7.56	14.28	3.36	0.84	0	2.52	50%	42%	9%
3 slices (84 g) bacon	131.52	10.32	8.64	.24	0	0	.24	71%	26%	3%
1 large (50 g) egg	72	5	6.5	0.5	0	0	0.5	63%	36%	1%
2 tbsp (30 g) heavy cream	102.63	11	0.63	0.88	0	0	0.88	96%	2%	1%
1 tbsp (14 g) bacon fat or butter	100	11	0	0	0	0	0	99%	0%	1%
Salt and pepper, to taste	0	0	0	0	0	0	0	0%	0%	0%
Totals (of 1 Serving):	800.9	65.05	42.55	12.98	5.34	0	7.64	73%	21%	6%
Per Serving:	800.9	65.05	42.55	12.98	5.34	0.00	7.64	73%	21%	6%

CA: Calories | **FAT:** Fat | **P:** Protein | **C:** Carbohydrates | **F:** Fiber | **SA:** Sugar Alcohols | **NC:** Net Carbs
FAT%: Calories from Fat | **P%:** Calories from Protein | **C%:** Calories from Carbohydrates

Pumpkin-Spice OMM with Maple Butter — P. 184

	CA	FAT	P	C	F	SA	NC	FAT%	P%	C%
Maple Butter										
1 tbsp (14 g) butter	100	11	0	0	0	0	0	99%	0%	1%
1/2 tbsp (8 g) sugar-free maple syrup	6.25	0	0	2.38	0	2.13	0.25	0%	0%	100%
Dash salt	0	0	0	0	0	0	0	0%	0%	0%
Pumpkin-Spice OMM										
2 tbsp (13 g) golden flaxseed meal	70	4.5	3	4	3	0	1	58%	17%	25%
2 tbsp (14 g) hazelnut flour	90	8.5	2	2.5	1.5	0	1	85%	9%	6%
2 tbsp (24 g) sugar replacement	0	0	0	24	0	24	0	0%	0%	100%
1/2 tsp (2 g) baking powder	2.5	0	0	0.5	0	0	0.5	0%	0%	100%
1/2 tsp (1 g) ground cinnamon	2.47	0.01	0.04	0.81	0.53	0	0.28	4%	6%	90%
1/4 tsp (.5 g) freshly ground nutmeg	2.63	0.18	0.03	0.25	0.11	0	0.14	62%	5%	34%
Dash ground cloves	0	0	0	0	0	0	0	0%	0%	0%
Dash dried powdered ginger	0	0	0	0	0	0	0	0%	0%	0%
Dash salt	0	0	0	0	0	0	0	0%	0%	0%
2 tbsp (31 g) mashed pumpkin	12.42	0	0.25	2.48	0.99	0	1.49	0%	8%	92%
1 large (50 g) whole egg	71.5	5	6.5	0.5	0	0	0.5	63%	36%	1%
Totals (of 1 Serving):	357.77	29.19	11.82	37.42	6.13	26.13	5.16	73%	13%	13%
Per Serving:	357.77	29.19	11.82	37.42	6.13	26.13	**5.16**	**73%**	13%	13%

Herby Sandwich Bread (Focaccia) — P. 190

	CA	FAT	P	C	F	SA	NC	FAT%	P%	C%
1 cup (104 g) golden flaxseed meal	560	36	24	32	24	0	8	58%	17%	25%
1 cup (112 g) almond flour	640	56	24	24	12	0	12	79%	15%	6%
1 1/2 tbsp (18 g) baking powder	22.5	0	0	4.5	0	0	4.5	0%	0%	100%
1 tbsp (2 g) fresh chopped rosemary	2.62	0.12	0.06	0.42	0.28	0	0.14	41%	9%	50%
1 tsp (2 g) crushed red chili flakes	6.36	0.34	0.24	1.14	0.54	0	0.6	48%	15%	37%
1 tsp (4 g) salt	0	0	0	0	0	0	0	0%	0%	0%
8 large (400 g) eggs	572	40	52	4	0	0	4	63%	36%	1%
1/4 cup + 2 tbsp (90 g) unsweetened almond milk	16.89	1.32	0.75	1.14	0.39	0	0.75	70%	18%	12%
1/4 cup (54g) extra-virgin olive oil	477.5	54	0	0	0	0	0	102%	0%	-2%
6 each (18 g) garlic cloves	24	0	0	6	0	0	6	0%	0%	100%
Totals (of 6 Servings):	2321.8	187.78	101.05	73.2	37.21	0	35.99	73%	17%	10%
Per Serving:	386.98	31.30	16.84	12.20	6.20	0.00	**6.00**	**73%**	17%	10%

CA: Calories | **FAT:** Fat | **P:** Protein | **C:** Carbohydrates | **F:** Fiber | **SA:** Sugar Alcohols | **NC:** Net Carbs
FAT%: Calories from Fat | **P%:** Calories from Protein | **C%:** Calories from Carbohydrates

Spiced Zucchini Bread OMM — P. 188

Ingredient	CA	FAT	P	C	F	SA	NC	FAT%	P%	C%
2 tbsp (13g) golden flaxseed meal	70	4.5	3	4	3	0	1	58%	17%	25%
2 tbsp (14 g) almond meal	80	7	3	3	1.5	0	1.5	79%	15%	6%
2 tbsp (24 g) sugar replacement	0	0	0	24	0	24	0	0%	0%	100%
1/2 tsp (2 g) baking powder	2.5	0	0	0.5	0	0	0.5	0%	0%	100%
1/2 tsp (1 g) ground cinnamon	2.47	0.01	0.04	0.81	0.53	0	0.28	4%	6%	90%
1/4 tsp (.5 g) freshly ground nutmeg	2.63	0.18	0.03	0.25	0.11	0	0.14	62%	5%	34%
Dash ground cloves	0	0	0	0	0	0	0	0%	0%	0%
Dash salt	0	0	0	0	0	0	0	0%	0%	0%
2 tbsp (23 g) grated zucchini	3.62	0.07	0.28	0.77	0.28	0	0.49	17%	31%	52%
1 tbsp (8 g) broken and toasted walnut halves	49.06	4.91	1.13	1	0.5	0	0.5	90%	9%	1%
1 large (50 g) whole egg	71.5	5	6.5	0.5	0	0	0.5	63%	36%	1%
1 tsp (5 g) melted butter	33.33	3.67	0	0	0	0	0	99%	0%	1%
1/2 tsp (2 g) vanilla extract	5.77	0	0	0.25	0	0	0.25	0%	0%	100%
Totals (of 1 Serving):	320.88	25.34	13.98	35.08	5.92	24	5.16	71%	17%	11%
Per Serving:	320.88	25.34	13.98	35.08	5.92	24.00	**5.16**	**71%**	17%	11%

Savory Zucchini, Bacon and Herb OMM — P. 186

Ingredient	CA	FAT	P	C	F	SA	NC	FAT%	P%	C%
2 tbsp (13g) golden flaxseed meal	70	4.5	3	4	3	0	1	58%	17%	25%
2 tbsp (14 g) almond meal	80	7	3	3	1.5	0	1.5	79%	15%	6%
2 tbsp (13 g) grated parmesan cheese	53.88	3.63	4.75	0.5	0	0	0.5	61%	35%	4%
1/2 tsp (2 g) baking powder	2.5	0	0	0.5	0	0	0.5	0%	0%	100%
Dash salt	0	0	0	0	0	0	0	0%	0%	0%
2 tbsp (23 g) grated zucchini	3.62	0.07	0.28	0.77	0.28	0	0.49	17%	31%	52%
1 tbsp (6 g) chopped toasted pecans	42.75	4.44	0.56	0.88	0.63	0	0.25	93%	5%	1%
1 large (50 g) whole egg	71.5	5	6.5	0.5	0	0	0.5	63%	36%	1%
1 tsp (5 g) melted bacon fat	33.33	3.67	0	0	0	0	0	99%	0%	1%
1 tbsp (7 g) real bacon bits	25	1.5	3	0	0	0	0	54%	48%	-2%
1/2 tsp (.5 g) chopped fresh thyme	0.51	0.01	0.03	0.12	0.07	0	0.05	18%	24%	59%
3 tbsp (43 g) full fat cream cheese	145.68	14.5	2.56	1.66	0	0	1.66	90%	7%	3%
Totals (of 1 Serving):	528.77	44.32	23.68	11.93	5.48	0	6.45	75%	18%	7%
Per Serving:	528.77	44.32	23.68	11.93	5.48	0.00	**6.45**	**75%**	18%	7%

THE FAKERY ~ NUTRITIONAL GRIDS

CA: Calories | **FAT:** Fat | **P:** Protein | **C:** Carbohydrates | **F:** Fiber | **SA:** Sugar Alcohols | **NC:** Net Carbs
FAT%: Calories from Fat | **P%:** Calories from Protein | **C%:** Calories from Carbohydrates

Blueberry, Lemon and Poppy Seed Muffins — P. 114

	CA	FAT	P	C	F	SA	NC	FAT%	P%	C%
1 cup + 2 tbsp (126 g) almond flour	720	63	27	27	13.5	0	13.5	79%	15%	6%
1/4 cup + 2 tbsp (42 g) coconut flour	186	4.5	10.5	27	18	0	9	22%	23%	56%
1/4 cup + 2 tbsp (72 g) sugar replacement	0	0	0	72	0	72	0	0%	0%	100%
3/4 tsp (3 g) baking soda	0	0	0	0	0	0	0	0%	0%	0%
3/4 tsp (3 g) salt	0	0	0	0	0	0	0	0%	0%	0%
1 lemon (108 g)	108	0	0	12	5	0	7	0%	0%	100%
6 large (300 g) eggs	428	30	13	3	0	0	3	63%	12%	25%
1/4 cup (60 g) unsweetened almond milk	11.25	0.88	0.5	0.75	0.25	0	0.5	70%	18%	12%
3 tbsp (42 g) melted butter	300	33	0	0	0	0	0	99%	0%	1%
1 cup (155 g) blueberries	79	1	1	19	4	0	15	11%	5%	84%
3 tbsp (27 g) poppy seeds	138	12	6	6	6	0	0	78%	17%	4%
Totals (of 6 Servings):	1970.2	144.38	58	166.75	46.75	72	48	66%	12%	22%
Per Serving:	328.38	24.06	9.67	27.79	7.79	12.00	**8.00**	**66%**	12%	22%

Crunchy Mocha-Zucchini Muffins — P. 128

	CA	FAT	P	C	F	SA	NC	FAT%	P%	C%
1 cup (112 g) hazelnut flour	720	68	16	20	12	0	8	85%	9%	6%
1/4 cup + 2 tbsp (42 g) coconut flour	186	4.5	10.5	27	18	0	9	22%	23%	56%
1/4 cup + 2 tbsp (72 g) sugar replacement	0	0	0	72	0	72	0	0%	0%	100%
1/4 cup + 2 tbsp (32 g) unsweetened cocoa powder	73.5	4.48	6.42	18.78	10.92	0	7.86	55%	35%	10%
1/4 cup (24 g) ground chia	112	7.2	3.2	11.2	9.6	0	1.6	58%	11%	31%
1 tbsp (14 g) baking powder	6	0	0	3.9	0	0	3.9	0%	0%	100%
3/4 tsp (3 g) salt	0	0	0	0	0	0	0	0%	0%	0%
4 large (200 g) eggs	285.33	20	8.67	2	0	0	2	63%	12%	25%
1 cup (180 g) grated zucchini	28.98	0.56	2.23	6.13	2.23	0	3.9	17%	31%	52%
2 tbsp (30 g) unsweetened almond milk	5.63	0.44	0.25	0.38	0.13	0	0.25	70%	18%	12%
3 tbsp (42 g) melted butter	300	33	0	0	0	0	0	99%	0%	1%
3 tbsp (16 g) cacao nibs	36	2.1	3.3	9.3	5.4	0	3.9	53%	37%	11%
3 tbsp (20 g) crushed, toasted, whole coffee beans	60	2	1	9	5	0	4	30%	7%	63%
1/2 cup (58 g) coarsely chopped hazelnuts	361	35	8.5	9.5	5.5	0	4	87%	9%	3%
Totals (of 6 Servings):	2174.4	177.28	60.07	189.19	68.78	72	48.41	73%	11%	16%
Per Serving:	362.41	29.55	10.01	31.53	11.46	12.00	**8.07**	**73%**	11%	16%

CA: Calories | **FAT:** Fat | **P:** Protein | **C:** Carbohydrates | **F:** Fiber | **SA:** Sugar Alcohols | **NC:** Net Carbs
FAT%: Calories from Fat | **P%:** Calories from Protein | **C%:** Calories from Carbohydrates

Cream Cheese Frosting — P. 196

	CA	FAT	P	C	F	SA	NC	FAT%	P%	C%
1/4 cup + 1 1/2 tsp (65 g) full-fat cream cheese	221.66	22.05	3.91	2.51	0	0	2.51	90%	7%	3%
3 tbsp (42 g) whole butter	300	33	0	0	0	0	0	99%	0%	1%
1/2 cup + 1 tbsp (108 g) powdered sugar replacement	0	0	0	108	0	108	0	0%	0%	100%
1/2 tsp (2 g) vanilla extract	5.77	0	0	0.25	0	0	0.25	0%	0%	100%
Dash salt	0	0	0	0	0	0	0	0%	0%	0%
Totals (of 6 Servings):	527.43	55.05	3.91	110.76	0	108	2.76	94%	3%	3%
Per Serving:	87.91	9.18	0.65	18.46	0.00	18.00	0.46	94%	3%	3%

Chocolate OMM — P. 166

	CA	FAT	P	C	F	SA	NC	FAT%	P%	C%
2 tbsp (13g) flaxseed meal	70	4.5	3	4	3	0	1	58%	17%	25%
2 tbsp (14g) almond meal	80	7	3	3	1.5	0	1.5	79%	15%	6%
1 tbsp (12 g) sugar replacement	0	0	0	12	0	12	0	0%	0%	100%
1 tbsp (5 g) unsweetened cocoa powder	12.25	0.75	1.07	3.13	1.82	0	1.31	55%	35%	10%
1/2 tsp (2g) baking powder	2.5	0	0	0.5	0	0	0.5	0%	0%	100%
Dash salt	0	0	0	0	0	0	0	0%	0%	0%
1 large (50g) egg	72	5	6.5	0.5	0	0	0.5	63%	36%	1%
1 tbsp (14 g) melted butter	100	11	0	0	0	0	0	99%	0%	1%
Totals (of 1 Serving):	336.75	28.25	13.57	23.13	6.32	12	4.81	76%	16%	8%
Per Serving:	336.75	28.25	13.57	23.13	6.32	12.00	4.81	76%	16%	8%

Italian Turkey Club Sandwich — P. 192

	CA	FAT	P	C	F	SA	NC	FAT%	P%	C%
1 sheet (624 g) Grain-Free Focaccia (p. 190)	1688.9	140.46	76.3	50.06	22.82	0	27.24	75%	18%	7%
1/2 cup (193 g) Pesto alla Genovese (p. 194)	853.15	89.83	11.62	6.81	0.26	0	6.55	95%	5%	-0%
1 1/2 lb (681 g) sliced turkey	681	13.62	122.58	13.62	0	0	13.62	18%	72%	10%
12 slices (96 g) cooked bacon	526.08	41.28	34.56	0.96	0	0	0.96	71%	26%	3%
1 medium (91 g) tomato	16	0	1	4	1	0	3	0%	25%	75%
Salt and pepper, to taste	0	0	0	0	0	0	0	0%	0%	0%
Totals (of 6 Servings):	3765.2	285.19	246.06	75.45	24.08	0	51.37	68%	26%	6%
Per Serving:	627.54	47.53	41.01	12.58	4.01	0.00	8.56	68%	26%	6%

INDEX

Note to Readers: Nutrient information page numbers are shown in *italics*.

A

agar-agar, 51
air (leavening agent), 57
almond flour
    a basic ingredient, 29
    see the effects, 67
almond milk
    substitutions, 80
apple
Cream Cheese-Filled Spiced Apple Muffins, 110–113
Arana, Karina
    her story, 6–11
arrowroot starch/flour, 55–56
    see the effects, 79

B

bacon
    Blue Cheese Lamburgers, 178–179
    Cheesy Bacon-Chive Muffins, 96–97
    Greasy Fried Pork Sandwich, 180–181
    Italian Turkey Club Sandwich, 192–193
    Savory Zucchini OMM, 186–187
Bacon and Orange Muffins, 148–151, *217*
bacon fat
    substituting for melted butter, 80–81
Bacon-Cheddar BBQ Pork Sliders, 174–175, *223*
baker's yeast, 60–61
baking
    pans, 135
    time and temperature, 89
baking powder, 59

baking soda, 58–59
bananas
    Chocolate-Banana Muffcakes, 124–125
basic equipment, 30
Basic Smappy Goodness, 64
Basic Tasty Smappy, 64
basil
    Pesto, Sausage and Parmesan Muffins, 102–103
    Pesto alla Genovese, 194–195
blob
    conceptually, 17–18
    gluten-free blobs, 24–25
blue cheese
    Pear Tart Fauxtan, 154–155
Blue Cheese Lamburgers, 178–179, *224*
blueberries
    Orange-Blueberry Chia Pudding, 38–39
Blueberry, Lemon and Poppy Seed Muffins, 114–115, *209*
Bonus Recipes 165–203
breads, savory
    Savory Quick-Bread Ratio, 23
    Grain-Free, Nut-Free Fauxcaccia, 106–108
    Herby Sandwich Bread, 190–191
    One-Minute Cheddar Bread, 172–173
    Poppy Seed OMMs, 178–179
    with Greasy Fried Pork Sandwich, 180–181
breads, sweet
    Sweet Quick-Bread Ratio, 23
    Fried Blob, 140–141
    Layered Eggnog Discs, 134–137
    Mini Gingerbread Loaves, 138–139
    Sour Cream Coffee Cake, 132–133
Brown Butter Ginger-Spice "Riddles & Games," 118–121, *210*
burger
    Blue Cheese Lamburgers, 178–179
butter, melted
    substitutions, 80

C

cacao nibs
    Chocolate-Chocolate Chunk Muffins, 126–127
    Crunchy Mocha-Zucchini Muffins, 128–129
    Mini Carrot Cake Muffins, 116–117
carbohydrate count, 61, 124, 126, 138
Carrot, Coconut & Macadamia Mega-Muffins, 122–123, *211*
carrots
    Frosted Carrot Cake OMM, 182–183
    Mini Carrot Cake Muffins, 116–117
    Sweet 'n' Creamy Coleslaw, 176–177
cassava flour, 53, 55
cheddar cheese
    Cheesy Bacon-Chive Muffins, 96–97
    Jalapeño Cheddar Muffins, 104–105
    One-Minute Cheddar Bread, 172–173
cheese. *See individual varieties*
cheesecake
    Pumpkin Cheesecake Swirl Muffin, 156–157
Cheesy Bacon-Chive Muffins, 96–97, *206*
chervil
    Muffin aux Fines Herbes, 100–101
chia eggs, 40–41, 81, 88, 107, 125
    substituting for eggs, 81
chia seed
    colors, 96
    Orange-Blueberry Chia Pudding, 38–39
chia seed flour, 36–41
    a basic ingredient, 29
    grind your own, 83
    see the effects, 69
    substituting for flaxseed meal, 81
chives
    Cheesy Bacon-Chive Muffins, 96–97
    Muffin aux Fines Herbes, 100–101
chocolate
    origin, 142–143, 163
    swirl idea, 156
    with chia, 40
    Crunchy Mocha-Zucchini Muffins, 128–129
    Mexican Chocolate Muffins, 142–143
    Mini Notella Muffins, 146–147
    Mocha-Mint Muffins, 144–145
    Notella, 198–199
Chocolate Ganache, 200–201, *219*
    with Chocolate Muffins, 126–127
    with Mini Coconut Muffaroons, 130–131
Chocolate OMM, 166–167, *221*
Chocolate-Banana Muffcakes, 124–125, *211*
Chocolate-Chocolate Chunk Muffins, 126–127, *212*
Chorizo, Cilantro and Cotija Muffins, 98–99, *206*
cilantro
    Chorizo, Cilantro and Cotija Muffins, 98–99
Cinnamon Roll OMM, 168–169, *222*
cocoa powder. *See also* chocolate
    see the effects, 77
coconut
    Carrot Mega-Muffins, 122–123
    Mini Coconut Muffaroons, 130–131
coconut flour, 33–36
    a basic ingredient, 29
    see the effects, 68
    with vanilla, 40
coconut oil
    substituting for melted butter, 80
coffee beans
    Crunchy Mocha-Zucchini Muffins, 128–129
colby cheese
    One-Minute Cheddar Bread, 172–173
Coleslaw, Sweet 'n' Creamy, 176–177
cornstarch
    in baking powder, 59
    compared with other starches, 55
Cotija cheese
    Chorizo, Cilantro and Cotija Muffins, 98–99
cranberries
    Orange-Cranberry Muffins, 152–153
cream cheese
    Savory Zucchini OMM, 186–187

Cream Cheese-Filled Spiced Apple Muffins, 110–113, *209*
Cream Cheese Frosting, 196–197, *228*
    with Cinnamon Roll OMM, 168–169
    with Frosted Carrot Cake OMM, 182–183
    with Mini Carrot Cake Muffins, 116–117
    with Mini Gingerbread Loaves, 138–139
Crunchy Mocha-Zucchini Muffins, 128–129, *212*

D

Dark Brown Smappy: Baking Mix, 65
Deep-Dish Pizza, 92, 94, *205*
doughnuts, doughnut holes
    Fried Blob, 140–141
    Mini Notella Muffins, 146–147
drinks
    Luxurious Eggnog, 202–203

E

eggnog
    Layered Eggnog Discs, 134–137
    Luxurious Eggnog, 202–203
eggs
    substituting chia, 40–41
    substituting chia egg, 81
erythritol
    grinding, 83
    Smappy recipes, 63–65

F

The Fakery
    welcome, 22
    why?, 16
fats, when grinding nuts, 84
fermentation, 45–46
fines herbes
    Muffin aux Fines Herbes, 100–101
flaxseed, flaxseed meal, 41–42
    colors, 96
    compared with chia, 40
    grind your own, 83
    see the effects, 70
    substituting chia seed, 81
Flours, 31–43
    blending, 35–36, 88–89
    flour or meal?, 32–33
    see the effects, 66–79
    chia seed flour, 36–41
    coconut flour, 33–36
    flaxseed meal, 41–42
    nut flours, 31–33
    protein powder, 42–43
focaccia
    Grain-Free, Nut-Free Fauxcaccia, 106–108
    Herby Sandwich Bread, 190–191
French Toast, OMM, 170–171
Fried Blob, 140–141, *215*
Frosted Carrot Cake OMM with Pecans, 182–183, *225*
frosting
    Chocolate Ganache, 200–201
    Cream Cheese Frosting, 196–197

G

garlic
    Herby Sandwich Bread, 190–191
gelatin, 49–50
    see the effects, 74
ghee
    substituting for melted butter, 80
ginger
    Mini Gingerbread Loaves, 138–139
    Riddles & Games, 118–121
glucomannan, 50–51
    see the effects, 75
Gluten Replacers, 44–52
    improving structure, 89
    agar-agar, 51
    gelatin, 49–50

glucomannan, 50–51
guar gum, 49
psyllium seed husk fiber, 51–52
xanthan gum, 45–47
goo, 54
Goodness sweeteners, 63–65
Grain-Free, Nut-Free Fauxcaccia, 106–108, *208*
    with Italian Turkey Club Sandwich, 192–193
grain-free baking, 16
Greasy Fried Pork Sandwich, 180–181, *225*
greens, mixed
    Blue Cheese Lamburgers, 178–179
Grind Your Own, 82–87
    grinders, *basic equipment*, 30
guar gum, 49
    see the effects, 73

H

ham
    Greasy Fried Pork Sandwich, 180–181
Hazelnut Streusel, 132–133, *214*
hazelnuts
    Crunchy Mocha-Zucchini Muffins, 128–129
    Notella, 198–199
hempseed milk
    substituting for almond milk, 80
Herby Sandwich Bread (Focaccia), 190–191, *227*
hygroscopic, *defined*, 52

I

inulin
    Smappy recipes, 65
isolate, *defined*, 43
Italian sausage
    Pesto, Sausage and Parmesan Muffins, 102–103
Italian Turkey Club Sandwich, 192–193, *228*

J

Jalapeño Cheddar Muffins, 104–105, *208*

L

lamb
    Blue Cheese Lamburgers, 178–179
Layered Eggnog Discs, 134–137, *214*
Leavening Agents, 57–61
    increasing the amount, 88
    air, 57
    baker's yeast, 60–61
    baking powder, 59
    baking soda, 58–59
    water, 57–58
lemon
    Blueberry Muffins, 114–115
Light Brown Smappy: Baking Mix, 65
linseed, 41
Luxurious Eggnog, 202–203, *229*

M

macadamia nuts
    Carrot Mega-Muffins, 122–123
macaroons
    Mini Coconut Muffaroons, 130
Maple Butter
    with Pumpkin-Spice OMM, 184–185, *226*
meal or flour?, 32–33
Meatza, 93
Mexican Chocolate Muffins, 142–143, *216*
microwave ovens and the OMM, 12–15
milk
    substituting for almond milk, 80
Mini Carrot Cake Muffins, 116–117, *210*
Mini Coconut Muffaroons, 130–131, *213*
Mini Notella Muffnuts, 146–147, *217*
Mini Gingerbread Loaves, 138–139, *215*
mint

Mocha-Mint Muffins, 144–145
mocha. *See* chocolate
Mocha-Mint Muffins, 144–145, *216*
molasses, 138–139
Mom and coffee story, 107
mozzarella
    Deep-Dish Pizza, 92, 94
muffaroons, 130–131
muffcakes, 124–125
Muffin aux Fines Herbes, 100–101, *207*
muffins. *See also* OMM
    ratio experiment, 66–79
muffins, savory
    Cheesy Bacon-Chive Muffins, 96–97
    Chorizo, Cilantro and Cotija Muffins, 98–99
    Jalapeño Cheddar Muffins, 104–105
    Muffin aux Fines Herbes, 100–101
    Pesto, Sausage and Parmesan Muffins, 102–103
    Savory Zucchini OMM, 186–187
muffins, sweet
    Bacon and Orange Muffins, 148–151
    Blueberry Muffins, 114–115
    Carrot Mega-Muffins, 122–123
    Chocolate-Banana Muffcakes, 124–125
    Chocolate-Chocolate Chunk Muffins, 126–127
    Cream Cheese Apple Muffins, 110–113
    Crunchy Mocha-Zucchini Muffins, 128–129
    Frosted Carrot Cake OMM, 182–183
    Mexican Chocolate Muffins, 142–143
    Mini Carrot Cake Muffins, 116–117
    Mini Coconut Muffaroons, 130–131
    Mini Notella Muffins, 146–147
    Mocha-Mint Muffins, 144–145
    Orange-Cranberry Muffins, 152–153
    Pumpkin Muffins, 156–157, 158–159
    Pumpkin-Spice OMM, 184–185
    Riddles & Games, 118–121
    Spiced Zucchini Bread OMM, 188–189
    Strawberry Yogurt Muffins, 160–161
    Vanilla Bean Muffcakes, 162–163
muffnuts, 146–147

N

Notella, 198–199, *228*
    with Mini Notella Muffins, 146–147
nut allergies, 32, 80, 85–86, 107
nut flours, 31–33
    a basic ingredient, 29
    grind your own, 83–87
    storing, 86
    substituting sunflower seed flour, 80
nutrient tables, 204–229
nuts with starches, 56

O

olive oil
    substituting for melted butter, 80
OMM (One-Minute Muffins)
    background, 12–15
    Chocolate OMM, 166–167
    Cinnamon Roll OMM, 168–169
    Frosted Carrot Cake OMM, 182–183
    OMM French Toast, 170–171
    Pumpkin-Spice OMM, 184–185
    Savory Zucchini OMM, 186–187
    Spiced Zucchini Bread OMM, 188–189
OMM French Toast, 170–171, *222*
One-Minute Cheddar Bread and Buns, 172–173, *223*
    with Sliders, 174–175
orange
    Bacon and Orange Muffins, 148–151
orange oil, 38
Orange-Blueberry Chia Pudding, 38–39, *205*
Orange-Cranberry Muffins, 152–153, *218*

P

pancakes and waffles
    blob, 24, 54
    Layered Eggnog Discs, 134–137
    psyllium seed husk fiber, 51
    quick-bread batter, 18
    Riddles & Games, 118–121
parmesan cheese
    Deep-Dish Pizza, 92, 94
    Pesto, Sausage and Parmesan Muffins, 102–103
    Pesto alla Genovese, 194–195
    Savory Zucchini OMM, 186–187
parsley
    Muffin aux Fines Herbes, 100–101
Pear, Walnut and Blue Cheese Tart Fauxtan, 154–155, *219*
Pecan Streusel, 148–151, *217*
pecans
    Frosted Carrot Cake OMM, 182–183
    Savory Zucchini OMM, 186–187
pecorino cheese
    Pesto alla Genovese, 194–195
peppermint
    Mocha-Mint Muffins, 144–145
pepperoni
    Deep-Dish Pizza, 92–94
Pesto, Sausage and Parmesan Muffins, 102–103, *207*
Pesto alla Genovese, 194–195
    with Italian Turkey Club Sandwich, 192–193
pie
    Spiced Pumpkin-Sour Cream Muffin Pies, 158–159
Pie Crust, 158–159, *220*
pine nuts
    Pesto alla Genovese, 194–195
pizza, pizza crust
    Deep-Dish Pizza, 92–94
polydextrose
    Smappy recipes, 64
Poppy Seed OMMs, 178–179, *224*
poppy seeds
    Blueberry Muffins, 114–115
pork
    Bacon-Cheddar Sliders, 174–175
porridge
    Orange-Blueberry Chia Pudding, 38–39
pound cake to quick bread, 19–21
protein powder, 42–43
    see the effects, 71
psyllium seed husk fiber, 51–52
    see the effects, 76
pudding
    Orange-Blueberry Chia Pudding, 38–39
Pumpkin Cheesecake Swirl Muffin, 156–157, *219*
Pumpkin Muffins, 156–157, 158–159, *220*
Pumpkin-Spice OMM, 184–185, *226*

Q

quick bread
    defined, 17–18
    pound cake to quick bread, 19–21
Quick Bread Recipes, 165–203

R

raisins
    Cinnamon Roll OMM, 168–169
    Mini Carrot Cake Muffins, 116–117
ratios
    overview, 19–21
    mixing, 111
    see the effects, 66–79
    sweet and savory ratios, 23
recipe size, 88
Recipes, Quick Breads, 165–203
Recipes, Savory, 91–108
Recipes, Sweet, 109–164
red chili flakes
    Herby Sandwich Bread, 190–191
Riddles & Games, 118–121

rosemary
    Herby Sandwich Bread, 190–191
Rules of thumb
    coconut flour, 34
    gluten replacers, 44–52

S

sandwiches
    Bacon-Cheddar Sliders, 174–175
    Blue Cheese Lamburgers, 178–179
    Greasy Fried Pork Sandwich, 180–181
    Italian Turkey Club Sandwich, 192–193
sauces
    Pesto alla Genovese, 194–195
sausage
    Deep-Dish Pizza, 92–94
    Pesto, Sausage and Parmesan Muffins, 102–103
Savory Recipes, 91–108
Savory Zucchini, Bacon and Herb OMM, 186–187, *226*
seeds
    grind your own, 83
    with starches, 56
sides
    Sweet 'n' Creamy Coleslaw, 176–177
sifters, basic equipment, 30
sifting ground nuts, 84–85
Smappy Goodness Baking Blend, 65
Smappy sweeteners, 63–65
Sour Cream Coffee Cake, 132–133, *213*
Sour Cream Glaze, 148–151, *218*
soy, 41
soy milk
    substituting for almond milk, 80
Spiced Pumpkin-Sour Cream Muffin Pies, 158–159
Spiced Zucchini Bread OMM, 188–189, *227*
Starches, 53–56
    a little bit, 89
    arrowroot starch/flour, 55–56
    tapioca starch/flour, 53–55, 56

stevia
    production, 46
    Smappy recipes, 63–65
Strawberry Yogurt Muffins, 160–161, *220*
streusel
    Hazelnut Streusel, 132–133
    Pecan Streusel, 148–151
structure, preserving. See under ratios
Stuff You'll Need
    generally, 27–30
    flours, 31–43
    gluten replacers, 44–52
    leavening agents, 57–61
    starches, 53–56
    sweeteners, 62–65
Substitutions, 80–81
    for baking powder, 59
sucralose
    Smappy recipes, 63–65
sugar consumption, 63
sugar replacements
    a basic ingredient, 29
    recipes, 63–65
sugar-free baking, 16
sunflower seed flour
    grind your own, 83, 85–86
    nut allergies, 32, 80, 85–86
    substituting for nut flours, 80
Sweet 'n' Creamy Coleslaw, 176–177, *224*
    with Sliders, 174–175
Sweet Recipes, 109–164
Sweeteners, 62–65
    a basic ingredient, 29
    blending, 88–89
    grind your own, 83

T

tapioca starch/flour, 53–55
    see the effects, 78

tarragon
    Muffin aux Fines Herbes, 100–101
tarts
    Pear Tart Fauxtan, 154–155
Tasty Smappy Baking Blend, 64
Tasty sweeteners, 63–65
The Blob that Ate Cincinnati, 17–18
turkey
    Italian Turkey Club Sandwich, 192–193

V

vanilla
    with coconut flour, 40
    origin, 163
Vanilla Bean Muffcakes, 162–163, *221*
Visualize, 66–79

W

waffles and pancakes
    blob, 24, 54
    Layered Eggnog Discs, 134–137
    psyllium seed husk fiber, 51
    quick-bread batter, 18
    Riddles & Games, 118–121
walnuts
    Cinnamon Roll OMM, 168–169
    Pear Tart Fauxtan, 154–155
    Spiced Zucchini Bread OMM, 188–189
water
    substituting for almond milk, 80
water (leavening agent), 57–58

X

xanthan gum, 45–47
    see the effects, 72

Y

yacón syrup
    Smappy recipes, 65
yeast, 60–61
yogurt
    Strawberry Yogurt Muffins, 160–161

Z

zucchini
    Crunchy Mocha-Zucchini Muffins, 128–129
    Savory Zucchini OMM, 186–187
    Spiced Zucchini Bread OMM, 188–189

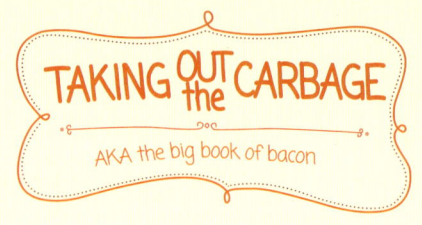

What if You Could Lose Weight and Dramatically Change Your Life. . . by Eating Delicious Food?

A perfect starting point; it contains not just recipes, but the rules and know-how to get you there. Far more than an ordinary cookbook, this one is all-in-one!

- 574 pages (a near 6 1/2 lb. (2.91^{kg}) behemoth!) and 226 delectable, low-carb, low-glycemic recipes, with a strong focus on REAL FOODS.

- Both metric and imperial measurements, to save you headaches in the kitchen

- An extremely detailed nutritional analysis of each recipe, broken down by ingredient, so you know exactly where your nutrients are coming from

- A complete two-week meal plan to take some of the work out of low-carb living, plus a secret third week and tips on how you can easily create your own meal plan

- Ingredient lists, organized by carb count, to help guide you as you're planning your meals

- A little something sweet... a comprehensive look at modern sugar alternatives

- Removable shopping lists with perforated edges for easy tearing, to save you some trouble when it's time to restock your kitchen with nutritious ingredients

- Easy-to-follow dietary guidelines, including which foods are okay to eat and which foods to avoid at all costs

- A foreword by celebrity chef and good friend George

- Stella, an influential voice in the low-carb lifestyle community

- Plenty of sound weight-loss advice, including snack ideas, exercise recommendations, and effective ways to deal with cravings

- A high-quality cookbook designed to withstand abuse in the kitchen, with a strong but flexible binding and specially-coated pages to minimize stains

- Loads of sage wisdom (and other nonsense!) from yours truly, DJ Foodie

- And much, MUCH more!

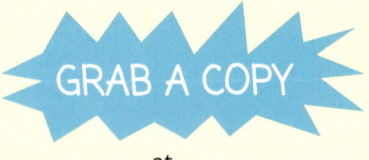

at
www.djfoodie.com